Mayo Clinic
Infectious Diseases Case Review

MAYO CLINIC SCIENTIFIC PRESS

Mayo Clinic Atlas of Regional Anesthesia and Ultrasound-Guided Nerve Blockade
Edited by James R. Hebl, MD, and Robert L. Lennon, DO

Mayo Clinic Preventive Medicine and Public Health Board Review
Edited by Prathibha Varkey, MBBS, MPH, MHPE

Mayo Clinic Infectious Diseases Board Review
Edited by Zelalem Temesgen, MD

Just Enough Physiology
By James R. Munis, MD, PhD

Mayo Clinic Cardiology: Concise Textbook, Fourth Edition
Edited by Joseph G. Murphy, MD, and Margaret A. Lloyd, MD

Mayo Clinic Electrophysiology Manual
Edited by Samuel J. Asirvatham, MD

Mayo Clinic Gastrointestinal Imaging Review, Second Edition
By C. Daniel Johnson, MD

Arrhythmias in Women: Diagnosis and Management
Edited by Yong-Mei Cha, MD, Margaret A. Lloyd, MD, and Ulrika M. Birgersdotter-Green, MD

Mayo Clinic Body MRI Case Review
By Christine U. Lee, MD, PhD, and James F. Glockner, MD, PhD

Mayo Clinic Gastroenterology and Hepatology Board Review, Fifth Edition
Edited by Stephen C. Hauser, MD

Mayo Clinic Guide to Cardiac Magnetic Resonance Imaging, Second Edition
Edited by Kiaran P. McGee, PhD, Eric E. Williamson, MD, and Matthew W. Martinez, MD

Mayo Clinic Critical Care Case Review
Edited by Rahul Kashyap, MBBS, J. Christopher Farmer, MD, and John C. O'Horo, MD

Mayo Clinic Medical Neurosciences, Sixth Edition
Edited by Eduardo E. Benarroch, MD, Jeremy K. Cutsforth-Gregory, MD, and Kelly D. Flemming, MD

Mayo Clinic Principles of Shoulder Surgery
By Joaquin Sanchez-Sotelo, MD

Mayo Clinic Essential Neurology, Second Edition
By Andrea C. Adams, MD

Mayo Clinic Antimicrobial Handbook: Quick Guide, Third Edition
Edited by John W. Wilson, MD, and Lynn L. Estes, PharmD

Mayo Clinic Critical and Neurocritical Care Board Review
Edited by Eelco F. M. Wijdicks, MD, PhD, James Y. Findlay, MB, ChB, William D. Freeman, MD, and Ayan Sen, MD

Mayo Clinic Internal Medicine Board Review, Twelfth Edition
Edited by Christopher M. Wittich, MD, PharmD, Thomas J. Beckman, MD, Sara L. Bonnes, MD, Nerissa M. Collins, MD, Nina M. Schwenk, MD, Christopher R. Stephenson, MD, and Jason H. Szostek, MD

Mayo Clinic Strategies for Reducing Burnout and Promoting Engagement
By Stephen J. Swensen, MD, and Tait D. Shanafelt, MD

Mayo Clinic General Surgery
By Jad M. Abdelsattar, MBBS, Moustafa M. El Khatib, MB, BCh, T. K. Pandian, MD, Samuel J. Allen, and David R. Farley, MD

Mayo Clinic Neurology Board Review, Second Edition
Edited by Kelly D. Flemming, MD

Mayo Clinic Illustrated Textbook of Neurogastroenterology
By Michael Camilleri, MD

Mayo Clinic Cases in Neuroimmunology
Edited by Andrew McKeon, MB, BCh, MD, B. Mark Keegan, MD, and W. Oliver Tobin, MB, BCh, BAO, PhD

Mayo Clinic Infectious Diseases Case Review

With Board-Style Questions and Answers

Editors

Larry M. Baddour, MD

Supplemental Consultant for Research,
Division of Infectious Diseases
Mayo Clinic, Rochester, Minnesota;
Professor Emeritus of Medicine
Mayo Clinic College of Medicine and Science

John C. O'Horo, MD, MPH

Consultant, Division of Infectious Diseases
Mayo Clinic, Rochester, Minnesota;
Associate Professor of Medicine
Mayo Clinic College of Medicine and Science

Mark J. Enzler, MD

Consultant, Division of Infectious Diseases
Mayo Clinic, Rochester, Minnesota;
Assistant Professor of Medicine
Mayo Clinic College of Medicine and Science

Rahul Kashyap, MBBS

Research Scientist, Department of
Anesthesiology and Perioperative Medicine
Mayo Clinic, Rochester, Minnesota;
Assistant Professor of Anesthesiology
Mayo Clinic College of Medicine and Science

MAYO CLINIC SCIENTIFIC PRESS

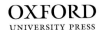

OXFORD
UNIVERSITY PRESS

Oxford University Press is a department of the University of Oxford. It furthers the University's objective of excellence in research, scholarship, and education by publishing worldwide. Oxford is a registered trade mark of Oxford University Press in the UK and certain other countries.

Published in the United States of America by Oxford University Press
198 Madison Avenue, New York, NY 10016, United States of America.

© 2022 by Mayo Foundation for Medical Education and Research.

Oxford is a registered trademark of Oxford University Press.

Library of Congress Cataloging-in-Publication Data
Names: Baddour, Larry M., editor. | O'Horo, John C., editor. | Enzler, Mark J., editor. | Kashyap, Rahul, editor.
Title: Mayo Clinic infectious diseases case review : with board-style questions and answers /
[edited by] Larry M. Baddour, John C. O'Horo, Mark J. Enzler, Rahul Kashyap.
Other titles: Infectious diseases case review | Mayo Clinic scientific press (Series)
Description: New York, NY : Oxford University Press, [2022] | Series: Mayo Clinic scientific press series |
Includes bibliographical references and index.
Identifiers: LCCN 2021042663 (print) | LCCN 2021042664 (ebook) | ISBN 9780190052973 (paperback) |
ISBN 9780190052997 (epub) | ISBN 9780190053000 (online)
Subjects: MESH: Communicable Diseases—diagnosis | Case Reports
Classification: LCC RC112 (print) | LCC RC112 (ebook) | NLM WC 100 | DDC 616.9/0475—dc23
LC record available at https://lccn.loc.gov/2021042663
LC ebook record available at https://lccn.loc.gov/2021042664

DOI: 10.1093/med/9780190052973.001.0001

Mayo Foundation does not endorse any particular products or services, and the reference to any products or services in this book is for informational purposes only and should not be taken as an endorsement by the authors or Mayo Foundation. The incidental appearance of brand names on any equipment or the mention of brand names in the narration in the accompanying videos has been avoided when at all possible; any occurrences were left to preserve the educational integrity of the videos and should not be taken as endorsement by the authors or Mayo Foundation. Care has been taken to confirm the accuracy of the information presented and to describe generally accepted practices. However, the authors, editors, and publisher are not responsible for errors or omissions or for any consequences from application of the information in this book and make no warranty, express or implied, with respect to the contents of the publication. This book should not be relied on apart from the advice of a qualified health care provider.

The authors, editors, and publisher have exerted efforts to ensure that drug selection and dosage set forth in this text are in accordance with current recommendations and practice at the time of publication. However, in view of ongoing research, changes in government regulations, and the constant flow of information relating to drug therapy and drug reactions, readers are urged to check the package insert for each drug for any change in indications and dosage and for added wordings and precautions. This is particularly important when the recommended agent is a new or infrequently employed drug.

Some drugs and medical devices presented in this publication have US Food and Drug Administration (FDA) clearance for limited use in restricted research settings. It is the responsibility of the health care providers to ascertain the FDA status of each drug or device planned for use in their clinical practice.

Printed by Integrated Books International, United States of America

Preface

The current COVID-19 pandemic highlights many aspects of infectious diseases that heretofore were unappreciated by many health care professionals and the public alike. Not only have detailed clinical features of illness been highlighted, but the various groups with increased risk of worse outcomes also have been identified. In addition, the safety and efficacy of COVID-19 treatments and prevention have been discussed extensively in most media venues, to the extent that societal measures used to control the pandemic are now well known and subject to political influence.

Pressing issues in infectious diseases existed before 2020 that needed to be addressed, and the effort to do so during the pandemic has been laudatory. Some important issues have been relevant during the pandemic as well, such as antimicrobial and diagnostic stewardship activities. For the former, the goals of reducing antimicrobial resistance, drug-related adverse events, and costs have been a focus for institutions and international programs. For the latter, health care costs have dramatically increased, and inappropriate use of all types of diagnostic procedures has spiraled out of control. As a related example, conundrums have developed about whether to provide secondary bacterial coverage in patients with COVID-19–related respiratory tract illness or about the optimal frequency, type, and timing of screening for microbiologic evidence of SARS-CoV-2 infection.

This textbook addresses many of the current-day illnesses seen by primary care clinicians and infectious diseases specialists. As its title indicates, a case presentation format is used for all 54 chapters, and this framework serves as a wonderful educational tool that mirrors, in many respects, the objectives of a "case conference" format. The dozens of authors from different areas of our specialty have ensured that a robust clinical examination of specific infection syndromes has been included. In addition, the Question and Answer section solidifies the educational benefits for all levels and types of clinicians who seek an understanding of disease diagnosis, management, and prevention.

A well-recognized characteristic of infectious diseases specialists is our focus on epidemiology, and this trait has served us well in developing successful clinical careers. Perhaps our *compulsive investigation* of a patient's illness has been key in the desire of our colleagues from other specialties to "get infectious diseases involved." This focus is evident in each chapter so that the reader will have a deeper understanding of the epidemiology of illness and its impact on early, pathogen-based diagnoses.

Advances in the microbiology laboratory have clearly been influential in the diagnosis and management of infectious diseases. Automated systems have revolutionized laboratory activities, and even work areas in the laboratory have evolved. This textbook addresses many of these laboratory tools and how to interpret laboratory test results, which now are often available in almost warp speed. As a result, the duration of empiric (and possibly incorrect) therapy is shortened with the subsequent initiation of specific treatment, to the benefit of the individual patient.

We expect that this book will be useful to busy clinicians who want to better understand key aspects of different infectious diseases syndromes in the daily application of patient care. The text will also be helpful for trainees who are preparing for board examinations that evaluate their knowledge base in infectious diseases.

Larry M. Baddour, MD, FIDSA, FAHA
Supplemental Consultant for Research
Division of Infectious Diseases, Mayo Clinic
Professor Emeritus of Medicine
Mayo Clinic College of Medicine and Science

Table of Contents

Contributors

Cybele L. Abad, MD
Research Collaborator in Infectious Diseases, Mayo Clinic School of Graduate Medical Education, Mayo Clinic College of Medicine and Science, Rochester, Minnesota

Jithma P. Abeykoon, MD
Fellow in Hematology and Oncology, Mayo Clinic School of Graduate Medical Education and Assistant Professor of Medicine and of Oncology, Mayo Clinic College of Medicine and Science, Rochester, Minnesota

Omar M. Abu Saleh, MBBS
Senior Associate Consultant, Division of Infectious Diseases, Mayo Clinic, Rochester, Minnesota; Assistant Professor of Medicine, Mayo Clinic College of Medicine and Science

Saira R. Ajmal, MD
Fellow in Clinical Microbiology, Mayo Clinic School of Graduate Medical Education, Mayo Clinic College of Medicine and Science, Rochester, Minnesota; now with Advocate Medical Group, Oak Lawn, Illinois

Tariq Azam, MD
Resident in Internal Medicine, Mayo Clinic School of Graduate Medical Education, Mayo Clinic College of Medicine and Science, Rochester, Minnesota; now with University of Michigan Medical School, Ann Arbor, Michigan

Larry M. Baddour, MD
Supplemental Consultant for Research, Division of Infectious Diseases, Mayo Clinic, Rochester, Minnesota; Professor Emeritus of Medicine, Mayo Clinic College of Medicine and Science

Caroline Ball, MD
Resident in Internal Medicine, Mayo Clinic School of Graduate Medical Education, Mayo Clinic College of Medicine and Science, Rochester, Minnesota; now with Loyola University Medical Center, Park Ridge, Illinois

Elena Beam, MD
Consultant, Division of Infectious Diseases, Mayo Clinic, Rochester, Minnesota; Assistant Professor of Medicine, Mayo Clinic College of Medicine and Science

Edison J. Cano Cevallos, MD
Fellow in Infectious Diseases, Mayo Clinic School of Graduate Medical Education and Assistant Professor of Medicine, Mayo Clinic College of Medicine and Science, Rochester, Minnesota

Natalia E. Castillo Almeida, MD
Fellow in Infectious Diseases, Mayo Clinic School of Graduate Medical Education and Assistant Professor of Medicine, Mayo Clinic College of Medicine and Science, Rochester, Minnesota

Kelly A. Cawcutt, MD
Fellow in Infectious Diseases, Mayo Clinic School of Graduate Medical Education, Mayo Clinic College of Medicine and Science, Rochester, Minnesota; now with University of Nebraska Medical Center, Omaha, Nebraska

Douglas W. Challener, MD
Fellow in Infectious Diseases, Mayo Clinic School of Graduate Medical Education and Assistant Professor of Medicine, Mayo Clinic College of Medicine and Science, Rochester, Minnesota

Sara L. Cook, MD, PhD
Resident in Anatomic and Clinical Pathology, Mayo Clinic School of Graduate Medical Education, Mayo Clinic College of Medicine and Science, Rochester, Minnesota

Nathan W. Cummins, MD
Consultant, Division of Infectious Diseases, Mayo Clinic, Rochester, Minnesota; Associate Professor of Medicine, Mayo Clinic College of Medicine and Science

Kathryn T. del Valle, MD
Resident in Pulmonary and Critical Care Medicine, Mayo Clinic School of Graduate Medical Education, Mayo Clinic College of Medicine and Science, Rochester, Minnesota

Daniel C. DeSimone, MD
Consultant, Division of Infectious Diseases, Mayo Clinic, Rochester, Minnesota; Associate Professor of Medicine, Mayo Clinic College of Medicine and Science

Maria V. Dioverti Prono, MD
Fellow in Infectious Diseases, Mayo Clinic School of Graduate Medical Education; Assistant Professor, Mayo Clinic College of Medicine and Science, Rochester, Minnesota; now with Johns Hopkins University School of Medicine, Baltimore, Maryland

Abdelghani El Rafei, MD
Research Fellow in Infectious Diseases, Mayo Clinic School of Graduate Medical Education, Mayo Clinic, Rochester, Minnesota; now with University of Minnesota Medical School, Minneapolis, Minnesota

Lina I. Elbadawi, MD
Resident in Internal Medicine, Mayo Clinic College of Medicine and Science, Rochester, Minnesota; now with Centers for Disease Control and Prevention, Atlanta, Georgia

Mark J. Enzler, MD
Consultant, Division of Infectious Diseases, Mayo Clinic, Rochester, Minnesota; Assistant Professor of Medicine, Mayo Clinic College of Medicine and Science

Zerelda Esquer-Garrigos, MD
Fellow in Infectious Diseases, Mayo Clinic School of Graduate Medical Education and Instructor in Medicine, Mayo Clinic College of Medicine and Science, Rochester, Minnesota; now with University of Mississippi Medical Center, Jackson, Mississippi

Jarrett J. Failing, MD
Fellow in Hematology and Oncology, Mayo Clinic School of Graduate Medical Education and Instructor in Medicine, Mayo Clinic College of Medicine and Science, Rochester, Minnesota; now with Sanford Health, Fargo, North Dakota

Madiha Fida, MBBS
Fellow in Infectious Diseases, Mayo Clinic School of Graduate Medical Education and Assistant Professor of Medicine, Mayo Clinic College of Medicine and Science, Rochester, Minnesota

Pooja R. Gurram, MBBS
Resident in Infectious Diseases, Mayo Clinic School of Graduate Medical Education and Assistant Professor of Medicine, Mayo Clinic College of Medicine and Science, Rochester, Minnesota

Alfonso Hernandez-Acosta
Visiting Medical Student, Mayo Clinic Alix School of Medicine, Mayo Clinic College of Medicine and Science, Rochester, Minnesota; now with Cook County Health, Chicago, Illinois

Alexandra S. Higgins, MD
Resident in Hematology, Mayo Clinic School of Graduate Medical Education, Mayo Clinic College of Medicine and Science, Rochester, Minnesota

Patrick S. Hoversten, MD
Resident in Gastroenterology, Mayo Clinic School of Graduate Medical Education, Mayo Clinic College of Medicine and Science, Rochester, Minnesota; now with University of Wisconsin School of Medicine and Public Health, Madison, Wisconsin

Anil C. Jagtiani, MD
Fellow in Infectious Diseases, Mayo Clinic School of Graduate Medical Education, Mayo Clinic College of Medicine and Science, Rochester, Minnesota; now with Kaiser Permanente Fontana Medical Center, Fontana, California

Joana Kang, MD
Senior Associate Consultant, Division of Hospital Internal Medicine, Mayo Clinic, Rochester, Minnesota; now with St. Luke's Clinic, Boise, Idaho

Mary J. Kasten, MD
Consultant, Division of Infectious Diseases, Mayo Clinic, Rochester, Minnesota; Associate Professor of Medicine, Mayo Clinic College of Medicine and Science

Sarwat Khalil, MBBS
Research Collaborator in Infectious Diseases, Mayo Clinic School of Graduate Medical Education, Mayo Clinic College of Medicine and Science, Rochester, Minnesota

Erica Lin, MD
Resident in Internal Medicine, Mayo Clinic School of Graduate Medical Education, Mayo Clinic College of Medicine and Science, Rochester, Minnesota; now with University of California—San Diego, Department of Medicine, San Diego, California

Jasmine R. Marcelin, MD
Fellow in Infectious Diseases, Mayo Clinic School of Graduate Medical Education, Mayo Clinic College of Medicine and Science, Rochester, Minnesota; now with University of Nebraska Medical Center, Omaha, Nebraska

Prasanna P. Narayanan, PharmD, RPh
Pharmacist, Mayo Clinic Hospital—Saint Marys Campus, Mayo Clinic, Rochester, Minnesota

Christina G. O'Connor, PharmD, RPh
Pharmacist, Mayo Clinic, Rochester, Minnesota; Assistant Professor of Pharmacy, Mayo Clinic College of Medicine and Science

John C. O'Horo, MD, MPH
Consultant, Division of Infectious Diseases, Mayo Clinic, Rochester, Minnesota; Associate Professor of Medicine, Mayo Clinic College of Medicine and Science

Caitlin P. Oravec, PA-C, MS
Physician Assistant, Division of Infectious Diseases, Mayo Clinic, Rochester, Minnesota

Douglas R. Osmon, MD
Consultant, Division of Infectious Diseases, Mayo Clinic, Rochester, Minnesota; Professor of Medicine, Mayo Clinic College of Medicine and Science

Poornima Ramanan, MD
Fellow in Infectious Diseases, Mayo Clinic School of Graduate Medical Education and Instructor in Medicine, Mayo Clinic College of Medicine and Science, Rochester, Minnesota; now with University of Colorado School of Medicine, Denver, Colorado

Raymund R. Razonable, MD
Consultant, Division of Infectious Diseases, Mayo
Clinic, Rochester, Minnesota; Professor of Medicine,
Mayo Clinic College of Medicine and Science

Talha Riaz, MBBS
Research Collaborator in Infectious Diseases, Mayo
Clinic School of Graduate Medical Education, Mayo
Clinic College of Medicine and Science, Rochester,
Minnesota

Candido E. Rivera, MD
Consultant, Division of Hematology and Oncology,
Mayo Clinic, Jacksonville, Florida; Assistant Professor
of Medicine, Mayo Clinic College of Medicine and
Science

Stacey A. Rizza, MD
Consultant, Division of Infectious Diseases, Mayo
Clinic, Rochester, Minnesota; Professor of Medicine,
Mayo Clinic College of Medicine and Science

Priya Sampathkumar, MD
Consultant, Division of Infectious Diseases, Mayo
Clinic, Rochester, Minnesota; Associate Professor of
Medicine, Mayo Clinic College of Medicine and Science

Jose J. Sanchez, MD
Resident in Internal Medicine, Mayo Clinic School of
Graduate Medical Education, Mayo Clinic College of
Medicine and Science, Rochester, Minnesota

Aditya S. Shah, MBBS
Senior Associate Consultant, Division of Infectious
Diseases, Mayo Clinic, Rochester, Minnesota; Assistant
Professor of Medicine, Mayo Clinic College of Medicine
and Science

Korosh Sharain, MD
Fellow in Cardiovascular Diseases, Mayo Clinic School
of Graduate Medical Education and Assistant Professor
of Medicine, Mayo Clinic College of Medicine and
Science, Rochester, Minnesota

FNU Shweta, MBBS
Fellow in Infectious Diseases, Mayo Clinic School
of Graduate Medical Education and Instructor in
Medicine, Mayo Clinic College of Medicine and
Science, Rochester, Minnesota

Irene G. Sia, MD
Consultant, Division of Infectious Diseases, Mayo
Clinic, Rochester, Minnesota; Professor of Medicine,
Mayo Clinic College of Medicine and Science

M. Rizwan Sohail, MD
Research Collaborator in Infectious Diseases, Mayo
Clinic School of Graduate Medical Education, Mayo
Clinic College of Medicine and Science, Rochester,
Minnesota

Eric C. Stone, MD
Fellow in Infectious Diseases, Mayo Clinic School of
Graduate Medical Education, Mayo Clinic College of
Medicine and Science, Rochester, Minnesota; now with
Long Beach Veterans Affairs Healthcare System, Long
Beach, California

Alan M. Sugrue, MB, BCh, BAO
Fellow in Cardiovascular Diseases, Mayo Clinic School
of Graduate Medical Education and Assistant Professor
of Medicine, Mayo Clinic College of Medicine and
Science, Rochester, Minnesota

Eugene M. Tan, MD
Fellow in Infectious Diseases, Mayo Clinic School of
Graduate Medical Education, Mayo Clinic College of
Medicine and Science, Rochester, Minnesota; now with
Sentara CarePlex Hospital, Hampton, Virginia

Nicholas Y. Tan, MD, MS
Fellow in Cardiovascular Diseases, Mayo Clinic School
of Graduate Medical Education and Assistant Professor
of Medicine, Mayo Clinic College of Medicine and
Science, Rochester, Minnesota

Aaron J. Tande, MD
Consultant, Division of Infectious Diseases, Mayo
Clinic, Rochester, Minnesota; Associate Professor
of Medicine, Mayo Clinic College of Medicine and
Science

Zelalem Temesgen, MD
Consultant, Division of Infectious Diseases, Mayo
Clinic, Rochester, Minnesota; Professor of Medicine,
Mayo Clinic College of Medicine and Science

Matthew J. Thoendel, MD, PhD
Senior Associate Consultant, Division of Infectious
Diseases, Mayo Clinic, Rochester, Minnesota; Assistant
Professor of Medicine, Mayo Clinic College of Medicine
and Science

Rodney L. Thompson, MD
Emeritus Member, Division of Infectious Diseases,
Mayo Clinic, Rochester, Minnesota; Emeritus Assistant
Professor of Medicine, Mayo Clinic College of Medicine
and Science

Prakhar Vijayvargiya, MBBS
Research Collaborator in Infectious Diseases, Mayo
Clinic School of Graduate Medical Education, Mayo
Clinic College of Medicine and Science, Rochester,
Minnesota

Abinash Virk, MD
Consultant, Division of Infectious Diseases, Mayo
Clinic, Rochester, Minnesota; Associate Professor
of Medicine, Mayo Clinic College of Medicine and
Science

Jennifer A. Whitaker, MD
Research Collaborator in Internal Medicine, Mayo
Clinic School of Graduate Medical Education, Mayo
Clinic College of Medicine and Science, Rochester,
Minnesota

Carilyn N. Wieland, MD
Consultant, Department of Dermatology, Mayo
Clinic, Rochester, Minnesota; Associate Professor of
Dermatology and of Laboratory Medicine & Pathology,
Mayo Clinic College of Medicine and Science

John W. Wilson, MD
Consultant, Division of Infectious Diseases, Mayo
Clinic, Rochester, Minnesota; Professor of Medicine,
Mayo Clinic College of Medicine and Science

Alan J. Wright, MD
Emeritus Member, Division of Infectious Diseases,
Mayo Clinic, Rochester, Minnesota; Emeritus Assistant
Professor of Medicine, Mayo Clinic College of Medicine
and Science

Joseph D. Yao, MD
Consultant, Division of Clinical Microbiology,
Rochester, Minnesota; Associate Professor of
Laboratory Medicine and of Medicine and Assistant
Professor of Microbiology, Mayo Clinic College of
Medicine and Science

John D. Zeuli, PharmD, RPh
Pharmacist, Mayo Clinic, Rochester, Minnesota

Cases

Pneumonia in a Patient With a Kidney Transplant

Nicholas Y. Tan, MD, MS, Omar M. Abu Saleh, MBBS, and Elena Beam, MD

Case Presentation

A 60-year-old man presented to the emergency department with a 2-week history of malaise, progressive cough with green sputum, dyspnea, and pleuritic chest pain. His medical history included adult-onset polycystic kidney disease, for which he underwent bilateral nephrectomy and deceased-donor kidney transplant 10 years prior. His medications included tacrolimus, mycophenolate mofetil, and prednisone. He denied exposure to farm animals but had a dog at home.

On admission, chest computed tomography (CT) showed a right upper-lobe consolidation with associated mediastinal lymphadenopathy (Figure 1.1). He started treatment with empiric, broad-spectrum antibiotics, including intravenous vancomycin, levofloxacin, and aztreonam. He remained hemodynamically stable and afebrile

Figure 1.1 Computed Tomographic Image of the Chest

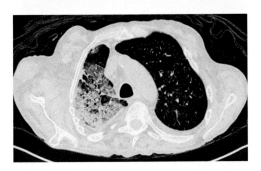

The image shows right upper-lobe consolidation.

on this regimen, with corresponding improvement in his cough and chest discomfort.

Blood cultures showed gram-positive rods after 18 hours of incubation, and these were later identified as *Rhodococcus equi*; adequate sputum cultures were not collected. When antibiotic susceptibilities were available, his treatment was changed to combination therapy with intravenous vancomycin, oral azithromycin, and minocycline. The bacteremia resolved after 12 days of antibiotic therapy and he was discharged, with close outpatient follow-up. A transesophageal echocardiogram did not show endocarditis, and a positron emission tomography—computed tomography (PET-CT) scan was consistent only with the known lung infection. Vancomycin was discontinued after 1 week of negative blood cultures; minocycline was later changed to moxifloxacin because of drug-related skin hyperpigmentation. A chest CT after 2 months of antibiotic therapy showed marked improvement in the pneumonia and mediastinal lymphadenopathy; oral antibiotic therapy was continued for an additional month (total duration of therapy was 3 months). He subsequently had complete resolution of his respiratory symptoms.

Discussion

R equi is a zoonotic organism that is a well-known cause of pneumonia for young horses.

The first report of *R equi* infection in a human was published in 1967; since then, it has become an increasingly common pathogen in immunocompromised populations, including transplant recipients and those with HIV (1).

R equi is a facultative, intracellular, nonmotile organism that is gram positive and weakly acid-fast. On solid media, it forms salmon-pink or red teardrop-shaped or coalescent mucoid colonies (Figure 1.2); in liquid media, it appears rod shaped and filamentous. Its ability to infect and persist in macrophages is a key aspect of its pathogenesis. Malacoplakia may be observed with tissue biopsy; it is characterized by the infiltration of foamy histiocytes and the presence of intracellular, concentric basophilic inclusions (Michaelis-Guttmann bodies) and coccobacilli. *R equi* has been isolated from soil and water, and high concentrations have been identified in areas with herbivore manure (eg, horse farms) (1).

The number of reported *R equi* infections in humans has risen dramatically in the past 30 years, likely because of the increasing prevalence of HIV-positive patients and transplant recipients. Modes of acquisition include inhalation or ingestion of the organism and direct inoculation of wounds or exposed mucous membranes. History of exposure to horses or pigs is a useful clinical clue; however, it is not always reported (only 39%-70% recall exposure to horses) (2,3). Among transplant recipients, *R equi* infection is associated with renal transplant, corticosteroid use, diabetes mellitus, recent opportunistic infection, and male sex. Trimethoprim-sulfamethoxazole use is not protective, likely due to a high resistance rate, with one study showing that 50% of a transplant cohort with *R equi* infection diagnosed in the first posttransplant year had received the drug prophylactically (2).

About 80% of patients present with pulmonary manifestations, with upper-lobe cavitary pneumonia being the most common radiographic finding; however, pleural effusion and nodular infiltrate also may be seen. Extrapulmonary disease due to *R equi* infection most often occurs through hematogenous spread; patients may have brain abscesses or osteomyelitis. Additionally, patients with hematopoietic stem cell transplant usually present sooner after transplant than solid-organ recipients with bacteremia (2). Constitutional symptoms, including fever, weight loss, and fatigue, may accompany respiratory findings and may thereby lead to a misdiagnosis of pulmonary tuberculosis. Additional differential diagnoses to consider include invasive mold infection, endemic fungal disease, and necrotizing bacterial pneumonia. The diagnosis is established by culture or by sequencing biopsy specimens or aspirates. Blood cultures are positive for 27% to 50% of reported cases, depending on their predisposing clinical condition (1).

Figure 1.2   Colonies on Solid Media

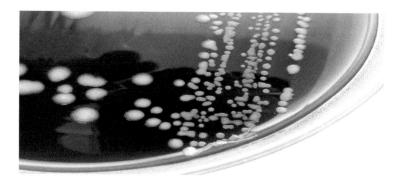

Agar plate showing coalescing coccoid colonies of *Rhodococcus equi* with a mucoid appearance.

No specific guidelines have been published to date for treating *R equi* infections. Generally, we recommend a 2- to 3-drug combination of antibiotics with intracellular activity, with selections guided by antimicrobial susceptibility testing (AST). For patients with severe infections, including bacteremia, intravenous therapy should be implemented first; transition to an oral regimen can be determined by the clinical response and AST results. Macrolides, glycopeptides, fluoroquinolones, and rifampin are commonly used initial agents; medications are then further tailored to match susceptibility patterns. Duration of antibiotic treatment depends on the patient's immune status, response rate, and site of infection (2-8 weeks appear adequate for immunocompetent

Table 1.1	**Gram-Positive or Gram-Variable Organisms Associated With Subacute Infections in Immunocompromised Hosts in the Setting of Environmental or Animal Exposures**			
Organism	**Morphology**	**Host Characteristics**	**Syndrome**	**Notes**
Actinomyces spp	Branched, filamentous Slow growing (14-21 days' incubation)	Immunosuppressed Diabetes mellitus, alcohol abuse	Suppurative infection, with abscess or fistula formation Pseudotumor	Susceptible to penicillins
Corynebacterium jeikeium	Palisading, club-shaped "Chinese letters"	Immunosuppressed Prosthetic heart valves	Line-related bacteremia Endocarditis Device infection	Susceptible to vancomycin
Erysipelothrix rhusiopathiae	Gram stain variable α-Hemolytic punctiform colonies	Can occur in immunocompetent hosts	Cutaneous infections Bacteremia, with high rates of endocarditis	Susceptible to penicillin Exposure to pigs, fish, wildlife; occupational exposures
Listeria monocytogenes	Small rods Tumbling or umbrella motility	Extremes of age Immunosuppressed Pregnant	Meningoencephalitis Rhombencephalitis Bacteremia Febrile gastroenteritis	Susceptible to TMP-SMX, less likely in those receiving prophylaxis Exposure to contaminated food
Nocardia spp	Branched, filamentous Weakly acid-fast	Immunosuppressed Chronic lung disease	Pulmonary, with or without CNS dissemination Skin and soft tissue abscesses	Certain species are TMP-SMX resistant Infection may occur despite prophylaxis
Nontuberculous mycobacterium	Acid-fast Slow growing Beaded gram positive	Immunosuppressed "Tea and toast syndrome"	Pulmonary infection most common; may also have bacteremia or line-related infection Constitutional symptoms (weight loss, fevers, night sweats)	Multidrug regimens required (eg, clarithromycin, rifampin, ethambutol) AST helpful for macrolide resistance
Rhodococcus equi	Coccobacilli Salmon-pink colonies	Immunosuppressed	Pulmonary infection Bacteremia	Exposure to horses in up to 70% of patients Treatment guided by AST

Abbreviations: AST, antimicrobial susceptibility testing; CNS, central nervous system; spp, species; TMP-SMX, trimethoprim-sulfamethoxazole.

patients, whereas 6 months or longer may be required for immunocompromised patients) (1-4). Surgical intervention may be required in refractory disease. Mortality rates are lower in immunocompetent individuals (~11%) compared with those with HIV (50%-55%) or non–HIV-related immunosuppression (20%-25%) (1).

The patient described above had several typical risk factors associated with *R equi* infection (male sex, history of corticosteroid use, and renal transplant). Although he had no exposure to farm animals such as horses or pigs, dogs are also recognized as a potential source of infection.

In general, when developing the differential diagnosis of subacute pulmonary infection in a transplant patient, several factors should be considered: 1) time since transplant, which can be a clue for donor-derived infection; 2) extent of immunosuppression; 3) use of chemoprophylaxis; 4) infectious exposure (within the community or through travel); and 5) recent stays in health care facilities. Table 1.1 summarizes gram-positive or gram-variable organisms that should be considered in immunocompromised individuals.

References

1. Yamshchikov AV, Schuetz A, Lyon GM. *Rhodococcus equi* infection. Lancet Infect Dis. 2010 May;10(5):350–9.
2. Vergidis P, Ariza-Heredia EJ, Nellore A, Kotton CN, Kaul DR, Morris MI, et al. Rhodococcus infection in solid organ and hematopoietic stem cell transplant recipients. Emerg Infect Dis. 2017 Mar;23(3):510–2.
3. Menon V, Gottlieb T, Gallagher M, Cheong EL. Persistent *Rhodococcus equi* infection in a renal transplant patient: case report and review of the literature. Transpl Infect Dis. 2012 Dec;14(6):E126-33. Epub 2012 Sep 26.
4. Topino S, Galati V, Grilli E, Petrosillo N. *Rhodococcus equi* infection in HIV-infected individuals: case reports and review of the literature. AIDS patient care STDS. 2010 Apr;24(4):211–22.

A Pregnant Pause

Jasmine R. Marcelin, MD, and Joseph D. Yao, MD

2

Case Presentation

A 26-year-old Ethiopian woman, gravida 2, para 1, who was 14 weeks pregnant with her second child, was referred to an infectious disease specialist for further evaluation of a positive HIV serologic screening test result. Her prior pregnancy was normal, resulting in a live birth by cesarean delivery. She had negative HIV serologic screening test results on 2 previous occasions, without a history of sexually transmitted infections. The patient was in a monogamous relationship with the father of both children.

Her current pregnancy was discovered when she presented to the emergency department with abdominal pain. She subsequently underwent routine prenatal screening: her fourth-generation HIV-1/HIV-2 antigen and antibody (Ag/Ab) screen was reactive, plus she had an indeterminate HIV-1 antibody result (reactive band for p31) in the reflexive HIV-1/HIV-2 antibody differentiation test. Additional HIV-2 antibody testing was negative.

Further testing with plasma HIV-1 RNA quantification showed an undetectable viral load, and her CD4+ count was 838 cells/mcL (reference range, 365-1,437 cells/mcL). She had no systemic signs or symptoms of HIV infection. She had never used injection drugs or required a blood transfusion. The father of her children was also Ethiopian, and his HIV-1/HIV-2 Ag/Ab screening test was negative. She underwent repeat HIV-1/HIV-2 Ag/Ab screening in the second and third trimesters, and both were negative. She did not require any antiretroviral therapy and successfully delivered her baby without incident.

Discussion

An estimated 14% of the 1.2 million HIV-infected teens and adults in the United States are unaware of their diagnosis. Current guidelines recommend universal HIV screening of all patients aged 13 to 65 years (1), but in this situation, epidemiologic risk factors also must be considered. Three-quarters of HIV infections worldwide are in sub-Saharan Africa, and more than 90% of pregnant women with HIV infection are from this geographic region (2). HIV-2 infection must also be considered. Although rare, it is most prevalent among individuals from West Africa, and HIV-2 infection should be considered in patients with positive initial HIV screening tests and indeterminate Western blots or if they are from high-risk regions (2). Our patient was from Ethiopia, which is on the east coast of Africa and is not a region with a high prevalence of HIV-2 infections.

The risk of perinatal transmission of HIV has decreased with the implementation of universal screening during pregnancy. Routine HIV screening, a recommended part of perinatal care (3), is typically performed during the first trimester at the initial visit. Women can decline such screening, but they should be encouraged to undergo testing at least once during every pregnancy and more frequently if they have risk of continued exposure to HIV, given the manageable risks of perinatal transmission. In addition, women with a high risk of seroconversion during pregnancy (eg, those with high-risk behaviors, discordant partners, living in high-prevalence countries) should be rescreened in the third trimester.

The current fourth-generation HIV-1 Ag/Ab screening tests are highly sensitive and specific. Although false-reactive results are uncommon, patients who are most likely to have such screening test results include pregnant women, patients with rheumatologic disorders, and patients with malignancies (4). One study indicated that greater parity also contributes to increased rates of false-reactive results (5).

An HIV screening algorithm is shown in Figure 2.1. When a person is screened with a fourth-generation HIV Ag/Ab test and has positive results, subsequent testing should include an HIV-1/HIV-2 antibody differentiation test and a qualitative and/or quantitative HIV RNA test (mainly for HIV-1) if the antibody differentiation test result is negative or indeterminate. Detectable plasma HIV RNA in the presence of a negative or indeterminate HIV antibody screen result would indicate an early HIV infection or acute retroviral syndrome. Early HIV infection can be asymptomatic, and acute retroviral syndrome can present with fever, viral respiratory–like symptoms, lymphadenopathy, and multiple nonspecific symptoms. When the HIV-1/HIV-2 antibody differentiation test result is indeterminate and HIV RNA is undetectable in the plasma, possible scenarios include a false-reactive HIV Ag/Ab screen, HIV-2 infection, or an incomplete antibody response in an HIV-infected individual. HIV-2 infection is suspected if the HIV-1/HIV-2 antibody differentiation test is positive for HIV-2 antibody with a negative reflexive HIV-1 RNA test result and the patient is from West Africa or in a sexual relationship with a person from West Africa.

Pregnant women are more likely to have a reactive HIV serologic screening test result with a negative or indeterminate HIV antibody differentiation test result. If a pregnant woman also has an undetectable HIV RNA level in the plasma during the first or second trimester, she should be retested at least 1 month later, but before delivery, to ascertain her true HIV infection status (6). Viral load testing should be pursued if the

Figure 2.1   Current Recommended HIV Testing Algorithm for All Adults (Pregnant and Nonpregnant)

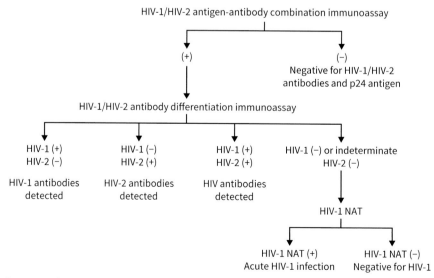

NAT indicates nucleic acid test; (+), reactive test result; (−), nonreactive test result.
Modified from Centers for Disease Control and Prevention and Association of Public Health Laboratories [6].

screening and supplemental serologic assays show discordant results. If a patient has a high risk of acquiring HIV, HIV serologic screening should be repeated during the third trimester. Sexual partners also should be screened for HIV infection.

References

1. Moyer VA; US Preventive Services Task Force. Screening for HIV: US Preventive Services Task Force Recommendation Statement. Ann Intern Med. 2013 Jul 2;159(1):51–60.
2. Ramjee G, Daniels B. Women and HIV in Sub-Saharan Africa. AIDS Res Ther. 2013 Dec 13;10(1):30.
3. HIV and pregnant women, infants, and children [Internet]. Atlanta (GA): Centers for Disease Control and Prevention [updated 2019 Mar 21; cited 2020 Feb 25]. Available from: https://www.cdc.gov/hiv/pdf/group/gender/pregnantwomen/cdc-hiv-pregnant-women.pdf.
4. Liu P, Jackson P, Shaw N, Heysell S. Spectrum of false positivity for the fourth generation human immunodeficiency virus diagnostic tests. AIDS Res Ther. 2016 Jan 5;13:1.
5. Celum CL, Coombs RW, Jones M, Murphy V, Fisher L, Grant C, et al. Risk factors for repeatedly reactive HIV-1 EIA and indeterminate Western blots: a population-based case-control study. Arch Intern Med. 1994 May 23;154(10):1129–37.
6. Centers for Disease Control and Prevention and Association of Public Health Laboratories [Internet]. Laboratory testing for the diagnosis of HIV infection: updated recommendations [updated 2014 Jun 27; cited 2020 Feb 25]. Available from: http://dx.doi.org/10.15620/cdc.23447.

What a Headache!

Eugene M. Tan, MD, Jasmine R. Marcelin, MD, and Zelalem Temesgen, MD

3

Case Presentation

A 70-year-old man presented to the emergency department with a fever of 38.6°C (101.5°F). He had a 6-month history of daily generalized headaches, neck stiffness, retro-orbital discomfort, night sweats, and fevers up to 37.8°C (100°F). He denied photophobia or any other visual or neurologic deficits. He had chronic lymphocytic leukemia and had been observed without any treatment for a 4-year period. A computed tomographic (CT) image of the head was normal. Cerebrospinal fluid (CSF) analysis showed 756 total nucleated cells/mcL (91% lymphocytes), decreased glucose (<20 mg/dL), and elevated protein (285 mg/dL). Opening pressure was not measured. Yeast and white blood cells were identified with a Gram stain of the CSF.

Because of concerns for fungal or bacterial meningitis, the patient initially received broad-spectrum antimicrobials (vancomycin, meropenem, liposomal amphotericin B). Cryptococcal antigen titer tests were positive for the CSF (>1:2,560) and serum (1:160). CSF fungal cultures grew *Cryptococcus neoformans*. His antimicrobial therapy was modified to liposomal amphotericin B (3-4 mg/kg per day, administered intravenously) plus flucytosine (25 mg/kg, administered orally every 6 hours). A subsequent CSF analysis showed an opening pressure of 11 cm H_2O, elevated protein (221 mg/dL), and decreased glucose (<20 mg/dL).

The patient was hospitalized for 4 days and was discharged with a plan to continue antimicrobial therapy on an outpatient basis. At the time of discharge, his serum creatinine was 1.2 mg/dL, which was considered a normal baseline value.

He had twice-weekly monitoring of his complete blood count and serum potassium and creatinine levels; he also had weekly liver function tests. Two weeks after discharge, his creatinine had increased to 2.2 mg/dL, and he had hypokalemia (3.4 mmol/L). Follow-up CSF studies after 2 weeks of combination therapy confirmed a similar opening pressure (12 cm H_2O), elevated protein (262 mg/dL), and decreased glucose (<20 mg/dL). A fungal smear and culture were negative.

At this point, flucytosine and liposomal amphotericin B were discontinued, and the patient was transitioned to an 8-week consolidation phase of fluconazole (400 mg, once daily). During a follow-up examination, 4 weeks into the consolidation phase, his creatinine had returned to 1.3 mg/dL. With potassium supplementation, his potassium normalized to 3.7 mmol/L. After completing 8 weeks of consolidation therapy with fluconazole (400 mg daily), his dose was decreased to 200 mg daily, with instructions to continue this medication lifelong for secondary prophylaxis.

The patient's history raised concerns regarding an underlying immunodeficiency. An HIV test had negative results, but during his initial hospitalization, laboratory tests showed that he had a low CD4 count (230 cells/mcL; reference range, 365-1,437 cells/mcL) and a low natural killer cell count (11 cells/mcL; reference range, 59-513 cells/mcL). Four months after he had recovered from the acute illness, repeat testing showed a normal CD4 cell count (553 cells/mcL), decreased natural killer cells (45 cells/mcL), decreased immunoglobulin (Ig) A (18 mg/dL; reference range, 61-356 mg/dL), decreased IgM (8 mg/dL; reference range, 37-286 mg/dL), and normal IgG (831 mg/dL; reference range, 767-1,590 mg/dL). He also had a poor response to the pneumococcal vaccine (only 6/23 serotype-specific IgG concentrations were ≥1.3 mcg/mL). He started receiving thrice-weekly prophylactic azithromycin and weekly subcutaneous immunoglobulin.

Discussion

C neoformans is a facultative, intracellular yeast that is found worldwide, often in avian feces. When inhaled, desiccated yeast cells or spores can cause a primary pulmonary infection; the infection can remain latent but may be activated when the host becomes immunocompromised. *C neoformans* then disseminates and traverses the blood-brain barrier to cause cryptococcal meningitis (CM) (1). Typical symptoms include fever, weight loss, night sweats, headache, and altered mental status (2). Cryptococcosis tends to occur in immunocompromised patients with HIV/AIDS, solid-organ transplant, or hematologic malignancy. However, 10% to 40% of HIV-negative patients with cryptococcosis have no apparent immunodeficiency.

A lumbar puncture is required for the diagnosis of CM. Lumbar puncture may show a high opening pressure (>25 cm H_2O), which may be associated with blurred vision, confusion, papilledema, and lower extremity clonus. In this setting, large volumes of CSF can be removed with daily serial lumbar punctures until the CSF pressure is less than 20 cm H_2O or decreases to 50% of the initial pressure. If opening pressures are severely elevated, a temporary lumbar drain can be inserted to remove 200 mL of CSF daily (3).

In CM, CSF analysis shows elevated protein, decreased glucose, and increased white blood cell count with lymphocytosis, but in HIV-associated CM, the CSF white blood cell count may be lower or normal. *C neoformans* will grow on most bacterial and fungal cultures (3). Cryptococcal polysaccharide antigen detection by rapid and simple

latex agglutination, lateral flow assay, or enzyme immunoassay have greater than 90% sensitivity for identifying *C neoformans*. CSF antigen titers can correlate with organism burden, and titers exceeding 1:1,024 may signify a poor prognosis (3). Imaging may assist with diagnosis. CT of the head can show meningeal enhancement, nodules (cryptococcomas), cerebral edema, or hydrocephalus, but images often may be normal as well. Magnetic resonance imaging is more sensitive than CT for detecting enhancing central nervous system nodules (3).

Treatment regimens for patients can differ, depending on whether they have HIV/AIDS, are receiving immunosuppressive medications (eg, after solid-organ transplant), or are immunocompetent. Antifungal therapy is generally the same for all categories of patients, but additional recommendations may apply to different subgroups. For example, immunosuppressive medications should be minimized for solid-organ transplant recipients, and patients with HIV/AIDS should adhere to their antiretroviral therapeutic regimen. Immunocompetent patients with CM should be evaluated for a potentially undiagnosed immunodeficiency (4).

Amphotericin B deoxycholate (0.7-1 mg/kg per day) is a polyene fungicidal agent that binds to ergosterol in the plasma membrane and increases permeability, but nephrotoxicity is a concern. However, liposomal amphotericin B is an alternative formulation that allows delivery of a much larger amphotericin dose with less nephrotoxicity. For the first 2 weeks of induction therapy, amphotericin B is combined with flucytosine (100 mg/kg per day in 4 divided doses), an anticancer drug that is converted to 5-fluorouracil and inhibits nucleic acid synthesis. In general, flucytosine dosing should be reduced by 50% for every 50% decline in creatinine clearance, and if flucytosine serum levels can be measured, they should be obtained 2 hours after the third to fifth dose, with a goal of 25 to 100 mg/L (5). After 2 weeks of combination therapy, a repeat lumbar puncture is performed to assess whether sterilization of the CSF has occurred (3).

Fluconazole is a fungistatic triazole that inhibits ergosterol synthesis. After 2 weeks of induction with amphotericin B and flucytosine, the next treatment phase is consolidation with fluconazole (400 mg daily) for 8 weeks. The rationale for switching to fluconazole is to avoid prolonged exposure to amphotericin B, which is nephrotoxic. After 8 weeks of consolidation therapy, fluconazole is decreased to a maintenance dose of 200 mg daily until immune reconstitution occurs. In patients with HIV, the CD4 count should be between 100 to 200 cells/mcL for 6 to 12 months (3).

Improvements in immune function can lead to immune reconstitution syndrome, which is a paradoxic worsening of symptoms due to excess inflammation directed at residual fungi. Generally, immune reconstitution syndrome can be treated with corticosteroids or, if life threatening, with adalimumab (4). In patients with newly diagnosed HIV/AIDS, deferring antiretroviral therapy for 2 to 10 weeks after the diagnosis of CM may improve survival because immune reconstitution syndrome occurs more commonly with earlier antiretroviral therapy (5,6).

References

1. Srikanta D, Santiago-Tirado FH, Doering TL. *Cryptococcus neoformans*: historical curiosity to modern pathogen. Yeast. 2014 Feb;31(2):47–60. Epub 2014 Jan 19.
2. Pappas PG, Perfect JR, Cloud GA, Larsen RA, Pankey GA, Lancaster DJ, et al. Cryptococcosis in human immunodeficiency virus-negative patients in the era of effective azole therapy. Clin Infect Dis. 2001 Sep 1;33(5):690–9. Epub 2001 Jul 26.
3. Bicanic T, Harrison TS. Cryptococcal meningitis. Br Med Bull. 2005 Apr 18;72:99–118.
4. Coelho C, Casadevall A. Cryptococcal therapies and drug targets: the old, the new and the promising. Cell Microbiol. 2016 Jun;18(6):792–9. Epub 2016 Apr 8.
5. Kaplan JE, Benson C, Holmes KK, Brooks JT, Pau A, Masur H; Centers for Disease Control and Prevention (CDC); National Institutes of Health; HIV Medicine Association of the Infectious Diseases Society of America. Guidelines for prevention and treatment of opportunistic infections in HIV-infected adults and adolescents: recommendations from CDC, the National Institutes of Health, and the HIV Medicine Association of the Infectious Diseases Society of America. MMWR Recomm Rep. 2009 Apr 10;58(RR-4):1–207.
6. Boulware DR, Meya DB, Muzoora C, Rolfes MA, Huppler Hullsiek K, Musubire A, et al; COAT Trial Team. Timing of antiretroviral therapy after diagnosis of cryptococcal meningitis. N Engl J Med. 2014 Jun 26;370(26):2487–98.

Retinal Lesions and Eye Pain

Prakhar Vijayvargiya, MBBS, and Jasmine R. Marcelin, MD

4

Case Presentation

A 39-year-old woman with a history of hypertension, nicotine and alcohol dependence, and intravenous (IV) drug use, plus a remote history of incarceration, woke up one morning with acute-onset pain in her right eye. She presented to the emergency department within 24 hours. She reported no antecedent eye trauma, and these symptoms had never occurred previously. She described the pain as pressure-like discomfort that worsened with eye movement, and she also had blurry vision, conjunctival redness, and photophobia. She did not use contact lenses. She worked in housekeeping but denied occupational exposure to chemicals and had no travel outside the United States. No other systemic signs of illness were present, and a chest radiograph did not show evidence of hilar lymphadenopathy or infiltrates. A funduscopic examination of the left eye showed 3+ cells and 1+ flare in the anterior chamber, with numerous scattered, fluffy, yellow-white retinal lesions and no evidence of hemorrhage or vasculitis. The findings were consistent with panuveitis in the left eye and intermediate uveitis in the right eye.

A number of laboratory tests were performed to determine the cause of uveitis (Table 4.1). The syphilis immunoglobulin (Ig) G antibody assay was positive, but the rapid plasma reagin (RPR) assay was negative. A second treponemal test, *Treponema pallidum* particle agglutination (TP-PA), was performed and was positive, confirming the diagnosis of syphilis. The patient denied having syphilis previously. She was in a monogamous relationship for the past 6 years, but before that relationship, she had multiple sexual partners and inconsistent condom use.

Her current sexual partner previously had been treated for gonorrhea but refused to be tested or presumptively treated for syphilis.

A diagnosis of syphilitic uveitis was made on the basis of the uveitis noted during the ocular examination, the positive treponemal tests, and the absence of a history of treatment for syphilis. Treatment with penicillin was recommended, but she refused because of financial and work-related issues. She took oral amoxicillin from a previous prescription for a few days, after which her symptoms improved. She was again seen in the clinic, 6 weeks later, with worsening eye symptoms that included burning, pain, and redness in her left eye. A funduscopic examination showed panuveitis of the left eye and intermediate uveitis of the right eye. She subsequently agreed to treatment with IV penicillin G (continuous infusion for 14 days). Her symptoms improved with therapy, and her vision returned to normal.

Discussion

Ocular syphilis is uncommon, but syphilis accounts for 1% to 5% of all uveitis cases at tertiary referral centers in the United States (1). Ocular syphilis can present as anterior uveitis (inflammation of the iris, ciliary body, or anterior chamber), intermediate uveitis (inflammation of the vitreous cavity), posterior uveitis (chorioretinitis), or panuveitis (inflammation of all layers of the uvea). In the literature, syphilitic uveitis most commonly manifests as panuveitis (2). Isolated anterior uveitis has primarily been reported in patients with HIV coinfection (3). Syphilitic uveitis can be seen in late latent or

Table 4.1.   Summary of Diagnostic Test Results Obtained With 2 Episodes of Eye Pain

Test	First Visit	6 Weeks Later	Reference Range
White blood cell count, ×10^9/L	7.5	6	3.5-10.5
Hemoglobin, g/dL	11.3	...	12.0-15.5
Platelet, ×10^9/L	386	...	150-450
Erythrocyte sedimentation rate, mm/h	42	...	0-29
C-reactive protein, mg/L	31.0	...	≤8.0 mg/L
Glucose, mg/dL	...	82	70-100
Angiotensin-converting enzyme, U/L	19	...	8-53
Antinuclear antibody, U	0.3	...	≤1
Anti-dsDNA antibody, IU/mL	≤12.3	...	≤30.0
Lyme disease (ELISA screen)	Negative	...	Negative
Syphilis IgG antibody	Positive	Positive	Negative
Syphilis antibody (TP-PA)	Positive	Positive	Negative
Rapid plasma reagin	Negative	Negative	Negative
QuantiFERON-TB test[a]	Negative	...	Negative
HIV fourth-generation antibody and p24 antigen screen	Negative	...	Negative
CMV antibody IgG	Positive	...	Negative
CMV antibody IgM	Negative	...	Negative
Chlamydia trachomatis amplified RNA	...	Negative	Negative
Neisseria gonorrhoeae amplified RNA	...	Negative	Negative
Cerebrospinal fluid			
Glucose, mg/dL	...	51	60% of plasma glucose
Protein, mg/dL	...	49	0-35
Total nucleated cells, per mcL	...	1	0-5
Venereal disease research laboratory	...	Negative	Negative

Abbreviations: CMV, cytomegalovirus; dsDNA, double-stranded DNA; ELISA, enzyme-linked immunosorbent assay; Ig, immunoglobulin; TP-PA, *Treponema pallidum* particle agglutination.

[a] Mayo Clinic does not endorse specific products or services.

tertiary stages of syphilis, but it can also be a manifestation of secondary syphilis (2).

Diagnosis of Syphilis

Panuveitis has a broad differential diagnosis of infectious and noninfectious causes, and extensive evaluation is necessary to identify the origin of disease. Common infectious causes include herpes simplex virus, varicella-zoster virus, cytomegalovirus, tuberculosis, syphilis, bartonellosis, and toxoplasmosis. Systemic inflammatory disorders that can cause panuveitis include sarcoidosis, Vogt-Koyanagi-Harada disease, Behçet disease, irritable bowel disease, and systemic lupus erythematosus. In addition, sympathetic ophthalmia is a posttraumatic granulomatous eye disorder that can cause panuveitis.

Syphilis can involve any ocular structure and is not limited to the uvea. An ophthalmologic examination can show conjunctivitis, episcleritis, scleritis, or interstitial scleritis. A posterior segment examination may show retinitis, chorioretinitis, vasculitis, serous retinal detachment, or acute syphilitic posterior placoid chorioretinopathy. Superficial retinal precipitates can be seen with optical coherence tomography. Enhanced imaging modalities such as indocyanine green angiography may help ophthalmologists confirm ocular syphilis in cases for which a fundus examination or fluorescein angiography cannot identify any retinochoroidal abnormality. Syphilitic

retinitis, however, responds promptly to treatment, with minimal disruption of retinal pigment epithelium.

Establishing the diagnosis of syphilitic uveitis requires serologic tests, in addition to the ophthalmologic evaluation. Treponemal tests (syphilis IgG, TP-PA, fluorescent treponemal antibody absorption) and nontreponemal tests (RPR, venereal disease research laboratory [VDRL]) need to be positive to confirm the diagnosis. If only the treponemal test is positive (ie, the nontreponemal test is negative, as was observed in the patient described above), a second treponemal test should be obtained (Figure 4.1).

A nontreponemal test can have a false-negative result in a patient with early stage syphilis or previous treatment for syphilis. In

Figure 4.1   Diagnostic Testing Algorithms for Syphilis

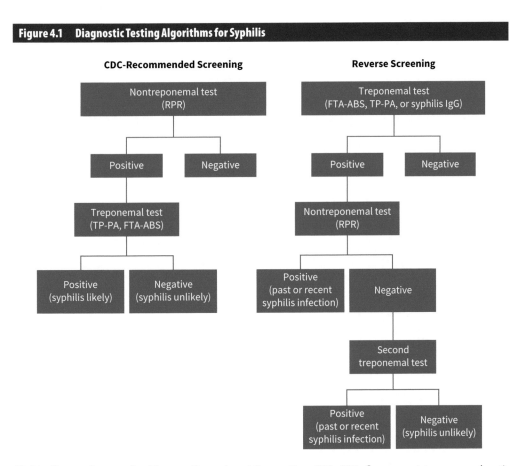

CDC indicates Centers for Disease Control and Prevention; FTA-ABS, fluorescent treponemal antibody absorption; Ig, immunoglobulin; RPR, rapid plasma reagin; TP-PA, *Treponema pallidum* particle agglutination.

rare cases, a positive nontreponemal test can become nonreactive over many years, even without any treatment. In late syphilis, the sensitivity of RPR is only 73% and VDRL is only 71% (4). Another reason for a false-negative nontreponemal test result can be the prozone phenomenon. Extremely high concentrations of syphilis antibodies can block formation of the antigen-antibody complex, thereby preventing development of a visible precipitate (which is required for the RPR test to be positive). This phenomenon affects 0.2% to 2% of cases and has been associated with pregnancy, secondary syphilis, and HIV (5). To bring the antibody concentration to a zone of equivalence so that a visible precipitate can form, the patient's serum sample must be diluted. In the above-discussed case, the patient's serum was diluted and the prozone effect was not observed. If a treponemal test result is believed to be false-negative, providers should request repeat testing if it can be performed with a diluted serum sample.

Treatment of Ocular Syphilis

It is not clear whether ocular syphilis represents secondary syphilis or neurosyphilis, but this distinction is important because it affects treatment decisions. In the absence of clinical trials, the recommendations for management of ocular syphilis are based on case reports and retrospective studies, and many experts suggest treating ocular syphilis as neurosyphilis because the eyes are contiguous with the brain. Treatment with IV penicillin G (3-4 million units every 4 hours or 18-24 million units per day by continuous infusion) for 10 to 14 days is considered first-line

therapy (6). Nevertheless, patients who receive IV penicillin therapy can have treatment failure or relapse. In a review of 143 reported cases of syphilitic uveitis from 1984 to 2008, no significant differences in clinical outcomes and follow-up serologic findings were noted between intramuscular and IV therapy, and treatment failures were observed even after IV therapy (3). If the initial cerebrospinal fluid study showed abnormal findings, then follow-up cerebrospinal fluid examinations should be performed every 6 months. The patient's response to treatment should be assessed until pleocytosis resolves.

References

1. Barile GR, Flynn TE. Syphilis exposure in patients with uveitis. Ophthalmology. 1997 Oct;104(10):1605–9.
2. Moradi A, Salek S, Daniel E, Gangaputra S, Ostheimer TA, Burkholder BM, et al. Clinical features and incidence rates of ocular complications in patients with ocular syphilis. Am J Ophthalmol. 2015 Feb;159(2):334–43.e1. Epub 2014 Nov 5.
3. Amaratunge BC, Camuglia JE, Hall AJ. Syphilitic uveitis: a review of clinical manifestations and treatment outcomes of syphilitic uveitis in human immunodeficiency virus-positive and negative patients. Clin Exp Ophthalmol. 2010 Jan;38(1):68–74.
4. Sena AC, White BL, Sparling PF. Novel *Treponema pallidum* serologic tests: a paradigm shift in syphilis screening for the 21st century. Clin Infect Dis. 2010 Sep 15;51(6):700–8.
5. Musher DM, Hamill RJ, Baughn RE. Effect of human immunodeficiency virus (HIV) infection on the course of syphilis and on the response to treatment. Ann Intern Med. 1990 Dec 1;113(11):872–81.
6. Workowski KA, Bolan GA; Centers for Disease Control and Prevention. Sexually transmitted diseases treatment guidelines, 2015. MMWR Recomm Rep. 2015 Jun 5;64(RR-03):1–137. Erratum in: MMWR Recomm Rep. 2015 Aug 28;64(33):924.

Ascites at the Border

5

Jasmine R. Marcelin, MD, and Abinash Virk, MD

Case Presentation

A 53-year-old man presented to the gastro-enterology outpatient clinic for evaluation of new-onset ascites. His medical history included diagnoses of chronic skin lesions, and 3 years before presentation, he had urinary retention with prostate hypertrophy. During the 6 months before presentation, he had a 60-pound weight loss with occasional night sweats, fatigue, and malaise. Three months before presentation, he noted abdominal distention and subsequently received a diagnosis of ascites of unknown cause. The patient resided in Texas but traveled to Mexico frequently; he underwent paracentesis in Mexico, and the procedure was reportedly unre-markable. One month before presentation, he had pain with defecation and orange-colored stool. He subsequently had left-sided, lower-quadrant pain in a band-like distribution, plus urinary frequency. He denied fever, chills, headache, diar-rhea, or respiratory symptoms. He was a former construction worker who lived near a farm but did not eat or drink any unpasteurized products. He denied alcohol or recreational drug use.

A physical examination showed that the patient's vital signs were normal, but he appeared chronically ill and emaciated. He had several flesh-colored skin lesions near his right eyelid and the nape of his neck. He had a markedly dis-tended abdomen with evidence of ascites but no cutaneous stigmata of cirrhosis. His other phys-ical examination findings were normal.

Magnetic resonance imaging of his abdomen showed a normal-appearing liver with ascites and marked bilateral adrenal thickening. A com-puted tomographic urogram showed diffuse omental and peritoneal carcinomatosis with multiple periaortic lymph nodes. He underwent

ultrasound-guided paracentesis, and the as-citic fluid had 5,931 total nucleated cells (36% neutrophils, 11% eosinophils). A lumbar punc-ture showed an opening pressure of 150 mm H_2O; cerebrospinal fluid (CSF) analysis showed a total protein level of 66 mg/dL, glucose level of 62 mg/dL, and total nucleated cell count of 1/mcL (17% neutrophils, 48% lymphocytes, 17% eosinophils). A CSF *Coccidioides immitis* antibody screen was positive, and a serum *Coccidioides* antibody screen was positive, with a titer of 1:128. A CSF fungal culture and fungal blood cultures were negative. Biopsy specimens from the facial skin lesions and omental thick-ening grew *Coccidioides posadasii* or *C immitis*; additionally, peritoneal fluid and urine also grew the same organism.

The patient recalled an episode of pneumonia 3 years before presentation, while he was a con-struction worker in Arizona, during which he received the diagnosis of disseminated coccidi-oidomycosis. Oral fluconazole was administered, with a loading dose of 1,200 mg, followed by 800 mg daily. Within weeks of initiating fluconazole therapy, the patient reported feeling improve-ment in his malaise, fatigue, and abdominal pain.

Discussion

Coccidioidal infection typically occurs after inhalation of arthroconidia of *C immitis* or *C posadasii*. The most common initial clinical presentation is a self-limited pneumonia, but disseminated disease can occur after hematoge-nous spread in about 1% of cases, with exposure typically occurring weeks to months before de-velopment of symptoms (1). The most common sites of dissemination include the skin and soft tissue, bones and joints, and the central nervous system. Other less-common sites of infection include the prostate, adrenal glands, and peritoneal cavity (2). Risk factors for dissemination include reduced cellular immunity (from HIV infection, transplant, or use of immunosuppressive agents), diabetes mellitus, pregnancy, African American race, and Filipino ancestry (3).

Disseminated coccidioidomycosis can be diagnosed by serologic screening with an enzyme immunoassay. If results are positive, immunodiffusion and complement fixation tests should follow (1). Serologic tests are positive in almost all cases of disseminated infection, except for patients who are immunocompromised. The diagnosis of coccidioidomycosis relies primarily on biopsy of clinical specimens. Histopathologically, thick-walled spherules are evident with Gomori methenamine silver stain. The organism can be cultured in a laboratory with appropriate precautions, and after growth, the organism can be further identified by morphology, nucleic acid hybridization probes, real-time polymerase chain reaction (PCR) sequencing, or mass spectrometry. Direct PCR of clinical specimens has 100% sensitivity and 98.4% specificity. Generally, the diagnosis can be made by sampling the most accessible involved tissue. Lumbar puncture is not recommended in patients without headache or meningeal symptoms because all patients with coccidioidal meningitis have central nervous system symptoms (4). This patient did not have central nervous system symptoms and likely did not have coccidioidal meningitis. His positive

antibody screen from the CSF likely was due to positivity in the peripheral serum.

Antifungal therapy is recommended for patients with extrapulmonary coccidioidomycosis. Fluconazole is the drug of choice, but itraconazole has equivalent activity and may have improved activity in osteoarticular infections (1). Both are preferred over amphotericin B products (which are recommended as first-line therapy only for women in the first trimester of pregnancy or for patients with life-threatening or refractory disease). Posaconazole and voriconazole have been used successfully, but the evidence supporting their use in coccidioidomycosis is limited to case reports. The typical duration of therapy for patients with extrapulmonary or disseminated disease is 6 to 12 months, although for meningitis, lifelong therapy is recommended.

References

1. Galgiani JN, Ampel NM, Blair JE, Catanzaro A, Geertsma F, Hoover SE, et al. 2016 Infectious Diseases Society of America (IDSA) clinical practice guideline for the treatment of coccidioidomycosis. Clin Infect Dis. 2016 Sep 15;63(6):e112–46. Epub 2016 Jul 27.
2. Odio CD, Marciano BE, Galgiani JN, Holland SM. Risk factors for disseminated coccidioidomycosis, United States. Emerg Infect Dis. 2017 Feb;23(2):308–11.
3. Brown J, Benedict K, Park BJ, Thompson GR 3rd. Coccidioidomycosis: epidemiology. Clin Epidemiol. 2013 Jun 25;5: 185–97.
4. Thompson G 3rd, Wang S, Bercovitch R, Bolaris M, Van Den Akker D, Taylor S, et al. Routine CSF analysis in coccidioidomycosis is not required. PLoS One. 2013 May 22;8(5):e64249.

A Lengthy Leg Problem

6

Jasmine R. Marcelin, MD, and Larry M. Baddour, MD

Case Presentation

A 50-year-old woman presented to her primary care physician in July after 2 days of right lower extremity erythema, pain, and warmth. She had a history of hypertension, varicose veins (including a vein-stripping procedure years earlier), and asthma. She did not have diabetes mellitus or peripheral vascular disease. The physical examination showed that she was afebrile and had stable vital signs. Her body mass index (BMI) was 48 kg/m^2. The erythema extended from her right ankle to her anterior midtibia area and was tender to palpation. There was no wound or evidence of purulence. She had bilateral tinea pedis, dry skin on her shins and soles of her feet, and bilateral varicose veins. A diagnosis of nonpurulent cellulitis was made, and she was prescribed a 7-day course of oral cephalexin (500 mg, every 6 hours; dose adjusted for weight).

With further discussion, she indicated that this was her fourth occurrence of right lower extremity cellulitis this year. Last year, she had 3 episodes, with 2 involving her left lower extremity. She had been treated with cephalexin, trimethoprim-sulfamethoxazole, cefadroxil, and doxycycline, and the episodes resolved each time.

After the presenting episode resolved, she initiated oral penicillin (500 mg, twice daily) for long-term secondary prophylaxis. During 1.5 years of follow-up, she had no recurrences.

Discussion

Nonpurulent cellulitis is a common clinical diagnosis. Cellulitis can occur without evidence of a portal of entry, and when it is nonpurulent, the most common pathogens are β-hemolytic streptococci (1). Damaged venous or lymphatic systems (or both), such as those seen with lymphedema, chronic venous insufficiency, and saphenous venectomy, are risk factors for nonpurulent cellulitis (2). Potential mechanisms of pathogenesis include easier propagation of bacterial infection through damaged lymph systems, dermal or subcutaneous fluid accumulation reducing local immunity, and further damage after infection. Additionally, stasis dermatitis can accompany venous insufficiency and further compromise the cutaneous barrier with fissures that serve as portals of entry for pathogens. The incidence of nonpurulent cellulitis is more common in warmer months, possibly because of increased risk of insect bites or skin maceration (3). Finally, ipsilateral tinea pedis is a risk factor for lower extremity cellulitis, and β-hemolytic streptococcal colonization of toe webs is thought to be important in the pathogenesis of nonpurulent cellulitis in the setting of underlying tinea pedis (1,4). One episode of cellulitis increases the risk of recurrent episodes; other risk factors for recurrence include lymphedema, peripheral vascular disease, and chronic venous insufficiency (5). Patients who have had 3 or more episodes of cellulitis per year are ideal candidates for pharmacologic prophylaxis, especially if they also have the above comorbid conditions (6).

Oral antibiotic prophylaxis is effective in preventing recurrent episodes of nonpurulent cellulitis (7). The recommended regimen is oral penicillin V (250 mg, twice daily). This regimen is cost effective, and in one study (8), it reduced the rate of cellulitis recurrence by 45% in a 12-month period. However, the protective effect was sustained only while patients were receiving prophylaxis, and patients had recurrence soon after prophylaxis was discontinued. Long-term prophylaxis was not associated with an increased frequency of adverse events, but prophylaxis was less likely to be successful in the long term for patients who had greater than 3 episodes, preexisting edema, or BMI greater than 33 kg/m^2 compared with patients who did not have those risk factors (8). Considering the risk factors for cellulitis and those for failure of prophylaxis, a successful antibiotic prophylaxis regimen likely requires inclusion of adjuvant nonpharmacologic methods such as weight loss, lymphedema management, skin moisturization, and treatment of tinea pedis.

References

1. Semel JD, Goldin H. Association of athlete's foot with cellulitis of the lower extremities: diagnostic value of bacterial cultures of ipsilateral interdigital space samples. Clin Infect Dis. 1996 Nov;23(5):1162–4.
2. Bjornsdottir S, Gottfredsson M, Thorisdottir AS, Gunnarsson GB, Ríkardsdottir H, Kristjansson M, et al. Risk factors for acute cellulitis of the lower limb: a prospective case-control study. Clin Infect Dis. 2005 Nov 15;41(10):1416–22. Epub 2005 Oct 13.
3. Marcelin JR, Challener DW, Tan EM, Lahr BD, Baddour LM. Incidence of and effects of seasonality on nonpurulent lower extremity cellulitis after the emergence of community-acquired methicillin-resistant *Staphylococcus aureus*. Mayo Clin Proc. 2017 Aug;92(8):1227–33. Epub 2017 Jul 8.
4. Baddour LM, Bisno AL. Recurrent cellulitis after coronary bypass surgery. Association with superficial fungal infection in saphenous venectomy limbs. JAMA. 1984 Feb 24;251(8):1049–52.
5. Tay EY, Fook-Chong S, Oh CC, Thirumoorthy T, Pang SM, Lee HY. Cellulitis recurrence score: a tool for predicting recurrence of lower limb cellulitis. J Am Acad Dermatol. 2015 Jan;72(1):140–5. Epub 2014 Oct 16.
6. Chen HM, Li YL, Liu YM, Liu CE, Cheng YR, Chen CH, et al. The experience of intramuscular benzathine penicillin for prophylaxis of recurrent cellulitis: a cohort study. J Microbiol Immunol Infect. 2017 Oct;50(5):613–18. Epub 2015 Sep 9.
7. Oh CC, Ko HC, Lee HY, Safdar N, Maki DG, Chlebicki MP. Antibiotic prophylaxis for preventing recurrent cellulitis: a systematic review and meta-analysis. J Infect. 2014 Jul;69(1):26–34. Epub 2014 Feb 24.
8. Thomas KS, Crook AM, Nunn AJ, Foster KA, Mason JM, Chalmers JR, et al; UK Dermatology Clinical Trials Network's PATCH I Trial Team. Penicillin to prevent recurrent leg cellulitis. N Engl J Med. 2013 May 2;368(18):1695–703.

A Filamentous Monster

7

Abdelghani El Rafei, MD, Daniel C. DeSimone, MD, Alan M. Sugrue, MB, BCh, BAO, and Rodney L. Thompson, MD

Case Presentation

A 62-year-old man was admitted to a tertiary care hospital with an 8-month history of fatigue and dry cough. The patient's clinical course is summarized in the timeline (Figure 7.1).

At admission, he was hemodynamically stable, afebrile, and had a normal respiratory rate. A physical examination showed that he had decreased breath sounds bilaterally, scattered crackles, and tenderness with palpation of the right chest wall. A complete blood count showed an elevated white blood cell count of

13.4×10^9/L (reference range, $3.5\text{-}10.6 \times 10^9$/L) with neutrophilia and normocytic anemia with a hemoglobin level of 10.4 g/dL (reference range, 13.5-17.5 g/dL). In addition, the C-reactive protein level was 173.4 mg/L (reference range, <8 mg/L) and his erythrocyte sedimentation rate was elevated at 130 mm/h (reference range, 0-22 mm/h). His electrolytes, lactate, creatinine, and troponin levels were all normal, as was his liver function.

He had a computed tomographic (CT) scan of the chest that showed bilateral cavitating lung lesions (Figure 7.2).

Figure 7.1 Patient Timeline

July
- Received a 7-day course of amoxicillin-clavulanic acid for presumed pneumonia, without improvement
- Repeat CXR showed 3-mm nodules in the RUL and LLL
- Given the chronic joint pain and fatigue, polymyalgia rheumatica was diagnosed, and he received oral prednisone (40 mg, once daily); joint pain improved

January
- Patient had generalized symptoms of fatigue, malaise, and shortness of breath

May
- Patient had nonproductive cough and chest pain with deep inspiration

September
- Patient admitted to a tertiary care hospital for further evaluation

March
- Evaluated by PCP
- Received antibiotic treatment for presumed pneumonia, without improvement

June
- CXR was unremarkable
- Received a 7-day course of levofloxacin for presumed pneumonia

August
- Received a fourth course of antibiotics for presumed pneumonia
- CT scan showed 2 nodules in the RUL and 1 in the LLL

CT indicates computed tomographic; CXR, chest radiograph; LLL, left lower lobe; PCP, primary care physician; RUL, right upper lobe.

Figure 7.2   Chest Computed Tomographic Scan Showing Bilateral Cavitary Areas of Mass-Like Consolidation

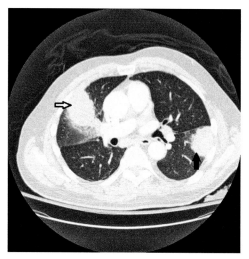

The lesion identified in the right upper lobe (hollow arrow) measured 5.9×4.1 cm, with possible chest wall involvement. The lesion in the superior segment of the left lower lobe (solid arrow) measured 4.5×4.5 cm.

He subsequently underwent a CT-guided biopsy of one of these lesions, and the biopsy specimen was cultured for aerobic and anaerobic bacteria, fungi, and mycobacteria. Cultures on day 5 showed gram-positive filamentous bacilli consistent with *Nocardia* (Figure 7.3).

Figure 7.3   Lung Tissue Culture Growing Filamentous Bacilli

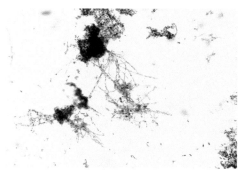

Modified acid-fast staining; original magnification, ×40.

The patient was discharged and was prescribed a treatment regimen of amikacin (950 mg, once daily, administered intravenously) and double-strength trimethoprim-sulfamethoxazole (TMP-SMX; 2 tablets, twice daily). He was scheduled to have follow-up with an infectious disease specialist in an outpatient setting. The sputum culture, obtained at admission, showed *Nocardia* on day 22.

Discussion

Nocardia is a gram-positive, weakly acid-fast, branching, aerobic bacilli that is ubiquitous in the environment. Since its first description by veterinarian Edmond Nocard in 1888, more than 50 species have been identified (1). Detection of these organisms by Gram stain is crucial for diagnosis. The acid-fast staining is characteristic and helps differentiate *Nocardia* from other bacteria with similar morphology (eg, *Actinomyces*). The modified Kinyoun method is preferred because it uses a weaker acid for decolorization compared with conventional acid-fast staining. Acid-fast staining should always be used in conjunction with Gram stain because the acid-fast characteristic of *Nocardia* is heavily dependent on the growth media used and the age of the culture. *Nocardia* may take up to 14 days to grow, thus culture media should be monitored for growth for more than 2 weeks if *Nocardia* infection is suspected (1). Invasive procedures are often needed for adequate sampling; in one series (2), 44% of cases required invasive measures to establish a diagnosis.

Nocardia most commonly affects the lungs because inhalation is the main route of infection (3). Risk factors for pulmonary nocardiosis include chronic pulmonary diseases that require long-term corticosteroid therapy (eg, chronic obstructive pulmonary disease, asthma, bronchiectasis). Patients with systemic immunodeficiency (eg, from HIV, immunosuppression after organ transplant, congenital immunologic disease, chemotherapy) also have increased risk of *Nocardia* infection (4). Nevertheless, others with no apparent risk factors also may be susceptible, with data suggesting that 10% to 40% of infected patients have no known immunodeficiency (3). Pulmonary nocardiosis often presents in a sub-acute or chronic manner. Symptoms are nonspecific and may include fever, night sweats, anorexia, weight loss, dyspnea, cough, hemoptysis, and pleuritic chest pain (5). Imaging findings include reticulonodular infiltrates, pleural effusion, and multiple or single nodules. Cavitation among nodules is common. Lesions in the lungs can invade the chest wall, often mimicking an underlying malignancy. The constellation of nonspecific symptoms and imaging findings often lead to delayed or missed diagnoses. The presented case was consistent with the published literature, with conventional radiographs failing to yield any clinically significant findings in the first 6 months of symptoms. Even after nodules were detected with conventional radiographs, the diagnosis was not established for another 3 months.

Extrapulmonary involvement occurs in up to 50% of cases and may even occur with a healed or asymptomatic pulmonary infection. Although *Nocardia* can spread to almost any organ, extrapulmonary disease most commonly involves the central nervous system (CNS) (3-5). Symptoms of CNS involvement are usually insidious and often resemble those of a brain tumor in immunocompetent patients. Patients usually present with headache, nausea, seizures, or altered mental status. CNS imaging is warranted in patients with neurologic symptoms, severe pulmonary nocardiosis, or the setting of immunocompromise (5).

For the past 50 years, sulfonamides (with or without trimethoprim) have been a cornerstone of therapy for most patients with *Nocardia* infection, but optimal antimicrobial therapy has yet to be established. Empiric antibiotic therapy includes TMP-SMX with parenteral amikacin or imipenem for severe or life-threatening infections. Combination therapy appears to be synergistic in several in vitro studies (4, 6). However, comparisons of clinical efficacy for specific drug regimens have not been reported in the literature. Most treatment recommendations are made on the basis of in vitro studies and expert opinion (3-5). TMP-SMX is typically used alone for cutaneous infections. For severe infections without CNS involvement, 2 antimicrobial agents are typically used (eg, TMP-SMX plus parenteral amikacin or TMP-SMX plus imipenem). If CNS involvement is suspected, treatment with 3 agents is suggested (eg, TMP-SMX, amikacin, and imipenem). Parenteral therapy is administered for 3 to 6 weeks, depending on the patient status and clinical response. After completion of parenteral therapy, antimicrobial drugs can be administered orally. Oral therapy is continued for 6 months for immunocompetent patients and for 12 months for immunocompromised patients (4,5).

References

1. Brown-Elliott BA, Brown JM, Conville PS, Wallace RJ Jr. Clinical and laboratory features of the *Nocardia* spp based on current molecular taxonomy. Clin Microbiol Rev. 2006 Apr;19(2):259–82.
2. Georghiou PR, Blacklock ZM. Infection with *Nocardia* species in Queensland: a review of 102 clinical isolates. Med J Aust. 1992 May 18;156(10):692–7.
3. Beaman BL, Beaman L. *Nocardia* species: host-parasite relationships. Clin Microbiol Rev. 1994 Apr;7(2):213–64.
4. Lerner PI. Nocardiosis. Clin Infect Dis. 1996 Jun;22(6): 891–903.
5. Wilson JW. Nocardiosis: updates and clinical overview. Mayo Clin Proc. 2012 Apr;87(4):403–7.
6. Gombert ME, duBouchet L, Aulicino TM, Berkowitz LB. Antimicrobial synergism in the therapy of experimental cerebral nocardiosis. J Antimicrob Chemother. 1989 Jul;24(1):39–43.

The Great Mimicker 8

Abdelghani El Rafei, MD, Korosh Sharain, MD, Kelly A. Cawcutt, MD, and Zelalem Temesgen, MD

Case Presentation

A 47-year-old woman from Arkansas was referred to the hematology clinic because of a 5-month history of bilateral lower extremity rash and constitutional symptoms of unknown origin. She was in her usual state of health until she noticed a purpuric, nonpruritic rash on her lower extremities that was associated with discomfort and swelling (Figure 8.1). Her medical history included a bicuspid aortic valve replacement with a St. Jude porcine aortic valve, 12 years before presentation.

At presentation, the patient was afebrile. Physical examination findings included a diffuse, erythematous lesion on her lower extremities, nontender splenomegaly with the spleen tip palpable at 4 cm below the costal margin, and a 4/6 systolic murmur that was best heard in the aortic region.

Laboratory evaluations showed microcytic anemia and thrombocytopenia (hemoglobin, 9.8 g/dL [reference range, 12.0-15.5 g/dL]; white blood cells, 3.1×10^9/L [reference range, $3.5\text{-}10.5\times10^9$/L]; platelets, 113×10^9/L [reference range, $150\text{-}450\times10^9$/L]). Liver function tests showed elevated results (alanine aminotransferase, 74 U/L [reference range, 7-45 U/L]; aspartate aminotransferase, 100 U/L [reference range, 8-43 U/L]), and the inflammatory marker C-reactive protein also was increased (13.1 mg/dL [reference range, ≤8.0 mg/dL]). A skin biopsy was consistent with leukocytoclastic vasculitis. Computed tomographic (CT) imaging of the abdomen showed hepatosplenomegaly. A liver biopsy showed panacinar hepatitis. Peripheral blood flow cytometry and T-cell rearrangement studies were ordered to determine whether a lymphoproliferative disease was present, and they were negative for any malignancy.

The patient was further evaluated for a possible autoimmune disease by specialists in rheumatology, gastroenterology, and dermatology. Additional laboratory investigations included antibody testing for lupus, rheumatic fever, antineutrophil cytoplasmic antibody (small-vessel vasculitis), autoimmune hepatitis, cryoglobulinemia, complement levels, hepatitis B antibodies, and hepatitis C antibodies. Polymerase chain reaction tests were performed for viral RNA and HIV screening. All test results

Figure 8.1 Lower Extremities With Purpuric Rash

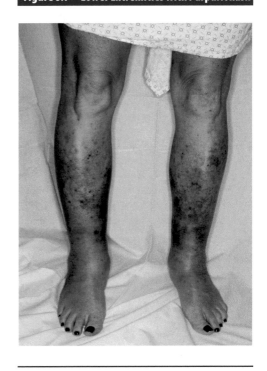

were normal, except for elevated rheumatoid factor (66 IU/mL [reference range, <15 IU/mL]). A fluorodeoxyglucose positron emission tomography–CT image showed a nodular infiltrate in the middle lobe of the right lung with moderate hypermetabolism that suggested a potential infectious or inflammatory process. The patient was referred to pulmonary and critical care specialists for further evaluation of the nodule. Serologic tests for endemic fungi and *Mycobacterium tuberculosis* were negative.

CT imaging of the chest showed consolidation surrounding the aortic graft, consistent with postoperative changes. The patient underwent transesophageal echocardiography to further evaluate the changes surrounding the aortic graft seen on CT; it showed a large, complex, multiloculated pseudoaneurysm involving the posterior aortic root.

On further questioning, the patient described driving by a cattle ranch on a daily basis with the windows open. General bacterial blood cultures were negative. Serologic tests for Q fever showed markedly elevated findings: immunoglobulin (Ig) G phase 1 antibody (1:16,384) and IgG phase II antibody (1:16,384). Altogether, the results of the evaluation supported a diagnosis of Q fever endocarditis, 6 months after the initial symptoms had developed.

Discussion

Q fever is a zoonotic infection caused by the bacterium *Coxiella burnetii*. The disease name honors Herald Rea Cox and Macfarlane Burnet, who identified the Q fever agent (1). Ruminants are the primary reservoirs for this zoonotic infection. Organisms are shed with parturition products, milk, feces, and other secretions of infected animals, and they can survive in nature for weeks. Inhalation of contaminated aerosols is the primary route of infection (2). Acute infection is typically asymptomatic but may present with an influenza-like illness, with evidence of pneumonia or hepatitis (or both). The diagnosis

is often missed because symptoms are nonspecific. Progression to chronic infection may occur in immunocompromised patients or those with underlying valve disease. Infective endocarditis is the most common form of chronic Q fever (3).

The difficulty of identifying Q fever endocarditis often leads to considerable delays in diagnosis. In a study of 15 cases of Q fever endocarditis, the mean period between symptom onset and diagnosis was 6 months (4). The delay in the case detailed above was due in part to the concern of possible hematologic or autoimmune disease. The most common presentation of Q fever endocarditis is a chronic, low-grade fever (70%) (3). Splenomegaly or hepatomegaly (or both) occur in 5% to 58% of patients. A purpuric rash may occur in up to 19% of patients and is often seen on the extremities corresponding to immunocomplex vasculitis (3). A review of the patient's cardiac and exposure history is crucial for making the diagnosis of Q fever endocarditis because it almost always occurs in the setting of an underlying valvular disease, particularly a prosthetic valve (3). Among patients with valvular disease, the risk of developing Q fever endocarditis after an acute infection is as high as 40%. Most patients (60%) in the acute, initial phase of illness are asymptomatic and the diagnosis may be easily missed; visceral involvement does not occur until late in the course of Q fever endocarditis (3,4). Thus, patients with underlying valve pathology, chronic fevers, and unexplained disease, and particularly patients with exposure to domestic and farm animals, should undergo Q fever serologic testing and echocardiography.

Serologic testing is the most valuable diagnostic tool. *C burnetii* expresses antigenic variation when cultured. Paradoxically, phase 1 antibodies are markers of chronic infection, whereas phase 2 antibodies are markers of acute infection (1). Dupont et al (1) demonstrated that a phase 1 IgG titer ≥800 has 100% sensitivity and a 99.8% positive predictive value for diagnosing chronic Q fever infection. As a result, the Duke criteria for infective endocarditis were modified to include positive Q fever serology as a major criterion (5). Echocardiography may demonstrate valve dehiscence or vegetations. Vegetations may be difficult to detect, although detection rates have improved to 86% (they were approximately 50% in earlier studies) (4).

References

1. Dupont HT, Thirion X, Raoult D. Q fever serology: cutoff determination for microimmunofluorescence. Clin Diagn Lab Immunol. 1994 Mar;1(2):189–96.

2. Hartzell JD, Wood-Morris RN, Martinez LJ, Trotta RF. Q fever: epidemiology, diagnosis, and treatment. Mayo Clin Proc. 2008 May;83(5):574–9.

3. Raoult D, Marrie T, Mege J. Natural history and pathophysiology of Q fever. Lancet Infect Dis. 2005 Apr;5(4):219–26.

4. Houpikian P, Habib G, Mesana T, Raoult D. Changing clinical presentation of Q fever endocarditis. Clin Infect Dis. 2002 Mar 1;34(5):E28–31. Epub 2002 Jan 23.

5. Fournier PE, Casalta JP, Habib G, Messana T, Raoult D. Modification of the diagnostic criteria proposed by the Duke Endocarditis Service to permit improved diagnosis of Q fever endocarditis. Am J Med. 1996 Jun;100(6):629–33.

Altered Mental Status After Hematopoietic Stem Cell Transplant

9

Jarrett J. Failing, MD, Omar M. Abu Saleh, MBBS, and Jennifer A. Whitaker, MD

Case Presentation

A 55-year-old woman from the upper Midwest presented with progressive confusion during the past 24 hours and possible visual hallucinations. She had myelodysplastic syndrome and had received an allogeneic bone marrow transplant 22 days earlier from an unrelated matched donor. Her posttransplant course had been complicated by neutropenic fever (due to periengraftment syndrome) that resolved with methylprednisolone. She was taking prophylactic tacrolimus, penicillin V potassium, pentamidine, fluconazole, and acyclovir.

A physical examination showed that she was alert but oriented only to person and had anterograde amnesia. No focal neurologic deficits were present. She was afebrile and had a normal leukocyte count. Brain magnetic resonance imaging (MRI) showed increased signal intensity in the mesial temporal lobes of both cerebral hemispheres on fluid-attenuated inversion recovery (FLAIR) and T2-weighted sequences (Figure 9.1). A lumbar puncture and analysis of the cerebrospinal fluid (CSF) showed a mild lymphocytic pleocytosis and elevated total protein. Polymerase chain reaction (PCR) testing of the CSF was negative for herpes simplex virus 1, herpes simplex virus 2, Epstein-Barr virus, cytomegalovirus, varicella-zoster virus, JC polyomavirus, and toxoplasmosis but was positive for human herpesvirus (HHV) 6. HHV-7 testing was not performed.

HHV-6 encephalitis was diagnosed after considering the recent allogeneic bone marrow transplant, altered mental status, the MRI showing hyperintense lesions bilaterally in the mesial temporal lobes, and identification of HHV-6 in the CSF. Treatment with ganciclovir was initiated (5 mg/kg, every 12 hours, administered intravenously). Her course was complicated by a generalized tonic-clonic seizure on posttransplant day 26. A repeat MRI showed posterior reversible encephalopathy syndrome, which was thought to be associated with tacrolimus. Her encephalitis

Figure 9.1   Magnetic Resonance Image of the Head

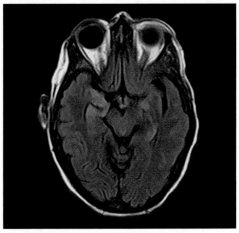

Increased signal intensity was observed in the mesial temporal lobes of both cerebral hemispheres.

improved with therapy and resolved on day 15, but she continued to have mild difficulty with short-term memory. She completed a 30-day course of ganciclovir; a repeat CSF analysis showed a normal cell count and total protein, and the PCR test was negative for HHV-6. She began prophylaxis with valganciclovir.

Discussion

For patients who have undergone allogeneic hematopoietic stem cell transplant (allo-HCT), the differential diagnosis for acute central nervous system (CNS) infection is broad. It includes non-infectious causes such as posterior reversible encephalopathy syndrome, bleeding, and adverse effects from medications, and it also includes a long list of possible viral, bacterial, and fungal infections. However, for the case described above, the combination of the clinical presentation and CSF and imaging findings led to the diagnosis of HHV-6 encephalitis.

HHV-6 is a member of the Betaherpesvirinae family. It is a ubiquitous virus; most children acquire the primary infection by age 2 to 3 years and 90% will have a latent infection (1,2). Approximately 1% of the population has HHV-6 integration into a somatic chromosome, which then can be passed to subsequent generations. People with chromosomal integration have high plasma levels of HHV-6, and these findings often are misinterpreted as a sign of active disease. However, a viral load exceeding 10^6 copies/mL usually raises suspicion for chromosomally integrated virus. There are 2 species of the virus, HHV-6A and HHV-6B, but most infections in allo-HCT patients are due to HHV-6B. Risk factors for activating a latent HHV-6 infection include severe immunosuppression, umbilical cord blood transplant, bone marrow transplant with an unrelated donor, and corticosteroid treatment (1). Among patients who undergo allo-HCT, 30% to 70% will have HHV-6 reactivation within 2 to 4 weeks after transplant (1). Although reactivation often can be asymptomatic, it is associated with an increased risk of subsequent cytomegalovirus reactivation, acute graft-versus-host disease, and nonrelapse mortality, especially for patients with high levels of viral DNA in the plasma (3).

HHV-6 encephalopathy is estimated to occur in less than 1% to 11.6% of allo-HCT patients, typically within 2 to 6 weeks after transplant (1). Patients with acute graft-versus-host disease, engraftment syndrome, bone marrow transplant with an unrelated donor, and umbilical cord blood transplant have higher risk (1,4). Symptoms include memory loss (classically anterograde amnesia), confusion, delirium, and loss of consciousness. Seizures occur in 40% to 70% of patients. The constellation of these classic findings is termed *posttransplant limbic encephalitis*. When the diagnosis of HHV-6 encephalitis is considered, CSF should be analyzed for HHV-6 DNA (PCR assay), and a brain MRI should be obtained. Imaging will often show hyperintense lesions in the bilateral medial temporal lobes on FLAIR and T2-weighted images (1). However, patients with HHV-6 encephalitis may not show changes with MRI, and the CSF can be positive for HHV-6 without the patient having encephalitis (2). High levels of plasma HHV-6 viremia (PCR assay) are associated with CNS involvement, but patients with negative plasma test results can still have CNS disease (1,2). In terms of prognosis, a case series of 44 patients reported that 43% of patients made a full recovery, 25% died of encephalitis, 14% showed initial improvement but then died, and 18% had lingering neurologic compromise (5).

The recommended first-line agents for treatment of HHV-6 encephalitis are ganciclovir or foscarnet for 3 to 6 weeks, but no controlled trials have been conducted. New agents such as HHV-6–specific T-cell therapy are being studied. Currently, no evidence supports prophylaxis for HHV-6 encephalitis in allo-HCT patients (1). More studies are needed to better understand the pathogenesis, prevention, and treatment of this disease.

References

1. Ogata M, Fukuda T, Teshima T. Human herpesvirus-6 encephalitis after allogeneic hematopoietic cell transplantation: what we do and do not know. Bone Marrow Transplant. 2015 Aug;50(8):1030–6. Epub 2015 Apr 27.

2. Hill JA, Boeckh MJ, Sedlak RH, Jerome KR, Zerr DM. Human herpesvirus 6 can be detected in cerebrospinal fluid without associated symptoms after allogeneic hematopoietic cell transplantation. J Clin Virol. 2014 Oct;61(2):289–92. Epub 2014 Jul 12.

3. Zerr DM, Boeckh M, Delaney C, Martin PJ, Xie H, Adler AL, et al. HHV-6 reactivation and associated sequelae after hematopoietic cell transplantation. Biol Blood Marrow Transplant. 2012 Nov;18(11):1700–8. Epub 2012 May 26.

4. Zerr DM, Fann JR, Breiger D, Boeckh M, Adler AL, Xie H, et al. HHV-6 reactivation and its effect on delirium and cognitive functioning in hematopoietic cell transplantation recipients. Blood. 2011 May 12;117(19):5243–9. Epub 2011 Mar 9.

5. Zerr DM. Human herpesvirus 6 and central nervous system disease in hematopoietic cell transplantation. J Clin Virol. 2006 Dec;37 Suppl 1:S52–6.

The Resistance

10

Jasmine R. Marcelin, MD, and Nathan W. Cummins, MD

Case Presentation

A 55-year-old asymptomatic woman from Africa received a diagnosis of HIV-1 infection with a routine physical examination. She had recently immigrated to the United States (within the past 3 years). She had no fever, chills, or any signs of systemic illnesses. Her medical history included a recent diagnosis of cervical intraepithelial neoplasia that eventually required a hysterectomy. She had never been tested for HIV. She was in a monogamous relationship with her husband, who was still in Africa. She was unaware of her husband's HIV status or whether he had other sexual partners. During her last contact with him, he had been doing well, without any "mysterious illnesses." The patient had never been exposed to blood product infusions, nor had she used intravenous drugs. At the time of diagnosis, her plasma HIV-1 viral load was 54,000 copies/mL and the CD4+ helper T-cell count was 52 cells/mcL (5%). Her HIV virus was wild type (no evidence of resistance mutations with genotypic drug-resistance testing). Tests for sexually transmitted diseases (chlamydia, gonorrhea, syphilis) had negative results.

She started treatment with tenofovir, emtricitabine, and efavirenz for HIV, trimethoprim-sulfamethoxazole for prophylaxis of pneumocystis pneumonia, and azithromycin for prophylaxis of disseminated *Mycobacterium avium* complex infection. She had no adverse reactions to this treatment, and her HIV viral load decreased to 1,130 copies/mL within 1 month of starting therapy. However, 2 months after starting therapy, her HIV viral load increased to 47,000 copies/mL and her CD4+ helper T-cell count was 102 cells/mcL (7%). She insisted that she had been completely adherent to her antiretroviral regimen, with no missed doses or adverse effects. She had no known absorption issues and no recent gastrointestinal infections. Repeat HIV-1 genotypic drug-resistance testing identified the following mutations: K103N, Y181C, M184V, V90I, and T215F. Her antiretroviral therapy (tenofovir, emtricitabine, efavirenz) was discontinued, and she began receiving combination therapy that included tenofovir plus emtricitabine, ritonavir-boosted atazanavir, and raltegravir. She tolerated this switch in therapy well, and 1 month later, her HIV viral load decreased to 143 copies/mL. After 1 year of receiving these medications, her treatment regimen was simplified to combination therapy with abacavir, lamivudine, and dolutegravir plus tenofovir (the HLA-B*57:01 genetic screen was negative), and she no longer required prophylaxis for opportunistic infections.

Discussion

Mutations in HIV genes that result in drug resistance can be caused by 1) antiretroviral drug selection pressure in treatment-experienced patients or 2) transmission of a resistant HIV strain in treatment-naive patients. Varying genetic barriers to resistance (ie, variation in the mutations needed to confer drug resistance) have been observed for some antiretroviral drug classes; consequently, certain resistance-conferring mutations in HIV may result in high-level resistance to one member of a drug class but spare others. Among transmitted HIV strains with drug-resistant mutations, the most common variants (eg, K103N/S) confer resistance to newer-generation nonnucleoside reverse transcriptase inhibitors (1). The M184V mutation is the most common nucleoside or nucleotide reverse transcriptase inhibitor resistance mutation. It confers complete resistance to emtricitabine and lamivudine but spares tenofovir; paradoxically, it increases susceptibility to tenofovir and zidovudine. Protease inhibitors (PIs) generally have a high genetic barrier to resistance, and currently, changes to PI regimens more commonly are because of adverse effects, rather than development of resistance. Acquired and transmitted resistance to integrase strand transfer inhibitors (INSTIs) currently is uncommon, but the Q148S mutation confers high-level resistance to elvitegravir and raltegravir. Dolutegravir resistance is uncommon but can occur with combinations of INSTI-resistance mutations. Table 10.1 shows commonly observed mutations in HIV that are associated with drug resistance.

When a patient has drug-resistance mutations in HIV, the provider must determine whether a resistant strain was acquired with the infection or if resistance developed with drug selection pressure. However, regardless of the cause of resistance, the first step is to assess the patient's adherence to the prescribed treatment regimen and identify any potential barriers affecting compliance. Next, all current and prior genotypic drug resistance testing must be carefully reviewed to identify current and archived drug-resistance mutations. Archived mutations are present in minority viral strains that are overcome by wild-type virus in the absence of antiretroviral treatment, but they can reemerge when relevant selective drug pressure is reapplied (2). Our patient appeared to have a wild-type virus at the time of diagnosis, but archived mutations became apparent during treatment with tenofovir, emtricitabine, and efavirenz. This scenario is inferred, as the development of primary resistance causing a viral rebound would be highly unusual within 1 month after initiating therapy and while maintaining good adherence.

Table 10.1	Common HIV Mutations Conferring Drug Resistance	
Mutation	**Antiretroviral Drug Class**	**Specific Medications**
M184V	NRTI	Emtricitabine, lamivudine Abacavir, low-level resistance Tenofovir and zidovudine, increased susceptibility
K65R	NRTI	All affected, except zidovudine
E138K	NNRTI	Rilpivirine
K103N/S	NNRTI	Nevirapine, efavirenz
K101P	NNRTI	All affected Phenotypic impact is variable
Y181C/I/V	NNRTI	All affected by varying degrees, including etravirine Phenotypic impact is variable
Y188L	NNRTI	All affected, except etravirine
Y143C/R/H	INSTI	Raltegravir
Q148H/R/K	INSTI	Raltegravir, elvitegravir Dolutegravir, low-level resistance Greater effect in conjunction with other INSTI-resistance mutations

Abbreviations: INSTI, integrase strand transfer inhibitor; NNRTI, nonnucleoside reverse transcriptase inhibitor; NRTI, nucleoside or nucleotide reverse transcriptase inhibitor.

Combination antiretroviral therapy should be selected to maximize use of effective agents and to avoid agents that are expected to be associated with resistance; however, this practice is controversial because it could enhance susceptibility to other agents or result in a less-fit virus (eg, M184V mutation) (3). Online tools exist that can help identify appropriate antiretroviral agents by analyzing genotypes and identifying regimens that would not be active (4). The goal is to construct a combination antiretroviral regimen with at least 3 drugs with expected activity against the virus. Therefore, optimal management of resistant HIV infection sometimes may include 4 or more antiretroviral drugs, and some patients may never achieve full virologic suppression. In such a situation, the goal is to maximize immunologic recovery, minimize toxicity, and prevent clinical progression (2). Optimal regimens change over time as more information about resistance becomes available. As seen in this case, the empiric regimens that were commonly used are changing to more active regimens.

References

1. Panichsillapakit T, Smith DM, Wertheim JO, Richman DD, Little SJ, Mehta SR. Prevalence of transmitted HIV drug resistance among recently infected persons in San Diego, CA 1996-2013. J Acquir Immune Defic Syndr. 2016 Feb 1;71 (2):228–36.
2. Panel on Antiretroviral Guidelines for Adults and Adolescents [Internet]. Guidelines for the use of antiretroviral agents in adults and adolescents with HIV. Department of Health and Human Services [cited 2020 Mar 6]. Available from: http://www.aidsinfo.nih.gov/ContentFiles/AdultandAdolescentGL.pdf.
3. Gallant JE. The M184V mutation: what it does, how to prevent it, and what to do with it when it's there. AIDS Read. 2006 Oct;16(10):556–9.
4. Rhee SY, Gonzales MJ, Kantor R, Betts BJ, Ravela J, Shafer RW. Human immunodeficiency virus reverse transcriptase and protease sequence database. Nucleic Acids Res. 2003 Jan 1;31(1):298–303.

Emergency Infectious Diseases

11

Douglas W. Challener, MD, Jasmine R. Marcelin, MD,
and John C. O'Horo, MD

Case Presentation

A 76-year-old man presented to the emergency department after 5 days of severe, left-sided neck pain and was admitted to the hospital. He was a retired butcher with a recent history of right vertebral artery dissection. His temperature was 37.8°C, peripheral white blood cell count was 14.0 cells/mcL, neutrophil count was 11.3 cells/mcL, erythrocyte sedimentation rate was 79 mm/h, and C-reactive protein was 186.5 mg/dL. Computed tomography (CT) of the neck identified a peripherally enhancing loculated fluid collection, consistent with an abscess, in the left paraspinal musculature. Fluid obtained during an ultrasonographically guided aspiration grew *Streptococcus anginosis* that was susceptible to penicillin and cephalosporins. Treatment with intravenous piperacillin-tazobactam was initiated. An otolaryngologist was consulted, and a series of soft tissue débridements of the neck confirmed necrotizing fasciitis. After 12 soft tissue débridements and a C3 to C6 laminectomy, no evidence of necrotizing fasciitis remained. A swallow study did not show evidence of aspiration, and a panoramic dental radiograph did not show an abscess. No evidence of endocarditis was present on a transesophageal echocardiogram. He was discharged home approximately 1 month after being hospitalized. At that point, intravenous antibiotics were discontinued, and he felt much better.

Discussion

Necrotizing fasciitis, first described by Hippocrates in the fifth century BC, is an infection of the tissues between the skin and the muscular fascia. It most commonly affects the superficial fascia, rather than the fascia overlying the muscles. The most common sites are the extremities, perianal region, and genitals (Fournier gangrene). Patients may have a high fever, severe pain, tense edema, dark discoloration of the skin, and lethargy. Often, the patient has a recent history of trauma or surgery that provided a portal of entry for bacteria. The break in the skin can be as small as an insect bite or an abrasion, and it may not be visible to the examiner.

Necrotizing fasciitis is a relatively rare infection, with an incidence rate of 500 to 1,500 cases per year in the United States. The infection progresses very quickly, and rapid identification and treatment are essential for the best outcomes. In the absence of rapid and appropriate care, mortality rates may be high (up to 76%) (1). Necrotizing fasciitis must be differentiated from cellulitis early in the disease course. The skin and underlying soft tissue in necrotizing fasciitis are hard (indurated), whereas subcutaneous tissue is soft in cellulitis. In necrotizing fasciitis, the hardened soft tissue makes it difficult to discern the fascial plane between the subcutaneous tissue and the underlying muscle, and it extends beyond the overlying erythema. Sometimes, an overlying erythematous region is present that tracks proximally as the infection advances. Subcutaneous crepitus occurs in some patients and suggests gas in the tissues (1).

Necrotizing fasciitis typically progresses through several clinical stages. Wong et al (1) proposed characterizing the clinical evolution with 3 stages: early, intermediate, and late. The early stage of infection has erythema, warmth, and swelling, with tenderness that extends beyond this erythematous area of skin. As the infection progresses to the intermediate stage, the overlying skin becomes indurated or fluctuant, and blisters or bullae can form. The late stage consists of crepitus, skin necrosis, and anesthesia. Hemorrhagic bullae also may be present. Systemic symptoms such as fever and hypotension are not reliable indicators of severe infection.

Diagnosis is challenging because patients often have no cutaneous findings, especially in the early stage of disease. The diagnosis is clinical and confirmed by surgical débridement and histologic examination. The appearance of the subcutaneous tissue and fascial planes during surgery confirms the diagnosis. Fascia characteristically appears swollen, gray, and necrotic. Also, fascia typically is nonadherent with blunt dissection and does not bleed. Sample specimens for culture and histologic examination should be obtained from the margins of infectious involvement. Culture findings can help guide antibiotic therapy, and outcomes of histologic examination can corroborate intraoperative findings and may have prognostic value (2). The typical histologic appearance of necrotizing fasciitis is superficial fascial necrosis, presence of bacteria within the tissue, necrosis of the vessel walls, and fibrinous thrombi within the vessels (1).

Imaging techniques such as CT, magnetic resonance imaging (MRI), and ultrasonography may be useful adjuncts when establishing the diagnosis of necrotizing fasciitis. Ultrasonographic findings include fluid collections in the deep fascia and abnormal thickening of the fascia. Advanced imaging with CT or MRI may show fascial plane infection. CT features include fluid and gas along the soft tissue planes around the superficial fascia and deep fascial thickening and enhancement. With MRI, the same findings, plus T2-weighted hyperintensities in the muscle, also suggest necrotizing fasciitis (1). The sensitivities and specificities of these imaging techniques are not well defined. Most importantly, the use of advanced imaging should not delay operative

management if the level of clinical suspicion for necrotizing fasciitis is sufficiently high (3).

A retrospective study described development of a risk-stratification tool, the Laboratory Risk Indicator for Necrotizing Fasciitis, and the authors proposed that it could be used to help distinguish necrotizing fasciitis from other soft tissue infections (4). It stratifies risk on the basis of laboratory findings, including C-reactive protein, white blood cell count, hemoglobin, sodium, creatinine, and glucose. Although this tool is helpful for excluding necrotizing fasciitis, it has not been prospectively validated by large studies. It cannot be overemphasized that any clinical suspicion of necrotizing fasciitis warrants prompt surgical consultation.

The infection that causes necrotizing fasciitis can be monomicrobial or polymicrobial. Monomicrobial infections are usually from group A, β-hemolytic streptococci (GAS), other β-hemolytic streptococci, or community-associated methicillin-resistant *Staphylococcus aureus.* Polymicrobial infections are most common and include a combination of anaerobic and aerobic bacteria. Usually, these infections consist of mixed bacteria from the gastrointestinal or genitourinary tracts. Putrid-smelling, "dishwater gray" pus is characteristically present in mixed infections (3).

First-line treatment is urgent surgical exploration and débridement. Serial débridements are typically necessary and continue until no necrotic tissue remains. The Infectious Diseases Society of America (IDSA) recommends antimicrobial therapy until the patient is clinically stable, afebrile for 48 to 72 hours, and no longer requires surgical débridement. Vancomycin or daptomycin, plus clindamycin, and either piperacillin-tazobactam, a carbapenem, or ceftriaxone and metronidazole are empiric regimens (Figure 11.1) that provide coverage against aerobes, anaerobes, methicillin-resistant *S aureus,* and GAS. If GAS is the causal organism in monomicrobial cases, treatment with penicillin and clindamycin is indicated. The use of intravenous immunoglobulin in these infections is being investigated. Currently, the IDSA does not recommend for or against its use (3).

Figure 11.1   Empiric Antimicrobial Therapy for Necrotizing Fasciitis

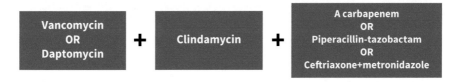

References

1. Wong CH, Chang HC, Pasupathy S, Khin LW, Tan JL, Low CO. Necrotizing fasciitis: clinical presentation, microbiology, and determinants of mortality. J Bone Joint Surg Am. 2003 Aug;85(8):1454–60.
2. Bakleh M, Wold LE, Mandrekar JN, Harmsen WS, Dimashkieh HH, Baddour LM. Correlation of histopathologic findings with clinical outcome in necrotizing fasciitis. Clin Infect Dis. 2005 Feb 1;40(3):410–4. Epub 2005 Jan 6.
3. Stevens DL, Bisno AL, Chambers HF, Dellinger EP, Goldstein EJ, Gorbach SL, et al. Practice guidelines for the diagnosis and management of skin and soft tissue infections: 2014 update by the Infectious Diseases Society of America. Clin Infect Dis. 2014 Jul 15;59(2):147–59. Epub 2014 Jun 18.
4. Wong CH, Khin LW, Heng KS, Tan KC, Low CO. The LRINEC (Laboratory Risk Indicator for Necrotizing Fasciitis) score: a tool for distinguishing necrotizing fasciitis from other soft tissue infections. Crit Care Med. 2004 Jul;32(7):1535–41.

Kidney Disease and HIV[a]

12

Eugene M. Tan, MD, Jasmine R. Marcelin, MD, and Stacey A. Rizza, MD

Case Presentation

A 30-year-old black woman with a diagnosis of HIV sought medical care after relocation to a different geographic area. For several years after her HIV diagnosis, she did not take any antiretroviral therapy (ART), but at an undisclosed time, the patient began treatment with elvitegravir, cobicistat, emtricitabine, and tenofovir. Within 1 month of starting ART, she self-discontinued her medications because of lower extremity muscle cramping. She did not have other medical care until the current presentation.

The patient was hospitalized for abdominal pain, nausea, and emesis. An esophagogastroduodenoscopy showed *Candida* esophagitis, which was treated with fluconazole for 14 days. Her CD4 T-cell count at that time was 256 cells/mcL (10%) and her HIV RNA level was 43,900 copies/mL.

Laboratory tests performed at the time of hospital admission showed acute kidney injury, with a serum creatinine level of 6.9 mg/dL. A urinalysis showed nephrotic-range proteinuria and a predicted urine protein level of 7.8 g per 24 hours. She underwent a kidney biopsy, which showed collapsing glomerulopathy that was consistent with advanced HIV-associated nephropathy (HIVAN). Because we noted decreasing urine output during hospitalization, she received a diagnosis of end-stage renal disease (ESRD) and intermittent hemodialysis was initiated. Her ESRD was complicated by anemia (treated with intravenous iron supplementation), secondary hyperparathyroidism, vitamin D deficiency (treated with vitamin D supplementation and phosphate binders), and hypertension (controlled with amlodipine, carvedilol, and furosemide).

After a thorough discussion, the patient agreed to reinitiate ART. Given her ESRD, a tenofovir-containing regimen was avoided. Her HLA-B*57:01 genetic test result was negative, so she initiated therapy with abacavir, lamivudine, and ritonavir-boosted darunavir. Because of her *Candida* esophagitis and CD4 T-cell percentage less than 14%, she also began *Pneumocystis* prophylaxis with monthly pentamidine (inhaled). Trimethoprim-sulfamethoxazole was avoided because of the ESRD.

She did not consistently adhere to her ART because of ongoing psychosocial stressors, and her CD4 T-cell count decreased to 197 cells/mcL (9%). When she became compliant with the ART medications, her CD4 T-cell count increased to a maximum of 306 cells/mcL (23%). After her renal function was stabilized with dialysis, once-weekly tenofovir was added back to her ART for maximum antiviral effects.

[a] Text from Lucas GM, Ross MJ, Stock PG, Shlipak MG, Wyatt CM, Gupta SK, et al; HIV Medicine Association of the Infectious Diseases Society of America. Clinical practice guideline for the management of chronic kidney disease in patients infected with HIV: 2014 update by the HIV Medicine Association of the Infectious Diseases Society of America. Clin Infect Dis. 2014 Nov 1;59(9):e96-138. Epub 2014 Sep 17; used with permission.

Discussion

Patients are considered to have chronic kidney disease (CKD) when markers of kidney damage are present for longer than 3 months. These markers are albuminuria, electrolyte dysfunction, structural abnormalities (detected histologically or with imaging), or history of kidney transplant. However, even in the absence of these markers, a glomerular filtration rate (GFR) persistently below 60 mL/min per 1.73 m^2 for longer than 3 months is also consistent with CKD (1).

Serum creatinine is most commonly used to estimate GFR, but levels can vary, depending on the patient's sex, race, age, muscle mass, and nutrition. Cystatin C has less variability with race, sex, or body composition, but it can be affected by thyroid disease, corticosteroid use, HIV RNA levels, and coinfection with hepatitis C. To estimate GFR in HIV-infected individuals, the CKD Epidemiology Collaboration recommends using the creatinine or cystatin C equations because they may be more accurate than the Modification of Diet in Renal Disease study equation (2).

HIV is a risk factor for CKD, and the prevalence of patients with GFR less than 60 mL/min per 1.73 m^2 ranges from 4.7% to 9.7% in North American and European individuals with HIV. Other risk factors for CKD include older age, female sex, diabetes mellitus, hypertension, injection drug use, lower CD4 T-cell counts, history of acute kidney injury, higher HIV RNA levels, coinfection with hepatitis C, and specific ART regimens. Risk factors for progression from CKD to ESRD include HIVAN, black race, family history of ESRD, magnitude of proteinuria, and severe immunosuppression (2).

The 2 major categories of HIV-related kidney disease include HIVAN and HIV-associated immune complex kidney disease. HIVAN is common in black patients and patients with untreated HIV or advanced immunosuppression. Clinically, HIVAN is characterized by severe proteinuria without hematuria or red blood cell casts, rapidly decreasing GFR, and echogenic kidneys. HIV can directly infect glomerular epithelial cells, collapse the glomerular capillary tuft, efface foot processes, form pseudocrescents, and thicken the glomerular basement membrane. Histologically, HIVAN appears as collapsing focal segmental glomerulosclerosis, microcystic tubular dilatation, and tubulointerstitial inflammation by macrophages and T lymphocytes (2).

HIV-associated immune complex kidney disease includes immune complex glomerulonephritis, immunoglobulin A nephropathy, and lupus-like nephritis. Antibodies bound to HIV antigens are deposited on capillary loops and the mesangium. Complement activation may result in a lupus-like pathology in the kidney. HIV-associated immune complex kidney disease may also be associated with tubulointerstitial inflammation with macrophages, eosinophils, and B cells (2).

Various ART regimens may affect renal function. Tenofovir, a nucleoside reverse transcriptase inhibitor, is recommended in various first-line ART regimens; however, it can cause nephrotoxicity because it accumulates in the proximal tubules, preventing transport of organic acid, and it can also cause interstitial nephritis or Fanconi syndrome (3). Atazanavir is a protease inhibitor that can increase risk of reduced GFR, nephrolithiasis, proximal tubular dysfunction, interstitial nephritis, and acute kidney injury. Cobicistat is a cytochrome P450 3A inhibitor that functions as a pharmacologic boosting agent for other antiretroviral agents. It is often combined with elvitegravir, emtricitabine, and tenofovir, but it is not recommended for patients with an estimated creatinine clearance less than 70 mL/min because of reduced tubular secretion and subsequent increase in serum creatinine. Rilpivirine, a nonnucleoside reverse transcriptase inhibitor, and dolutegravir, an integrase strand transfer inhibitor, also inhibit creatinine secretion by renal transport proteins within tubular epithelial cells (2).

Patients with HIV should be monitored with a creatinine-based estimated GFR, urinalysis, and quantitative measure of albuminuria or proteinuria whenever ART is initiated or changed.

Otherwise, in patients with stable HIV, serum creatinine should be obtained at least twice yearly and urinalysis should be obtained at least annually. These screening tests are recommended to detect drug nephrotoxicity and estimate GFR for proper dose adjustment of drugs that are renally metabolized. Measuring albuminuria or proteinuria can identify HIVAN earlier and allow time for treatment. If abnormalities are detected with these screening tests, further evaluation should be performed with renal function testing, complete urinalysis, quantification of albuminuria, blood pressure and glucose measurement, renal sonography, and a thorough review of medications. Referral to a nephrologist should be considered for patients with a marked decline in GFR (>25% from baseline or <60 mL/min per 1.73 m^2), albuminuria (>300 mg/d), combined hematuria and proteinuria, and increasing blood pressure (2).

Patients with HIVAN should receive ART to reduce the risk of ESRD progression. ART is associated with a lower incidence of HIVAN and ESRD and with improved kidney function (1). Commonly used ART drugs that require dose adjustment for renal insufficiency include emtricitabine, lamivudine, tenofovir, and zidovudine (4). Angiotensin-converting enzyme inhibitors or angiotensin receptor blockers should be used in patients with HIVAN. The optimal goal for blood pressure is less than 140/90 mm Hg in the presence of normal or mild albuminuria (<30 mg/d), but for patients with moderate to severe albuminuria (>30-300 mg/d), the goal for blood pressure is less than 130/80 mm Hg.

Statins and aspirin can be used to reduce risk of cardiovascular events (2). Corticosteroids may be beneficial in reducing serum creatinine, proteinuria, and interstitial inflammation. Prednisone may be tapered for a 2- to 9-month period and may be associated with an increased risk of avascular necrosis of the femoral head (4). For patients with HIVAN that progresses to ESRD, kidney transplant can be considered, but candidates should have a CD4 T-cell count exceeding 200 cells/mcL, undetectable plasma HIV RNA, and a stable ART regimen (2).

References

1. Stevens PE, Levin A; Kidney Disease: Improving Global Outcomes Chronic Kidney Disease Guideline Development Work Group Members. Evaluation and management of chronic kidney disease: synopsis of the kidney disease: improving global outcomes 2012 clinical practice guideline. Ann Intern Med. 2013 Jun 4;158(11):825–30.
2. Lucas GM, Ross MJ, Stock PG, Shlipak MG, Wyatt CM, Gupta SK, et al; HIV Medicine Association of the Infectious Diseases Society of America. Clinical practice guideline for the management of chronic kidney disease in patients infected with HIV: 2014 update by the HIV Medicine Association of the Infectious Diseases Society of America. Clin Infect Dis. 2014 Nov 1;59(9):e96–138. Epub 2014 Sep 17.
3. Marcelin JR, Berg ML, Tan EM, Amer H, Cummins NW, Rizza SA. Is abnormal urine protein/osmolality ratio associated with abnormal renal function in patients receiving tenofovir disoproxil fumarate? PLoS One. 2016 Feb 12;11(2):e0149562.
4. Kalayjian RC. The treatment of HIV-associated nephropathy. Adv Chronic Kidney Dis. 2010 Jan;17(1):59–71.

Constitutional Symptoms in a Patient After Cardiovascular Surgery

13

Joana Kang, MD, and Daniel C. DeSimone, MD

Case Presentation

A 37-year-old man from Wisconsin presented for evaluation of a 2-week history of fever. Blood cultures obtained at another medical center had grown *Cutibacterium acnes*. His medical history included congenital heart disease and extensive cardiac surgery, previous transient ischemic attacks (TIAs), and migraines. His surgical history included repair for narrowing of the ascending aorta (1988); aortic valve replacement with his own pulmonary valve plus cadaveric pulmonary allograft to replace the pulmonary valve (Ross procedure) for aortic regurgitation (1990); aortic valve replacement with a mechanical heart valve and vascular graft placement in the ascending aorta, aortic arch, and innominate and left common carotid arteries (2002); aortic valve replacement with a mechanical heart valve for paravalvular leak (2008); and closure of an ascending aortic pseudoaneurysm with a septal occluder device (2014).

The patient was in his usual state of health until 2 weeks before being seen at our institution. At that time, he had a fever, headache, and malaise. He experienced a sensation of drifting to the right and presented to a local hospital with concern that he was having a TIA. A computed tomographic (CT) scan of the head did not show evidence of a stroke, and his symptoms resolved. A few days later, preliminary results of blood cultures obtained during his evaluation showed an anaerobic, gram-positive bacilli. Chest CT showed a filling defect within the aortic arch

that was larger than what had been previously observed and raised concerns about growth of a known thrombus.

He was transferred to Mayo Clinic for further evaluation. He was initially treated empirically with intravenous vancomycin and piperacillin-tazobactam. His antibiotics were narrowed to ceftriaxone when the isolate was identified as *C acnes*. Transesophageal echocardiography revealed tiny strands (Lambl excrescences) on the prosthetic aortic valve but no definite evidence of infective endocarditis. Transthoracic echocardiography was similarly unremarkable. A fluorodeoxyglucose (FDG) positron emission tomography (PET)–CT scan was performed and showed marked circumferential FDG activity, associated with the ascending aortic arch graft, that tracked proximally along the proximal left common carotid and right brachiocephalic grafts (Figure 13.1). These findings were highly suggestive of infection of the ascending aortic graft.

The patient underwent surgical exploration, which showed infection of the arch and distal ascending aortic portions of the graft, with a large vegetation at the origin of the innominate artery graft. The infected portions of the graft were resected and replaced. Intraoperative cultures of the graft tissue grew *C acnes*, confirming the diagnosis of vascular graft infection (VGI). He was treated postoperatively with intravenous ceftriaxone for 6 weeks and then transitioned to amoxicillin for lifelong oral suppressive therapy. He is currently doing well, without evidence of

Figure 13.1   FDG PET-CT of the Chest

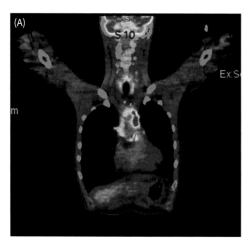
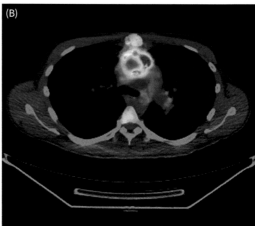

Image shows circumferential FDG activity associated with the ascending aortic arch graft. A, Coronal view. B, Cross-sectional view. CT indicates computed tomography; FDG, fluorodeoxyglucose; PET, positron emission tomography.

infection relapse at 23 months after the surgical débridement.

Discussion

VGI is an infrequent complication of aortic repair, with an estimated incidence rate of approximately 1.4%. However, mortality rates from VGI range from 25% to 75%, and clinician awareness of the syndrome and quick, reliable diagnostic methods are critical for improving clinical outcomes (1,2).

The diagnosis of VGI is made by considering a combination of clinical symptoms, laboratory studies, microbial cultures, and imaging studies. This approach, as highlighted in a recently proposed case definition (3,4), is similar to the modified Duke criteria (5) that are used to define cases of infective endocarditis. The imaging modalities currently available for diagnosis of aortic graft infections include ultrasonography, CT angiography (CTA), magnetic resonance imaging (MRI), and FDG PET-CT (6). Although ultrasonography is the least invasive of these tests, it is limited by low sensitivity and specificity because

of factors associated with the ultrasound operator and patient body size. CTA is the most commonly used imaging modality, and it has high sensitivity and specificity in high-grade graft infections. However, CTA has less sensitivity for low-grade infections and difficulty differentiating between expected postoperative changes and graft infection during the first 6 weeks after surgery (2). MRI and CTA have similar sensitivity and specificity for diagnosing aortic graft infections. FDG PET-CT has more recently become an important method for diagnosing graft infections because it can show the physical boundaries of the infection and the metabolic severity of the infection. The combination of focal FDG uptake and irregular graft boundaries on FDG PET-CT can accurately predict graft infection in 97% of cases (7). FDG PET-CT is especially useful in detecting low-grade graft infections that are not seen with CTA, and it can be used when CTA is negative but a high level of suspicion for infection remains (6).

Although a broad array of pathogens can cause VGI, the most common ones are gram-positive bacteria, including staphylococcal and streptococcal species (1). Infection with high-virulence organisms such as *Staphylococcus aureus* is usually associated with more severe infections that occur early after graft placement, and they have higher rates of morbidity and mortality. Lower-virulence organisms also cause prosthetic VGIs, as seen in our patient. *C acnes* is a gram-positive bacillus that is part of the normal skin flora, and it is most commonly associated with acne vulgaris. Aortic VGIs with *C acnes* is exceedingly rare, and a review of the literature identified only 3 previously reported cases (8,9). Prosthetic VGIs are categorized as early infections if they occur within 4 months after surgery, whereas they are categorized as late infections if they occur more than 4 months after surgery (2). Late infections (as occurred with our patient) may involve less-virulent organisms such as coagulase-negative staphylococci, *Corynebacterium* species, and *Cutibacterium* species; if they are recovered from multiple blood cultures, they should not be considered contaminants from skin flora (2).

References

1. Pettersson J, Daryapeyma A, Gillgren P, Hultgren R. Aortic graft infections after emergency and non-emergency reconstruction: incidence, treatment, and long-term outcome. Surg Infect (Larchmt). 2017 Apr;18(3):303–10. Epub 2017 Jan 27.

2. Fujii T, Watanabe Y. Multidisciplinary treatment approach for prosthetic vascular graft infection in the thoracic aortic area. Ann Thorac Cardiovasc Surg. 2015;21(5):418–27. Epub 2015 Sep 8.

3. Tokuda Y, Oshima H, Araki Y, Narita Y, Mutsuga M, Kato K, et al. Detection of thoracic aortic prosthetic graft infection with 18F-fluorodeoxyglucose positron emission tomography/computed tomography. Eur J Cardiothorac Surg. 2013 Jun;43(6):1183–7. Epub 2013 Jan 18.

4. Lyons OT, Baguneid M, Barwick TD, Bell RE, Foster N, Homer-Vanniasinkam S, et al. Diagnosis of aortic graft infection: a case definition by the Management of Aortic Graft Infection Collaboration (MAGIC). Eur J Vasc Endovasc Surg. 2016 Dec;52(6):758–63. Epub 2016 Oct 19.

5. Li JS, Sexton DJ, Mick N, Nettles R, Fowler VG Jr, Ryan T, et al. Proposed modifications to the Duke criteria for the diagnosis of infective endocarditis. Clin Infect Dis. 2000;30(4):633–8.

6. Censullo A, Vijayan T. Using nuclear medicine imaging wisely in diagnosing infectious diseases. Open Forum Infect Dis. 2017 Feb 3;4(1):ofx011.

7. Spacek M, Belohlavek O, Votrubova J, Sebesta P, Stadler P. Diagnostics of "non-acute" vascular prosthesis infection using 18F-FDG PET/CT: our experience with 96 prostheses. 2009;36(5):850–8.

8. Harlock JA, Qadura M, Lee G, Szalay DA. Infected aortic stent graft with *Propionibacterium acnes*. Vasc Endovascular Surg. 2013 Jul;47(5):394–6. Epub 2013 Apr 29.

9. Pineda DM, Tyagi S, Dougherty MJ, Troutman DA, Calligaro KD. Thoracic aortic graft infections secondary to *Propionibacterium* species: two cases and review of the literature. Vasc Endovascular Surg. 2016 Aug;50(6):431–4. Epub 2016 Jul 5.

Piggyback Ride Anyone?

Maria V. Dioverti Prono, MD, and M. Rizwan Sohail, MD

14

Case Presentation

A 29-year-old man from Micronesia presented to the emergency department with a headache, neck pain, chills, and rigors. He had a history of leprosy, which was treated with clofazimine, dapsone, and clarithromycin for approximately 1.5 years before presentation. His treatment course was complicated by erythema nodosum leprosum and iridocyclitis that required long-term corticosteroid therapy. The patient had exacerbation of erythema nodosum leprosum while attempting to taper the corticosteroid therapy and needed high-dose prednisone (80 mg/d) for several weeks before presentation.

The patient was febrile but hemodynamically stable. A physical examination showed that he had neck stiffness, and skin findings were consistent with dermatologic sequela from leprosy. The patient was admitted to the hospital. A computed tomographic scan of his head was negative for any mass lesions. Cerebrospinal fluid analysis showed a total nucleated cell count of 8,748/mm^3 with 75% neutrophils, glucose of 22 mg/dL, and protein level of 615 mg/dL, consistent with bacterial meningitis. Cerebrospinal fluid cultures grew *Enterococcus faecalis*. Blood and urine cultures were negative. The patient was treated with intravenous ampicillin for 2 weeks and intravenous gentamicin during the first week. His symptoms resolved.

Given the unusual causative agent for meningitis and the patient's country of origin, *Strongyloides* serologies and stool cultures were obtained, and both yielded positive results (Figure 14.1). The patient received 2 doses of oral ivermectin (0.2 mg/kg each, separated by a week). He recovered without sequelae.

Discussion

Strongyloides stercoralis is an intestinal nematode that is endemic in tropical and subtropical areas (including the southeastern United States). It has a unique ability to fully replicate inside its host (autoinfection) and can cause overwhelming infections in immunocompromised patients (1). *Strongyloides* has a complex life cycle that includes free-living and parasitic cycles (Figure 14.2). During the initial exposure, larvae penetrate through intact human skin, and the site of entry may have a localized, pruritic rash. Pulmonary symptoms may occur as larvae migrate through the lungs to their final destination in the gastrointestinal tract (2). Chronic infection is typically asymptomatic or mildly symptomatic (diarrhea, constipation, and dermatologic manifestation) and may be associated with intermittent eosinophilia (1, 2).

Figure 14.1   *Strongyloides stercoralis* in Stool Culture

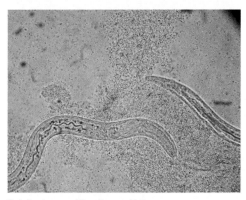

Original magnification, ×400.

Figure 14.2   Strongyloides Life Cycle

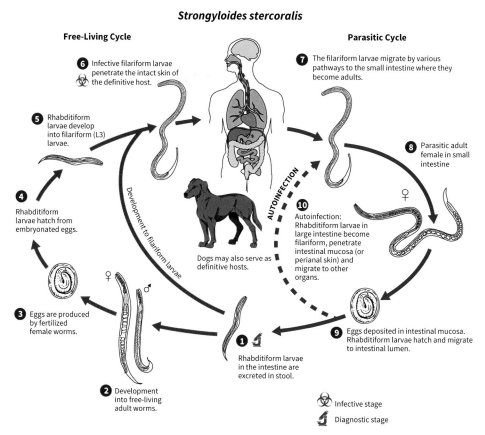

Strongyloides stercoralis

Free-Living Cycle

6 Infective filariform larvae penetrate the intact skin of the definitive host.

5 Rhabditiform larvae develop into filariform (L3) larvae.

4 Rhabditiform larvae hatch from embryonated eggs.

Development to filariform larvae

3 Eggs are produced by fertilized female worms.

2 Development into free-living adult worms.

Parasitic Cycle

7 The filariform larvae migrate by various pathways to the small intestine where they become adults.

8 Parasitic adult female in small intestine

AUTOINFECTION

10 Autoinfection: Rhabditiform larvae in large intestine become filariform, penetrate intestinal mucosa (or perianal skin) and migrate to other organs.

Dogs may also serve as definitive hosts.

9 Eggs deposited in intestinal mucosa. Rhabditiform larvae hatch and migrate to intestinal lumen.

1 Rhabditiform larvae in the intestine are excreted in stool.

Infective stage

Diagnostic stage

From the Centers for Disease Control and Prevention [cited 2021 Apr 12]. Available from: https://www.cdc.gov/dpdx/strongyloidiasis.

In immunocompromised hosts, enhanced autoinfection can lead to hyperinfection syndrome, a massive invasion by filariform larvae. The term *disseminated disease* has been used when worms are observed outside the lungs and intestines. It can be difficult to distinguish between disseminated disease and hyperinfection (3). Up to 39% of cases are associated with a bacterial or yeast infection, and bacteremia may often lead to purulent meningitis. Most bloodstream infections in this scenario are caused by gram-negative organisms because migrating larvae penetrating through the intestinal wall can carry organisms with them (2).

Most reported cases of hyperinfection have been associated with oral corticosteroid use,

with a mean dosage equivalent to prednisone at 52 mg/d (3). However, hyperinfection can occur regardless of the dose, duration, or route of corticosteroid administration (2). Another well-described risk factor for hyperinfection is coinfection with human T-cell leukemia virus type 1 (HTLV-1). Augmentation of regulatory T cells by HTLV-1 infection is hypothesized to downregulate the inflammatory response to *Strongyloides* infection (as evidenced by lower interleukin 5 levels and eosinophil counts), thereby allowing massive replication; this mechanism is supported by the higher parasitic burden in coinfected patients (4). Hyperinfection syndrome also has been associated with numerous drugs and biologic agents, hypogammaglobulinemia, hematologic malignancies, and solid-organ and hematopoietic stem cell transplant (2).

The diagnosis of a *Strongyloides* infection classically is established by serial stool examinations. Assay sensitivity reaches 92% when 3 different stool samples are analyzed (2). The parasite can also be isolated from sputum, bronchoalveolar lavage, or duodenal aspirate specimens, and rarely from skin, peritoneal fluid, and cerebrospinal fluid (3). Enzyme-linked immunosorbent serologic assays show positive results by about 4 to 6 weeks after the initial infection. Polymerase chain reaction assays are currently used as a research tool. Newer immunologic techniques, such as the luciferase immunoprecipitation system assay, may be useful, particularly for monitoring the response to treatment (2). Peripheral eosinophilia is uncommon and usually absent when the infection is limited to the gastrointestinal tract (1, 3). Chest radiographs show a pulmonary infiltrate in most patients with hyperinfection syndrome.

The recommended treatment for *Strongyloides* infection is ivermectin (200 mcg/kg daily, for 2 consecutive days), and repeat dosing can be considered 1 week after the initial treatment (5). For patients with hyperinfection or disseminated *Strongyloides* infection, experts recommend treatment with ivermectin (200 mcg/kg daily) until stool culture results are negative for 2 weeks (2). Reduction of immunosuppression should be strongly considered, if at all possible. For patients with severe infection, a combination of ivermectin and albendazole may be considered (2).

The mortality rate with hyperinfection syndrome is high (59% of cases in 1 study), and the mortality rate is 100% if the disease is left untreated (2, 3). Diagnosis is frequently delayed, and targeted therapy therefore may not start until late in the disease course, which likely contributes to the high mortality rate. Gram-negative bacteremia and sepsis also contribute to high death rates.

Screening for *Strongyloides* infection should be considered for any individual from an endemic area who is going to receive corticosteroids or another form of immunosuppression, and it should also be considered for patients with HTLV-1 infection (2).

References

1. Bennett JE, Dolin R, Blaser MJ, editors. Mandell, Douglas, and Bennett's principles and practice of infectious diseases. 9th ed. Philadelphia (PA): Elsevier; c2020. 3839 p.
2. Mejia R, Nutman TB. Screening, prevention, and treatment for hyperinfection syndrome and disseminated infections caused by *Strongyloides stercoralis*. Curr Opin Infect Dis. 2012 Aug;25(4):458–63.
3. Fardet L, Genereau T, Poirot JL, Guidet B, Kettaneh A, Cabane J. Severe strongyloidiasis in corticosteroid-treated patients: case series and literature review. J Infect. 2007 Jan;54(1):18–27. Epub 2006 Mar 14.
4. Montes M, Sanchez C, Verdonck K, Lake JE, Gonzalez E, Lopez G, et al. Regulatory T cell expansion in HTLV-1 and strongyloidiasis co-infection is associated with reduced IL-5 responses to *Strongyloides stercoralis* antigen. PLoS Negl Trop Dis. 2009 Jun 9;3(6):e456.
5. Dykewicz CA, Jaffe HW, Kaplan JE; Guidelines Working Group Members from CDC, the Infectious Disease Society of America, and the American Society of Blood and Marrow Transplantation. Guidelines for preventing opportunistic infections among hematopoietic stem cell transplant recipients. MMWR Recomm Rep. 2000 Oct 20;49(RR10);1–128.

Premature Closure

15

Douglas W. Challener, MD, Jasmine R. Marcelin, MD, and Aaron J. Tande, MD

Case Presentation

A 51-year-old man with a long-term diagnosis of autoimmune hepatitis was transferred to our hospital for evaluation of a fever of unknown origin (FUO). He was a never-smoker and reported being otherwise healthy until a year ago, when he had fevers, night sweats, and pruritus that were associated with elevated liver enzyme levels and presumed to be attributable to autoimmune hepatitis. An oncologist at another institution evaluated the patient for a possible lymphoma diagnosis, but this diagnosis was ruled out after a liver biopsy and peripheral blood flow cytometry test were negative. In the year before his presentation at our facility, he had been treated several times with long courses of high-dose oral corticosteroids (>30 mg of prednisone daily). Three months before his current presentation, he had fever, night sweats, and tachycardia, and he was prescribed prednisone and mycophenolate mofetil as empiric treatment for autoimmune hepatitis. He did not receive prophylactic antibiotics for *Pneumocystis jirovecii* pneumonia (PCP).

A chronic, nonproductive cough developed and was associated with an unintentional 25-pound weight loss. He was hospitalized at another facility. Computed tomographic (CT) imaging of his chest showed diffuse, bilateral, ground-glass opacities. Bronchoscopy was unremarkable, and cultures from a bronchoalveolar lavage were negative. Despite these negative results, he was treated with broad-spectrum antimicrobial agents, including vancomycin, piperacillin-tazobactam, azithromycin, and acyclovir, but he did not improve. After a 2-week hospitalization, he requested a transfer to our hospital for further evaluation. On arrival, he was alert, oriented, and in no distress. His heart rate was tachycardic, but his cardiac examination was otherwise unremarkable. We noted diffuse crackles throughout the lungs that were worse in the bases. There was no lymphadenopathy, rash, or splenomegaly, and the rest of his physical examination findings were normal.

Given his recent treatment with empiric corticosteroids, there was a concern for PCP, and empiric antibiotic treatment was initiated with trimethoprim-sulfamethoxazole. He underwent bronchoscopy with bronchoalveolar lavage plus lung biopsy. The trimethoprim-sulfamethoxazole was discontinued 4 days later, when a polymerase chain reaction assay for *Pneumocystis* was negative. Six days after the biopsy, the pathologic evaluation ultimately identified diffuse large B-cell lymphoma. Staging with positron emission tomography–CT showed fluorodeoxyglucose-avid regions in the lungs, liver, para-aortic lymph nodes, and bones. Chemotherapy was initiated. He tolerated it very well and showed improvement in his oxygen requirements and liver function.

Discussion

Broad differential diagnoses are fundamental to providing excellent patient care and avoiding diagnostic errors. This case illustrates shortcuts in clinical reasoning that delayed the accurate diagnosis and resulted in inappropriate treatment. Psychologists have described these shortcuts as *heuristics* and have created a classification system for these errors. The defined heuristics include premature closure, anchoring bias, blind obedience, the availability heuristic, and framing effects (1). With greater knowledge of the common diagnostic pitfalls, physicians can attempt to avoid these errors.

A common error is premature closure, which occurs when a firm belief in a single diagnosis prevents the clinician from considering other diagnostic possibilities. For example, a patient with known coronary disease presenting with chest pain and an elevated troponin level may tempt a clinician to immediately diagnose and treat acute coronary syndrome, without considering competing diagnoses such as pulmonary embolism. To avoid this pitfall, the clinical case should be routinely readdressed with a fresh perspective by asking, "What is the one diagnosis that should not be missed?" or "What is the worst possible diagnosis?" (1). Additionally, practitioners should be asking themselves if the diagnosis is still reasonable as new information becomes available. Interestingly, the risk of succumbing to premature closure appears to increase with an increasing number of potential diagnoses. Physicians are inclined to exclude alternative diagnoses when few are available. The costs associated with ruling out diagnoses can seem insurmountable when the differential diagnosis is broad (1).

An FUO is particularly ripe for diagnostic errors, especially premature closure. The differential diagnosis for the syndrome of FUO is among the most extensive and includes infections, malignancies, noninfectious inflammatory diseases, genetic disorders, and various miscellaneous conditions (2). For this patient, lymphoma had previously been considered and reportedly excluded. The clinicians then appropriately considered infectious causes for his fever. However, despite negative microbiologic test results at the other institution, the patient continued to receive broad-spectrum antimicrobials. The outside hospital had failed to expand the differential diagnoses beyond infection. However, PCP was a logical possibility because the patient had received high doses of

systemic glucocorticoids without appropriate antibiotic prophylaxis. Additionally, other potential causes of his syndrome were considered, leading to appropriate diagnostic testing with lung biopsy.

Anchoring bias is related to premature closure and describes the physician's reluctance to fully consider competing diagnoses after a diagnosis exists. It is caused by focusing exclusively on the initial impression of the patient and can lead to insufficient data gathering and not incorporating new information as it becomes available. Early career physicians are especially susceptible to premature closure and to anchoring bias (3). Physicians should always seek to include new diagnostic data to prevent anchoring bias. One could ask, "If the patient were to die today, what would it be from?" (1). Another potential way to avoid anchoring bias is to continually consider the probabilities and likelihoods of diagnoses for a given clinical setting.

Another logical pitfall is blind obedience, defined as the error of expressing deference to authority or a diagnostic result. For the patient described above, blind obedience was shown with the initial acceptance of the negative results of the lymphoma evaluation from an outside institution. The best way to avoid this error is through verification and reevaluation of diagnostic studies that may not be consistent with the clinical situation (1). Clinicians should adopt the "trust but verify" approach when interpreting data, especially if the data are incomplete. For this patient, pulmonary testing was appropriate and helped establish the correct diagnosis.

This case description also provides an example of the availability heuristic, which refers to the clinicians' tendency to diagnose entities that they see often and to neglect less frequently encountered diagnoses. Subspecialists are especially prone to this error. If physicians often see immunosuppressed patients with PCP, they are more likely to make this diagnosis when a new, similar clinical scenario is presented. A nephrologist seeing a patient with edema may immediately think of nephrotic syndrome, whereas a cardiologist might first consider heart failure.

The clinical maxim to help avoid this pitfall is "Hoofbeats are more likely to be from horses than zebras" (1). Clinicians should attempt to determine the most likely diagnoses, independent of their area of expertise.

This case includes a particularly interesting scenario of FUO plus hepatitis, and it includes some of the diagnostic pitfalls that commonly affect clinicians. Ultimately, the patient's diagnosis of autoimmune hepatitis was revised when the liver histopathology was reviewed again and shown to be consistent with B-cell lymphoma. If the initial diagnostic errors had not occurred, perhaps he would have received more timely treatment for lymphoma. Physicians must remain vigilant and aware of how they may be taking diagnostic shortcuts. Although these shortcuts are often effective and efficient, there are situations in which the shortcuts do not pay off. This case is a reminder of those situations.

References

1. Redelmeier DA. Improving patient care. The cognitive psychology of missed diagnoses. Ann Intern Med. 2005 Jan 18;142(2):115–20.
2. Efstathiou SP, Pefanis AV, Tsiakou AG, Skeva II, Tsioulos DI, Achimastos AD, et al. Fever of unknown origin: discrimination between infectious and non-infectious causes. Eur J Intern Med. 2010 Apr;21(2):137–43. Epub 2009 Dec 6.
3. Rylander M, Guerrasio J. Heuristic errors in clinical reasoning. Clin Teach. 2016 Aug;13(4):287–90. Epub 2015 Sep 23.

Disclosure

16

Eugene M. Tan, MD, Jasmine R. Marcelin, MD,
and Zelalem Temesgen, MD

Case Presentation

A 47-year-old woman with a 10-year history of HIV, most recently treated with tenofovir, emtricitabine, and efavirenz, presents for a general medical examination. She is asymptomatic. Her CD4 count is 418 cells/mcL, and she has no detectable HIV RNA. She has been sexually active with 1 male partner for the past 4 years. They consistently use condoms. He is not aware of her HIV status. She is not sure if he has ever been tested for HIV. She is afraid to disclose her HIV status to him because she does not know how he will react.

Discussion

US state laws vary with regard to notifying partners of persons living with HIV (PLWH). Some states have expanded confidentiality laws protecting sensitive health information. Other states have HIV-specific criminal laws, which impose penalties on HIV-infected individuals who knowingly expose others to HIV without first disclosing their status. In 1988, the federal government issued the Presidential Commission on the Human Immunodeficiency Virus Epidemic Report (1), which stated that criminal sanctions for HIV transmission should be directed only toward behavior that is scientifically proven to be a mode of transmission. In 1990, the Ryan White Comprehensive AIDS Resources Emergency Act (PHL101-881) (2) required states to have criminal laws that could adequately prosecute individuals who knowingly exposed

another person to HIV. In 2010, the President's National HIV/AIDS Strategy questioned whether existing HIV-specific criminal laws continue to further public interest (3).

HIV-specific criminal laws may have unintended consequences of increasing HIV-related stigma and may decrease the willingness of PLWH to disclose their status. PLWH may also be reluctant to disclose their HIV status because of fear of domestic partner violence and retaliation (3). A 2012 study of PLWH in New Jersey showed that 51% knew about the state's HIV exposure law, which requires PLWH to disclose their positive serostatus and receive informed consent from sexual partners. However, this knowledge was not associated with seropositive status disclosure, sexual abstinence, or condom use. The study concluded that HIV exposure laws do not appear to reduce sexual risk behavior or HIV transmission (4).

As of 2019, 34 states had laws that criminalize HIV exposure. In 21 states, persons who are aware that they have HIV are legally required to disclose their status to sexual partners, and 12 states require disclosure to needle-sharing partners. Some states classify HIV-specific criminal laws as felonies; several states criminalize one or more behaviors that pose a low or negligible risk for HIV transmission, such as oral sex, biting, spitting, or throwing bodily fluids (3).

Different obligations to disclose HIV status exist, apart from sexual relationships. For example, guardians or caregivers of young HIV-positive children may have an obligation to disclose the child's HIV status to him or her (5). Intravenous drug users may have an obligation to disclose their HIV status to fellow needle-sharers (6). The ethics of disclosure become even more ambiguous in other situations, such as an HIV-positive surgeon performing a procedure on patients. Such ethical questions have not been fully answered yet.

References

1. The Presidential Commission on the Human Immunodeficiency Virus Epidemic Report. ERIC number: ED299531. 1988 Jun 24. 202 p.
2. The Ryan White HIV/AIDS Treatment Extension Act of 2009. H.R.3792 111th Congress (2009-2010) [cited 2020 Aug 4]. Available from: https://www.congress.gov/bill/111th-congress/house-bill/3792.
3. Centers for Disease Control and Prevention [Internet]. HIV and STD criminal laws [cited 2020 Aug 4]. Available from: https://www.cdc.gov/hiv/policies/law/states/exposure.html.
4. Galletly CL, Glasman LR, Pinkerton SD, Difranceisco W. New Jersey's HIV exposure law and the HIV-related attitudes, beliefs, and sexual and seropositive status disclosure behaviors of persons living with HIV. Am J Public Health. 2012 Nov;102(11):2135–40. Epub 2012 Sep 20.
5. Dusabe-Richards E, Rutakumwa R, Zalwango F, Asiimwe A, Kintu E, Ssembajja F, et al. Dealing with disclosure: perspectives from HIV-positive children and their older carers living in rural south-western Uganda. Afr J AIDS Res. 2016 Dec;15(4):387–95.
6. Johannson A, Vorobjov S, Heimer R, Dovidio JF, Uuskula A. The role of internalized stigma in the disclosure of injecting drug use among people who inject drugs and self-report as HIV-positive in Kohtla-Järve, Estonia. AIDS Behav. 2017 Apr;21(4):1034–43.

Acute Respiratory Failure in a Patient With a Methicillin-Resistant *Staphylococcus aureus* Bloodstream Infection

Erica Lin, MD, Omar M. Abu Saleh, MBBS,
and Christina G. O'Connor, PharmD, RPh

Case Presentation

A 67-year-old man presented with a history of coronary artery disease that was complicated by ischemic cardiomyopathy and required placement of a dual-chamber implantable cardioverter-defibrillator. His primary concern was a possible infection of his cardiac implantable electronic device (CIED). He recently had been hospitalized for treatment of a methicillin-resistant *Staphylococcus aureus* (MRSA) bloodstream infection from a right axilla abscess. He initially was treated with intravenous vancomycin. A transesophageal echocardiogram did not show evidence of lead or valvular endocarditis. Computed tomography (CT) of the chest, abdomen, and pelvis showed bilateral pleural effusions. Thoracentesis showed transudative effusions, and cultures were negative for microbial growth. At discharge, he was transitioned from vancomycin to daptomycin for convenience, and he planned to complete a 6-week course of antimicrobial therapy.

Fifteen days after discharge, he had progressive dyspnea, pleuritic chest pain, and cough. On arrival to the hospital, he was febrile (38.5°C) and hypoxic (oxygen saturation, 82%). He also was noted to have increased work of breathing and required emergent intubation. Laboratory studies were notable for acute kidney injury. His creatinine level was 1.9 mg/dL (reference range, 0.8-1.3 mg/dL), and he had elevated brain-type natriuretic peptide (2,000 pg/mL). Intravenous furosemide was administered for diuresis, given the concern about an exacerbation of his congestive heart failure. A chest radiograph showed bilateral pulmonary infiltrates (Figure 17.1). Repeat blood cultures grew MRSA. Because he had persistently positive blood cultures even while receiving daptomycin therapy, he was transitioned to vancomycin. Shortly after this

Figure 17.1 Chest Radiograph at Presentation

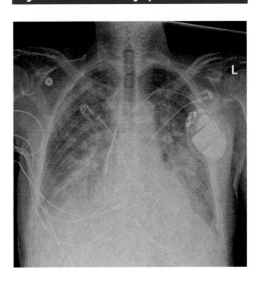

transition, he was extubated to a high-flow nasal cannula and transferred to the cardiac intensive care unit at our facility. The persistent MRSA bloodstream infection suggested a CIED infection that warranted device explantation.

Upon arrival to the cardiac intensive care unit, he was febrile (38.9°C), tachycardic (116 beats/min), and hypertensive (179/88 mm Hg). He required ongoing oxygen supplementation with a high-flow nasal cannula. A chest radiograph showed extensive patchy bilateral interstitial and alveolar infiltrates. A subsequent CT of the chest showed an increase in patchy and confluent consolidation, with ground-glass opacities, bronchiectasis, and bilateral pleural effusions. Bronchoscopy was performed, and bronchoalveolar lavage (BAL) showed 22% eosinophils. Given the concern for daptomycin-induced acute eosinophilic pneumonia (AEP), he received intravenous methylprednisolone, which was eventually tapered to oral prednisone. After glucocorticoids were initiated, his oxygen requirements markedly decreased. A chest radiograph, obtained after initiation of corticosteroids and withdrawal of daptomycin, showed improvement in the infiltrates (Figure 17.2). The patient's bloodstream infection resolved after device removal and completion of vancomycin therapy, and he received a new CIED.

Discussion

Pulmonary toxicity of antimicrobial agents is well described. For example, nitrofurantoin is associated with acute and chronic pulmonary toxicities, isoniazid is associated with lung fibrosis, and many other antibiotics, including daptomycin, have been reported to cause eosinophilic pneumonia.

AEP is characterized by pulmonary infiltrates and an excess of eosinophils with a BAL differential cell count or lung biopsy. Various factors such as medications and toxins have been implicated in AEP causation. Daptomycin-induced

Figure 17.2   Chest Radiograph After Initiation of Corticosteroids and Withdrawal of Daptomycin

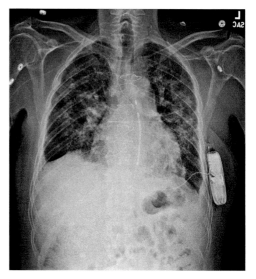

The patient had a newly implanted device.

AEP was first mentioned in 2007 (1) and has since been described in case reports and case series (2). Daptomycin is a cyclic lipopeptide antibiotic with activity against drug-resistant, gram-positive bacteria, including MRSA and vancomycin-resistant *Enterococcus*.

The pathophysiology of medication-induced AEP is still unknown. Allen (3) hypothesized that an eosinophil-mediated immune response is triggered by the offending agent. Activation of alveolar macrophages causes T helper 2 cells to produce interleukin 5. This cytokine promotes eosinophil production and migration in pulmonary alveoli. Other theories focus on the binding of daptomycin by pulmonary surfactant, resulting in its accumulation in the alveolar space and eventual epithelial injury.

Diagnosis of AEP is established on the basis of the following criteria: acute onset of febrile illness with respiratory manifestations, hypoxemia, diffuse infiltrates on imaging, an excess of eosinophilia with either greater than 25% eosinophils with a BAL differential cell count or eosinophilic pneumonia on biopsy, in the absence of other causes (4). Note that the absence of peripheral eosinophilia does not exclude the diagnosis. One limitation of this diagnostic approach is that many cases do not meet the 25% eosinophil threshold criterion. Therefore, several studies have proposed modifications to these diagnostic criteria (5,6). Kim et al (5) suggested classifying cases into definite, probable, possible, or unlikely events; the patient described above had a Naranjo score of 7, consistent with a probable adverse event. Solomon and Schwarz (6) proposed that diagnostic criteria for AEP induced by specific medications also include exposure to the agent in an appropriate timeframe, improvement after its withdrawal, and recurrence upon rechallenge.

Our patient's presentation was suggestive of daptomycin-induced AEP. Initially, his differential diagnosis was broad and included infectious and noninfectious causes such as cardiogenic pulmonary edema, acute respiratory distress syndrome, and antineutrophil cytoplasmic antibody–related pulmonary manifestation. However, the AEP diagnosis was strongly supported by the timing of his respiratory illness (2 weeks after initiation of daptomycin), the excess eosinophils with a BAL differential cell count, and his clinical improvement after transitioning to vancomycin and initiating corticosteroids. Of note, our patient did not meet all the diagnostic criteria suggested by Philit et al (4); his BAL differential cell count showed 22% eosinophils, which might be because the BAL was performed 2 days after daptomycin withdrawal. In a published case series, only 50% of patients met the 25% threshold (3).

Classically, medication-induced AEP is associated predominantly with male patients (mean age, 65 years) (2). Most patients present within the first 2 weeks of exposure to the inciting agent (2,3). The most common clinical presentation is fever, followed by dyspnea (3). Radiologic findings include infiltrates, opacities, and pleural effusions (2,3).

Management includes withdrawal of the inciting agent and close observation (6). Corticosteroids are often administered to suppress inflammation (6). Although some patients may require a trial of respiratory support with supplemental oxygenation or mechanical ventilation, almost all patients have symptomatic resolution with no residual deficits or fatalities.

In conclusion, health care providers should be able to recognize and manage the serious adverse effects of daptomycin. Specifically, they should have a high level of clinical suspicion for daptomycin-induced AEP if patients have new respiratory symptoms while receiving daptomycin. Prompt cessation of the offending agent can result in symptomatic improvement.

References

1. Hayes D Jr, Anstead MI, Kuhn RJ. Eosinophilic pneumonia induced by daptomycin. J Infect. 2007 Apr;54(4):e211-3. Epub 2007 Jan 17.
2. Uppal P, LaPlante KL, Gaitanis MM, Jankowich MD, Ward KE. Daptomycin-induced eosinophilic pneumonia: a systematic review. Antimicrob Resist Infect Control. 2016 Dec 12;5:55.
3. Allen JN. Drug-induced eosinophilic lung disease. Clin Chest Med. 2004 Mar;25(1):77–88.
4. Philit F, Etienne-Mastroianni B, Parrot A, Guerin C, Robert D, Cordier JF. Idiopathic acute eosinophilic pneumonia: a study of 22 patients. Am J Respir Crit Care Med. 2002 Nov 1;166(9):1235–9.
5. Kim PW, Sorbello AF, Wassel RT, Pham TM, Tonning JM, Nambiar S. Eosinophilic pneumonia in patients treated with daptomycin: review of the literature and US FDA adverse event reporting system reports. Drug Saf. 2012 Jun 1;35(6):447–57.
6. Solomon J, Schwarz M. Drug-, toxin-, and radiation therapy-induced eosinophilic pneumonia. Semin Respir Crit Care Med. 2006 Apr;27(2):192–7.

More Than One Problem

Douglas W. Challener, MD, and Jasmine R. Marcelin, MD

18

Case Presentation

A 40-year-old man presented to the clinic to establish care for known diagnoses of HIV and hepatitis C virus (HCV), genotype 1A. He did not have clinical stigmata of liver disease or radiographic evidence of cirrhosis. He had hemophilia A and had received many blood transfusions during childhood, which were thought to be the source of his coinfection. More recently, he had been receiving weekly factor VIII replacement for his hemophilia. His current antiretroviral therapy (ART) regimen consisted of nevirapine, indinavir, and ritonavir, and he reported good compliance with this regimen for the past 8 years. His most recent tests showed undetectable viral loads and CD4 T-cell counts that were consistently between 200 and 300 cells/mcL.

He had never received treatment for HCV. His ART regimen was changed to tenofovir disoproxil fumarate, emtricitabine, and efavirenz for the convenience of a single-pill regimen and in anticipation of potentially treating the HCV. Several months after this regimen change, his CD4 T-cell count was 208 cells/mcL (34%), with a leukocyte count of 3.1×10^9/L. His CD4 T-cell counts remained steady (in the mid 100s to low 200s cells/mcL). The CD4 T-cell count percentages were steady (range, 35%-45%) and indicated good overall immune control. His low absolute CD4 T-cell counts were attributed to late-stage chronic HCV. His HIV viral loads were consistently undetectable.

He was treated with ledipasvir-sofosbuvir for 12 weeks. At completion of therapy, he showed a sustained viral response (SVR), with no evidence of HCV viremia.

Discussion

Coinfection with HIV and HCV is common. Approximately a third of patients in the United States with HIV are coinfected with either hepatitis B virus or HCV. The high prevalence of coinfection has clinically significant implications for the course of HIV and HCV.

HIV and HCV are RNA viruses with considerable genetic variability that is caused by high mutation rates. Their replication patterns are also similar, with short half-lives and rapid virion exchange rates. HIV is capable of being assimilated by the host's genome, but HCV has no genomic integration and replicates in the cytoplasm. For these reasons, blocking viral replication may eradicate HCV infection but will cause HIV to go only into a latent, nonreplicative phase (1).

Rates of sexually transmitted HCV are low in HIV-negative patients. Studies examining serodiscordant patients in heterosexual relationships have failed to show substantially elevated HCV transmission in this group (2,3). HIV-positive patients, however, have markedly increased risk of infection, which possibly is associated with the number of sexual partners and high-risk behaviors (4).

HCV infection precedes HIV infection in most coinfected individuals. The acute infection by HCV in HIV-coinfected patients does not manifest with increased symptoms or an increase in complications when compared with infection in immunocompetent patients. However, chronic infection by HCV has different clinical features in HIV-infected versus HIV-negative individuals. These complications worsen as CD4 T-cell counts decrease.

Chronically coinfected persons have higher rates of cirrhosis, hepatic insufficiency, and hepatocellular carcinoma compared with HIV-negative individuals (5-7). The increased risk of liver disease in coinfected patients is likely multifactorial and may be due to increased alcohol use, immunosuppression, and iatrogenesis caused by antiretroviral drugs (8).

Because of the high prevalence of HIV-HCV coinfection, all patients with HIV diagnoses should be screened for HCV infection. This screening consists of an initial test for the presence of immunoglobulin G to HCV. If the patient is seropositive, the diagnosis should be confirmed with a quantitative HCV RNA assay. Often, this screening is automatically performed with a reflexive laboratory test and is the same test that would be performed in HIV-negative patients. If test results are positive, patients should be counseled to avoid alcohol and risky behaviors that promote transmission, and they should be evaluated for treatment of HCV (9).

The primary therapeutic goal in patients with HIV-HCV coinfection is to eradicate the HCV and limit progression of liver disease and complications. Clearance of HCV is associated with a regression of fibrosis and a reduced risk of hepatotoxicity. For those reasons, treatment of HCV is a priority in these patients (1). Treatment of HCV has advanced markedly in recent years with approval of direct antiretroviral agents (eg, sofosbuvir, telaprevir, boceprevir). Previously, a combination of peginterferon and ribavirin was the mainstay of treatment. This combination, however, was not very effective and had rates of SVR that were near 10%. With current therapies, SVR rates exceed 95%. Although plasma HCV RNA viral loads do not correlate with disease severity, they are helpful in tracking response to antiviral treatment (10).

ART should be started in all patients with HCV, regardless of the CD4 count. ART may slow the progression of liver disease, which is accelerated by HCV-HIV coinfection. The initial ART regimen does not necessarily change for patients with HCV coinfection. The prescriber should be cognizant of potential interactions between HCV and HIV medications. Also, the prescriber should be vigilant for hepatotoxicity caused by antiretroviral medications (1).

Treatment recommendations for HCV have evolved over time as new drugs entered the market. Physicians should review treatment guidelines from the American Association for the Study of Liver Diseases and the Infectious Diseases Society of America (www.hcvguidelines.org) for the most recent recommendations.

References

1. Operskalski EA, Kovacs A. HIV/HCV co-infection: pathogenesis, clinical complications, treatment, and new therapeutic technologies. Curr HIV/AIDS Rep. 2011 Mar;8(1):12–22.
2. Vandelli C, Renzo F, Romano L, Tisminetzky S, De Palma M, Stroffolini T, et al. Lack of evidence of sexual transmission of hepatitis C among monogamous couples: results of a 10-year prospective follow-up study. Am J Gastroenterol. 2004 May;99(5):855–9.
3. Marincovich B, Castilla J, del Romero J, Garcia S, Hernando V, Raposo M, et al. Absence of hepatitis C virus transmission in a prospective cohort of heterosexual serodiscordant couples. Sex Transm Infect. 2003 Apr;79(2):160–2.
4. Frederick T, Burian P, Terrault N, Cohen M, Augenbraun M, Young M, et al. Factors associated with prevalent hepatitis C infection among HIV-infected women with no reported history of injection drug use: the Women's Interagency HIV Study (WIHS). AIDS Patient Care STDS. 2009 Nov;23(11):915–23.
5. Graham CS, Baden LR, Yu E, Mrus JM, Carnie J, Heeren T, et al. Influence of human immunodeficiency virus infection on the course of hepatitis C virus infection: a meta-analysis. Clin Infect Dis. 2001 Aug 15;33(4):562–9. Epub 2001 Jul 6.
6. Ramachandran P, Fraser A, Agarwal K, Austin A, Brown A, Foster GR, et al. UK consensus guidelines for the use of the protease inhibitors boceprevir and telaprevir in genotype 1 chronic hepatitis C infected patients. Aliment Pharmacol Ther. 2012 Mar;35(6): 647–62. Epub 2012 Feb 1.
7. Romeo R, Rumi MG, Donato MF, Cargnel MA, Vigano P, Mondelli M, et al. Hepatitis C is more severe in drug users with human immunodeficiency virus infection. J Viral Hepat. 2000 Jul;7(4):297–301.

8. Soto B, Sanchez-Quijano A, Rodrigo L, del Olmo JA, Garcia-Bengoechea M, Hernandez-Quero J, et al. Human immunodeficiency virus infection modifies the natural history of chronic parenterally-acquired hepatitis C with an unusually rapid progression to cirrhosis. J Hepatol. 1997 Jan;26(1):1–5.

9. Cengiz C, Park JS, Saraf N, Dieterich DT. HIV and liver diseases: recent clinical advances. Clin Liver Dis. 2005 Nov;9(4):647–66.

10. Liang TJ, Ghany MG. Current and future therapies for hepatitis C virus infection. N Engl J Med. 2013 May 16;368(20):1907–17.

19

Raised, Purplish, Papular Mass in the Oral Cavity of a Patient Receiving Therapy for HIV/AIDS

Jithma P. Abeykoon, MD, Omar M. Abu Saleh, MBBS,
and Jose J. Sanchez, MD

Case Presentation

A 36-year-old man presented with a progressively enlarging purple mass near his left maxillary alveolar ridge (Figure 19.1). He denied having any symptoms such as pain, bleeding, or difficulty breathing or swallowing. He had no systemic symptoms; specifically, he had no fevers, chills, or night sweats. His oral examination was also notable for thrush. The remainder of his physical examination was otherwise unremarkable.

Five weeks before his current presentation, he received a diagnosis of AIDS due to HIV-1 infection, when he presented with a subacute respiratory illness caused by pneumocystis pneumonia. His HIV load was 79,000 copies/mL, and his CD4 count was 3 cells/mcL. He was treated with trimethoprim-sulfamethoxazole and prednisone. He began treatment with azithromycin for *Mycobacterium avium* complex prophylaxis, and within 2 weeks of receiving the AIDS diagnosis, he began combination antiretroviral therapy (cART) with efavirenz, emtricitabine, and tenofovir disoproxil fumarate. Within 4 weeks of therapy, his CD4 count increased to 34 cells/mcL.

Given his advanced immunosuppression and the clinical features of the lesion, the index of suspicion for Kaposi sarcoma (KS) was high. A biopsy of the mass confirmed the diagnosis of KS, with immunohistochemical stains showing expression of CD31 and human herpesvirus 8 (HHV-8). The patient had no evidence of visceral involvement, and the KS stage was T1 I1 S1. No specific treatment for KS was provided other than continuing cART.

Despite the poor prognosis predicted by his CD4 count at diagnosis and prior opportunistic infection, the initiation of cART early in the course of illness improved his outcome. Six months after initiating antiretroviral therapy (ART), the KS appeared to be in complete remission clinically. The patient continued with cART, was feeling well, and returned to work.

Figure 19.1   A Purple, Papular, Raised Lesion Near the Left Alveolar Region of the Mandible

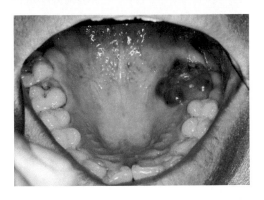

Discussion

KS is an angioproliferative disease that requires HHV-8 infection. It was first described by Moritz Kaposi in 1872 (1,2). The development of KS appears to depend on the viral homologs of human genes that are carried by HHV-8 (and eventually incorporated into the host genome). These genes promote angiogenesis and uncontrolled cell proliferation, and they also have antiapoptotic effects. Other diseases associated with HHV-8 include body cavity–based lymphoma (also termed *primary effusion lymphoma*) and Castleman disease (3). Four types of KS have been recognized: classic or sporadic, endemic or African, iatrogenic or immunosuppression-related, and AIDS-associated KS.

Classic KS is associated with older age (>60 years), male sex, and a Mediterranean, Central or Eastern European, or Middle Eastern origin. It usually has an indolent course, most commonly presenting as cutaneous disease affecting the lower extremities, with rare visceral involvement. Endemic KS is primarily seen in equatorial Africa. Cutaneous manifestations can be similar to those of classic KS but tend to be more aggressive. It can be associated with lower extremity lymphedema, especially in adults. In children, visceral organ involvement (including lymph nodes) can occur, indicating aggressive disease. Iatrogenic KS is seen primarily in solid-organ transplant recipients with considerable immunosuppression. Cyclosporine A treatment is a reported risk factor. Cutaneous manifestations are more common than visceral involvement in iatrogenic KS. AIDS-associated KS is seen in patients with HIV infection. Although cutaneous disease is common, visceral involvement can occur with poorly controlled HIV infection. KS is an AIDS-defining illness, but it can occur in patients with high CD4 counts. The severity of AIDS-associated KS depends on the patient's CD4 count and performance status, as well as organ involvement by KS (Table 19.1).

Regarding the differential diagnosis, bacillary angiomatosis attributable to bartonellosis can manifest with lesions that appear similar to those of KS. Other skin lesions, such as angiomas, hematomas, pyogenic granuloma, and nevi, should also be considered in the differential diagnosis. Biopsy of the lesion should be performed when possible because histopathologic examination is required to differentiate between these entities. The diagnosis of KS is confirmed if the biopsy specimen shows the HHV-8 latency-associated nuclear antigen (6).

Table 19.1. Staging of AIDS-Associated KS (4,5)[a]		
Factor	**Risk Level[b]**	
	Good	**Poor**
Tumor (T)	Confined to skin or LNs Nonnodular KS that is confined to the palate	Edema or ulcers associated with KS Gastrointestinal manifestation, extensive oral KS, and KS other than LN involvement in the viscera
Immune system (I)	CD4 count ≥150 cells/mcL	CD4 count <150 cells/mcL
Systemic illness (S)	No history of thrush, "B" symptoms,[c] and Karnofsky performance status ≥70%	Presence of thrush, other HIV-related illnesses, or Karnofsky performance status <70%

Abbreviations: KS, Kaposi sarcoma; LN, lymph node.

[a] The table was developed before the era of highly effective combination antiretroviral therapy.

[b] Risk is assigned a score of 0 (good risk) or 1 (poor risk).

[c] "B" symptoms are unexplained fever, night sweats, >10% involuntary weight loss, or diarrhea persisting for >2 weeks (5).

The incidence of KS is higher within the first 6 months after ART initiation, and it has been attributed to immune reconstitution inflammatory syndrome (7). In our patient, the diagnosis of KS was also made within 6 months of ART commencement.

The main treatment for AIDS-associated KS is cART. The goal of treatment should be symptom palliation and disease remission (4). For patients with advanced disease (T1 stage), cART combined with either liposomal anthracycline or paclitaxel is indicated (4). For patients with a heavy tumor burden and visceral manifestation, systemic chemotherapy, immunotherapy with interferon-α, and radiotherapy may be used (4).

References

1. Sternbach G, Varon J. Moritz Kaposi: idiopathic pigmented sarcoma of the skin. J Emerg Med. 1995 Sep-Oct;13(5):671–4.

2. Gao SJ, Kingsley L, Hoover DR, Spira TJ, Rinaldo CR, Saah A, et al. Seroconversion to antibodies against Kaposi's sarcoma-associated herpesvirus-related latent nuclear antigens before the development of Kaposi's sarcoma. N Engl J Med. 1996 Jul 25;335(4):233–41.

3. Cathomas G. Kaposi's sarcoma-associated herpesvirus (KSHV)/human herpesvirus 8 (HHV-8) as a tumour virus. Herpes. 2003 Dec;10(3):72–7.

4. Bower M, Collins S, Cottrill C, Cwynarski K, Montoto S, Nelson M, et al; AIDS Malignancy Subcommittee. British HIV Association guidelines for HIV-associated malignancies 2008. HIV Med. 2008 Jul;9(6):336–88.

5. Krown SE, Metroka C, Wernz JC; AIDS Clinical Trials Group Oncology Committee. Kaposi's sarcoma in the acquired immune deficiency syndrome: a proposal for uniform evaluation, response, and staging criteria. J Clin Oncol. 1989 Sep;7(9):1201–7.

6. Schneider JW, Dittmer DP. Diagnosis and treatment of Kaposi sarcoma. Am J Clin Dermatol. 2017 Aug;18(4):529–39.

7. Yanik EL, Napravnik S, Cole SR, Achenbach CJ, Gopal S, Olshan A, et al. Incidence and timing of cancer in HIV-infected individuals following initiation of combination antiretroviral therapy. Clin Infect Dis. 2013 Sep;57(5):756–64. Epub 2013 Jun 4.

Transplant Headaches

20

Eugene M. Tan, MD, Jasmine R. Marcelin, MD, and Stacey A. Rizza, MD

Case Presentation

A 72-year-old man with a history of type 1 diabetes mellitus underwent pancreas-alone transplant 13 years before his current presentation. His immunosuppression regimen at the time of admission consisted of prednisone, mycophenolate mofetil, and tacrolimus. He was admitted with headache, altered mentation, and fever, but computed tomography of his head showed normal findings. Cerebrospinal fluid (CSF) analysis showed an opening pressure of 31.5 mm Hg, a total nucleated cell count of 297 cells/mcL (46% polymorphonuclear cells), glucose level of 38 mg/dL, and protein level of 93 mg/dL. CSF cryptococcal antigen was positive, with a titer greater than 1:2,560; a concomitant serum cryptococcal antigen titer was 1:640. CSF cultures yielded *Cryptococcus neoformans*; blood and urine cultures were negative. He received induction treatment with liposomal amphotericin B and flucytosine for 2 weeks and had marked improvement. He then received consolidation treatment with fluconazole (800 mg daily) after hospital discharge.

One week after hospital discharge, the patient was readmitted with increasing fatigue, nausea, bilateral lower extremity swelling, tremors, and acute kidney injury. Laboratory evaluation showed a creatinine level of 3.3 mg/dL (last measurement was 2.0 mg/dL). His serum tacrolimus level was markedly elevated at 28.1 ng/mL (reference range, 5-15 ng/mL). He received a diagnosis of tacrolimus toxicity, and the drug was withheld. His renal function improved, and he was discharged after tacrolimus dosing was adjusted.

Discussion

Cryptococcal infections account for approximately 8% of all invasive fungal infections in solid-organ transplant recipients and typically occur 16 to 21 months after transplant (1). In addition, up to 62% of all cryptococcal infections in solid-organ transplant recipients affect the central nervous system (CNS) (2). In our patient, infection occurred many years after transplant, highlighting the fact that ongoing immunosuppression is a risk factor for cryptococcal infection, which can occur as a primary infection or reactivation of a latent infection. When infection presents early after transplant (within the first 30 days), the possibility of donor-derived infection must be considered (1). Given our patient's late presentation, we hypothesized that he may have had a recent environmental exposure, such as close contact with birds or bird droppings (3). However, he could not recall such exposure, as is common with most patients.

The diagnosis of cryptococcal infection should be considered for any transplant recipient who presents with altered sensorium and fever because the overall mortality rate is reported to be as high as 50% in a series of 28 solid-organ transplant recipients with cryptococcal meningitis; prompt initiation of antifungal treatment is imperative (3). CSF should be analyzed for any transplant recipients who present with a non-CNS cryptococcal infection, particularly if they have positive blood cultures, serum antigen titers greater than 1:64, late-onset disease, or altered sensorium, because any of these signs are predictors of CNS involvement (2). It is imperative to know whether the CNS is involved for diagnostic purposes and to guide treatment (eg, need for polyene antifungals, intracranial pressure monitoring) (2). Analysis should include opening pressure measurement, cryptococcal antigen testing, cell count with differential, and glucose and protein levels.

Initial treatment for invasive cryptococcal infection should consist of a lipid formulation of amphotericin B and flucytosine for at least 2 weeks. Lipid formulations of amphotericin B have been associated with better outcomes and reduced toxicity compared with the deoxycholate formulation (2). This treatment regimen is followed by a consolidation phase with high-dose fluconazole for 8 weeks and then maintenance therapy with lower doses of fluconazole for 6 to 12 months or possibly longer (1, 4). Immunosuppressive drugs should be minimized, if possible, without risking organ rejection. Intracranial pressure monitoring in the early phase of therapy is of utmost importance, with prompt external drainage, if needed (4). Risk factors associated with higher mortality rates during cryptococcal infection include altered mentation, absence of headache, liver failure, CSF showing a high opening pressure, low glucose levels, fewer than 20 leukocytes/mcL, and high antigen titers (3, 5).

Immune reconstitution inflammatory syndrome should be considered for those patients who initially respond to therapy but subsequently present with worsening symptoms that mimic the initial presentation. This syndrome may be precipitated by withdrawal of immunosuppressive medications in conjunction with antifungal treatment, typically after 4 to 6 weeks (1, 6). Antifungal therapy should not be discontinued. Corticosteroids have been used in those with severe symptoms.

Drug interactions should always be considered before initiating therapy with fluconazole, particularly for patients receiving calcineurin or mTOR inhibitors. Azole antifungals inhibit the metabolism of mTOR inhibitors, resulting in elevated levels that may lead to renal failure, cardiac arrhythmias, and CNS toxicity. Hence, dose reduction should be considered when fluconazole is initiated, with careful monitoring of drug serum levels (7).

References

1. Baddley JW, Forrest GN; AST Infectious Diseases Community of Practice. Cryptococcosis in solid organ transplantation. Am J Transplant. 2013 Mar;13 Suppl 4: 242-9.
2. Osawa R, Alexander BD, Lortholary O, Dromer F, Forrest GN, Lyon GM, et al. Identifying predictors of central nervous system disease in solid organ transplant recipients with cryptococcosis. Transplantation. 2010 Jan 15;89(1):69-74.
3. Wu G, Vilchez RA, Eidelman B, Fung J, Kormos R, Kusne S. Cryptococcal meningitis: an analysis among 5,521 consecutive organ transplant recipients. Transpl Infect Dis. 2002 Dec;4(4):183-8.
4. Bennett JE, Dolin R, Blaser MJ, editors. Mandell, Douglas, and Bennett's principles and practice of infectious diseases. 9th ed. Philadelphia (PA): Elsevier; c2020. 3839 p.
5. Diamond RD, Bennett JE. Prognostic factors in cryptococcal meningitis: a study in 111 cases. Ann Intern Med. 1974 Feb;80(2):176-81.
6. Singh N, Perfect JR. Immune reconstitution syndrome associated with opportunistic mycoses. Lancet Infect Dis. 2007 Jun;7(6):395-401.
7. Trofe-Clark J, Lemonovich TL; AST Infectious Diseases Community of Practice. Interactions between anti-infective agents and immunosuppressants in solid organ transplantation. Am J Transplant. 2013 Mar;13 Suppl 4: 318-26.

Neurologic Lesions Acquired Abroad

21

Caroline Ball, MD, and Kelly A. Cawcutt, MD

Case Presentation

A 34-year-old woman presented to a local hospital with a 2-month history of cough, left-sided headache, and left arm numbness. Originally from Ghana, she had a history of peripartum cardiomyopathy. She was prescribed an unknown antibiotic for a presumed bacterial upper respiratory tract infection. The following day, she had bilateral cranial nerve VII palsies and was admitted to the hospital for evaluation. She was switched to doxycycline for presumed Lyme disease. However, the Lyme serology was negative and doxycycline was discontinued. She became progressively fatigued, and marked hypercalcemia was observed (serum calcium, >14 mg/dL; parathyroid hormone, <6 pg/mL; parathyroid hormone–related peptide, 0.6 pmol/L) that was resistant to intravenous (IV) fluids. Lumbar puncture and cerebrospinal fluid (CSF) analysis showed a glucose level of 42 mg/dL, protein level of 118 mg/dL, and white blood cell count of 44/mcL (66% lymphocytes). The CSF cytology report noted "atypical cytology." The CSF was negative for venereal disease research laboratory (VDRL), Lyme disease by enzyme-linked immunosorbent assay, *Cryptococcus*, herpes simplex virus (HSV) 1 and 2, and varicella-zoster virus. Blood and CSF cultures were negative. A chest radiograph and computed tomographic image of the chest were unremarkable. Magnetic resonance imaging (MRI) of the brain showed multiple enhancing lesions. Given her hypercalcemia, demographic characteristics, and enhancing lesions on MRI, she had a presumed diagnosis of neurosarcoidosis, and treatment

with high-dose IV corticosteroids was initiated (1 g methylprednisolone, daily for 5 days). A subsequent prednisone taper was planned, beginning at 60 mg (oral) daily.

Three days after initiation of corticosteroids, a vesicular rash developed across her buttocks. A culture was positive for HSV-2, and she began treatment with acyclovir and was dismissed from the hospital. Despite the acyclovir, a secondary, unique, maculopapular rash developed across her lower extremities. The lower extremity rash caused a constant burning sensation and was exquisitely painful to palpation.

She was subsequently admitted to a tertiary referral center and underwent evaluation by the infectious diseases, dermatology, and rheumatology services. Initial laboratory studies at her second admission showed hypercalcemia (10.2 mg/dL) and a low level of angiotensin-converting enzyme (6 U/L).

Her lower extremity rash was biopsied. Although biopsy results were not immediately available, the preliminary results were not suggestive of HSV or sarcoidosis. Acyclovir was discontinued because of concern that her rash was an acyclovir-based drug eruption.

The patient continued to have pain and progression of her lower extremity rash. The prednisone taper for neurosarcoidosis continued in the setting of concurrent hypercalcemia. One month after initiating corticosteroids, a repeat MRI showed that the prior hyperintensities had increased in size and new punctate hyperintensities were visible. A repeat lumbar puncture showed a glucose level of 41 mg/dL, protein level of 154 mg/dL, total nucleated cell count of 17/mcL (predominantly lymphocytes), and negative cytology, including flow cytometry.

During her hospitalization, her cranial nerve VII palsies improved. However, she had progressive anorexia, fatigue, and night sweats. The hypercalcemia persisted and peaked at 15.1 mg/dL, despite IV fluids, calcitonin, and IV bisphosphonate therapy. She continued her prednisone taper. A positron emission tomographic scan was obtained and showed multiple fluorodeoxyglucose-avid lymph nodes. She underwent excisional biopsy of an inguinal lymph node, which showed peripheral T-cell lymphoma.

She prepared to undergo chemotherapy with cyclophosphamide, doxorubicin, vincristine, and prednisone, plus high-dose methotrexate. Unfortunately, before initiating chemotherapy, she had cardiac arrest and died despite aggressive attempts at resuscitation. Postmortem antibody screening and confirmation tests for human T-lymphotropic virus (HTLV) 1 and 2 were positive. Discrimination testing indicated infection with HTLV-1.

Discussion

Our patient presented with acute T-cell lymphoma (ATL) caused by HTLV-1. ATL is 1 of 2 clinical disease processes attributed to HTLV-1; the other, HTLV-1–associated myelopathy/tropical spastic paraparesis, is beyond the scope of this discussion.

HTLV-1 is estimated to affect 5 to 20 million individuals worldwide (1). HTLV-1 is endemic in southwestern Japan, the Caribbean, tropical Africa, the Middle East, South America, and Papua New Guinea (2,3). Transmission of HTLV-1 occurs through sexual intercourse (most commonly from men to women), from mother to child (predominantly through breastfeeding), and through blood transfusions. Most carriers are asymptomatic (2). The lifetime risk of developing ATL for carriers of HTLV-1 is 3% to 5%.

Viral, epigenetic, and genetic factors contribute to an HTLV-1–infected individual's risk of developing ATL (3). There is no evidence that supports screening asymptomatic carriers of HTLV-1 for ATL (2).

Four clinical subtypes of ATL are defined by the Japan Clinical Oncology Group, although the subtypes are generally categorized as *aggressive* or *indolent* ATL (4). Symptoms of all subtypes are diverse and can include generalized lymphadenopathy, skin lesions, hepatosplenomegaly, leukocytosis with abnormal lymphocytes, hypercalcemia, and frequent opportunistic infections.

Treatment is determined on the basis of the ATL category. Several treatment protocols have been described for aggressive ATL, including chemotherapy, antiretroviral therapy, and hematopoietic stem cell transplant (2, 4). Aggressive ATL has a poor prognosis, regardless of the treatment modality used. Indolent ATL is treated with interferon α and zidovudine if the patient is symptomatic, whereas watchful waiting is appropriate if the patient is asymptomatic. Skin lesions can be treated with locally directed therapy. Hypercalcemia in ATL, such as that observed with our patient, should be treated with hydration, IV bisphosphonates, calcitonin, and glucocorticoids, and it should be treated as an oncologic emergency (2).

References

1. Marano G, Vaglio S, Pupella S, Facco G, Catalano L, Piccinini V, et al. Human T-lymphotropic virus and transfusion safety: does one size fit all? Transfusion. 2016 Jan;56(1):249–60. Epub 2015 Sep 21.
2. Ishitsuka K, Tamura K. Human T-cell leukaemia virus type I and adult T-cell leukaemia-lymphoma. Lancet Oncol. 2014 Oct;15(11):e517–26.
3. Tsukasaki K, Tobinai K. Human T-cell lymphotropic virus type I-associated adult T-cell leukemia-lymphoma: new directions in clinical research. Clin Cancer Res. 2014 Oct 15;20(20):5217–25.
4. Katsuya H, Yamanaka T, Ishitsuka K, Utsunomiya A, Sasaki H, Hanada S, et al. Prognostic index for acute- and lymphoma-type adult T-cell leukemia/lymphoma. J Clin Oncol. 2012 May 10;30(14):1635–40. Epub 2012 Apr 2.

Fifty-Year-Old Man With Diabetes Mellitus and Sinusitis

Douglas W. Challener, MD, Jasmine R. Marcelin, MD,
and Jennifer A. Whitaker, MD

Case Presentation

A 50-year-old man with uncontrolled type 2 diabetes mellitus and severe persistent asthma requiring frequent systemic corticosteroids presented to the emergency department (ED) with sinus pressure, a headache, swelling of his left cheek, and diarrhea for 3 days. A computed tomographic scan of the sinuses showed mucosal thickening of the bilateral frontal and sphenoid sinuses. Soft tissue stranding was noted in the retromaxillary fat pad, extending inferiorly into the buccal space and masticator space. Mild proptosis with skin thickening over the globe also was observed. An otolaryngologist who performed nasopharyngoscopy in the ED had no concerns about invasive fungal disease.

The patient was admitted to the hospital for management of diabetic ketoacidosis (DKA), sinusitis, and preseptal cellulitis. The DKA resolved, but he had worsening facial pain and swelling, despite initiation of intravenous (IV) ampicillin-sulbactam (3 g every 6 hours). The patient underwent a second otolaryngologic examination. Eschars in the sinuses were discovered, and histopathologic examination of surgical specimens showed wide, aseptate, hyaline hyphae with evidence of angioinvasion, consistent with fungi in the order Mucorales. Fungal cultures eventually grew *Rhizopus* species. The patient required repeat surgical débridement and was initially treated with IV liposomal amphotericin B. However, an acute kidney injury developed, and he subsequently was transitioned to oral posaconazole, which

was continued after discharge. He received counseling on risk factor modification, including improved asthma control (as a means of avoiding systemic glucocorticoids) and optimizing glycemic control. He did well in the following year, without relapse of infection, before he was lost to follow-up.

Discussion

The first case of infection due to Mucorales fungi was reported in 1885. Infections with Mucorales were previously termed *zygomycosis*, but in the contemporary literature, the term *mucormycosis* is preferred (on the basis of molecular studies). Mucorales are wide (6-16 μm), aseptate, and wide-branching (right-angle branching) pathogens; genera within the Mucorales order include *Mucor*, *Rhizopus*, *Rhizomucor*, *Absidia*, *Cunninghamella*, and *Saksenaea*. *Rhizopus* fungi cause approximately half of human infections by Mucorales, with most of the remaining caused by *Mucor* species (1). The hallmark of these diseases is angioinvasion, often resulting in vessel thrombosis and tissue necrosis. Although mucormycosis can cause severe illness, it is relatively rare, with about 500 cases occurring in the United States each year (2).

These fungi are ubiquitous in the environment, but they are typically more likely to be pathogenic in patients with certain risk factors (1). The typical patient with mucormycosis has uncontrolled diabetes mellitus and often is in

DKA. Mucorales fungi require iron-enriched environments for growth and replication, and higher serum iron levels increase the risk of infection. Some researchers have theorized that at the low blood pH observed in DKA, iron-binding proteins in the blood can denature and increase serum iron levels (3). Likewise, patients with iron-overload disorders have increased risk of infection. Interestingly, patients using iron chelators, such as deferoxamine, also have greater risk of infection. For these patients, the chelator acts as a siderophore for the Mucorales fungi, effectively providing a microenvironment of heavily concentrated iron (1). Other high-risk groups are immunosuppressed patients, patients with hematologic malignancies, and injection drug users.

The most common mechanism of exposure is inhalation. The fungi can also enter the host through breaks in the skin or through ingestion. The most common clinical syndrome, especially for patients with DKA, is a rhinocerebral infection, which presents as facial and eye pain and facial numbness (1). The disease may progress to conjunctival suffusion, blurred vision, periorbital soft tissue edema, and eventual spread into the orbit, with dysfunction of the extraocular muscles and proptosis. Invasive sinusitis is present most often with an invasion of the paranasal sinuses. Palate eschars are sometimes present. If the skull base is eventually involved, cranial nerve palsies can result.

Mucorales infections also cause several other less common clinical syndromes. Lung imaging can show a localized infiltrate with pulmonary infection. Infection can also mimic a pulmonary embolism with angioinvasion and resultant hemoptysis. Agricultural workers who have inhaled the fungi may present with an allergic hypersensitivity pneumonitis, without invasive disease. Gastrointestinal infection is associated with a high risk of death; these infections most commonly occur in immunocompromised patients and present as abdominal pain or gastrointestinal bleeding. Cutaneous infections are most common in patients with an underlying skin condition and are often located at sites of cutaneous trauma. They can range from simple erythema to necrotizing fasciitis. Disseminated disease can cause scattered tissue infarctions due to angioinvasion and, ultimately, multisystem organ failure (1).

Diagnosis of mucormycosis relies on histopathologic identification of the characteristic angioinvasion and fungi with silver stain. It can be difficult to differentiate Mucorales from other hyaline septated molds (*Fusarium*, *Scedosporium*) on the basis of morphology alone. Advanced laboratory techniques such as immunohistochemistry or polymerase chain reaction are important for diagnosis (4). Tissue samples in suspected cases require careful processing. If mucormycosis is a concern, the microbiology laboratory should be asked to prepare the sample in a way that does not disrupt the fungal structure. Tissue cultures are also often used to identify fungal growth, but blood cultures are not useful for diagnosis. Advanced imaging modalities help determine the extent of disease. For example, magnetic resonance imaging of the head with gadolinium contrast is often performed to define the scope of rhinocerebral disease.

Treatment of mucormycosis requires surgical resection and antifungal pharmacologic therapy. The approach to treatment varies slightly, depending on the location of the infection. Patients with rhinocerebral disease need an urgent otolaryngology consultation for surgical débridement. Pulmonary infection may also require surgical evaluation and resection, particularly if it is limited to 1 lobe and the patient has massive hemoptysis. Pharmacologic treatment consists of IV liposomal amphotericin B for longer than 6 weeks. Oral posaconazole is also effective, but echinocandins, fluconazole, and voriconazole are not. Case reports have indicated that hyperbaric oxygen therapy may be a useful adjunct therapy. Cutaneous infection also requires surgery with resection to healthy tissue. Immunocompetent patients with cutaneous infections do not necessarily require systemic antifungal therapy because topical natamycin or ketoconazole often is sufficient. For all patients with mucormycosis, risk factor reduction is necessary to resolve the infection and prevent recurrence (5).

References

1. Farmakiotis D, Kontoyiannis DP. Mucormycoses. Infect Dis Clin North Am. 2016 Mar;30(1):143–63.

2. Chayakulkeeree M, Ghannoum MA, Perfect JR. Zygomycosis: the re-emerging fungal infection. Eur J Clin Microbiol Infect Dis. 2006 Apr;25(4):215–29.

3. Ibrahim AS, Spellberg B, Walsh TJ, Kontoyiannis DP. Pathogenesis of mucormycosis. Clin Infect Dis. 2012 Feb;54 Suppl 1:S16–22.

4. Guarner J, Brandt ME. Histopathologic diagnosis of fungal infections in the 21st century. Clin Microbiol Rev. 2011 Apr;24(2):247–80.

5. Spellberg B, Edwards J Jr, Ibrahim A. Novel perspectives on mucormycosis: pathophysiology, presentation, and management. Clin Microbiol Rev. 2005 Jul;18(3):556–69.

John C. O'Horo, MD, and Mark J. Enzler, MD

Case Presentation

A 19-year-old man from Nairobi, Kenya, presented to the clinic in 2009 with a chief concern of lower extremity swelling, with his left leg being much bigger than his right. Six years earlier, he had experienced left-sided tinea pedis, which resolved after treatment with a topical antifungal agent. When the swelling first occurred several years earlier, he locally received a diagnosis of psoriatic arthritis, but his condition did not improve after treatment with methotrexate. He moved to the United States in 2008. Now, the edema in his left calf had markedly progressed and evolved to include arthralgias and nail dystrophy. He had been seen at another institution and had undergone serologic evaluation for several parasites, including *Wuchereria bancrofti*; however, all the tests showed negative results. He had no history of intravenous drug use, transfusions, sexual activity, or exposure to persons with similar symptoms.

The patient presented to our clinic for further evaluation. He had massive lower extremity edema, with the left leg larger than the right, and patchy purplish skin discoloration (Figure 23.1). He also indicated that he had intermittent scrotal swelling and nocturnal itching. He had no chyluria, and the physical examination showed no hydrocele.

Filarial blood smears, performed at midday and in the evening, were negative, as were filarial immunoglobulin (Ig) G and IgE serologic studies. Ultrasonography of his scrotum and legs did not show live parasites. Histopathology of shave and punch biopsies of the skin from the left leg showed spindle-shaped tumor cells pushing through collagen, consistent with sarcoma (Figure 23.2).

In situ hybridization identified human herpesvirus 8 (HHV-8) (Figure 23.3), leading to a diagnosis of endemic (African) Kaposi sarcoma (KS). An HIV test was negative, but his CD4 count was depressed (113 cells/mcL). He started therapy with trimethoprim-sulfamethoxazole for *Pneumocystis jirovecii* prophylaxis.

The patient underwent a fludeoxyglucose (FDG)–positron emission tomographic scan, which showed multiple FDG-avid nodes in the iliac, femoral, axillary, and pericardial regions,

Figure 23.1 Patient's Left Leg With Lymphedema and Overlying Skin Changes

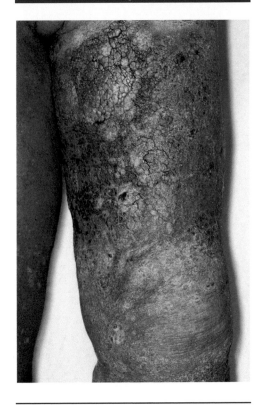

Figure 23.2   Skin Punch Biopsy Specimen

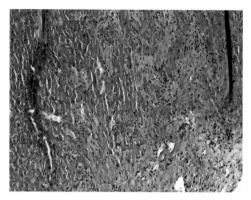

A histopathologic slide shows proliferation of spindle-shaped tumor cells pushing through the collagen (hematoxylin-eosin, original magnification ×20).

which were thought to be due to KS. He returned to his referring facility to start chemotherapy with liposomal doxorubicin. Unfortunately, he had a poor response to chemotherapy, with leukopenia, thrombocytopenia, and anemia, and he had a clinically significant tumor burden after 6 cycles of treatment. A repeat biopsy showed plasmablastic lymphoma. His disease was believed to be too advanced for treatment, and the patient ultimately died.

Figure 23.3   Skin Punch Biopsy Specimen

In situ hybridization is positive for human herpesvirus 8.

Discussion

At first glance, this patient's case appeared to be consistent with lymphatic filariasis (LF). The marked lower extremity lymphedema observed in a patient from a country where the disease is endemic raised clinical suspicion for that diagnosis, as did the intermittent scrotal swelling and nocturnal itching. However, several features argued against this diagnosis and provided a reason to dig deeper.

First, although this patient was from Kenya, central Nairobi is not an endemic area for lymphatic or Bancroftian filariasis. Even in LF-endemic areas, repeat exposure to a large number of filarial parasites is needed to cause the massive lower extremity lymphedema that was seen in this patient, which is why LF more commonly affects older adults. Second, the skin changes overlying the patient's lymphedema were not typical of LF. Third, the absence of hydrocele and chyluria, although not diagnostic, also did not support the LF diagnosis. Fourth, the patient's negative filarial blood smears and serologies argued against an LF diagnosis (1).

KS is broadly differentiated into 4 types: 1) epidemic (HIV related), 2) immunocompromised (iatrogenic immunosuppression related), 3) classic (most commonly affecting middle-aged Mediterranean men), and 4) endemic. Endemic KS is common in Africa and accounts for 2% to 10% of all pediatric cancers and 25% to 50% of soft tissue sarcomas in children. Males are more commonly affected than females overall, but women and children have a higher incidence of endemic KS, rather than classic or epidemic KS. The typical presentation of endemic KS is chronic lymphedema primarily affecting the feet and legs, and the skin changes seen with our patient are common.

The geographic distribution of endemic KS closely corresponds to volcanic regions. Volcanic silicates may be absorbed through the feet and can cause lymphedema, independent of infection. Persons with lymphedema in these areas often have evidence of silicates in lymphatic vessels and lymph nodes. Some have theorized that the lymphedema results in local cell-mediated immunosuppression and makes the host more susceptible to circulating HHV-8 infection. HHV-8–associated sarcoma, in turn, can worsen the lymphedema and immune function, allowing for more viral and tumor replication and proliferation (2).

Endemic KS is not associated with HIV, and it follows a different disease course than epidemic (HIV-associated) KS. Patients with endemic (African) KS have a median survival of months to years, whereas patients with epidemic KS have a poorer median survival of weeks to months (3). In epidemic KS, the main treatment is antiretroviral therapy targeting HIV and immune reconstitution. Sarcoma-directed chemotherapy, while used, is typically not effective. In contrast, endemic KS is chemosensitive, and several different therapeutic options are available. Antiviral therapy directed at HHV-8 has been tested, but it has not shown a consistent benefit and currently is not part of established treatment guidelines (4). Local radiotherapy and surgery can be used to treat limited disease. HHV-8 has been implicated in other cancers, including plasmablastic lymphoma in patients with HIV (5); however, for our patient, we do not know whether the lymphoma was HHV-8 related because HHV-8 in situ hybridization of lymph nodes was not performed.

References

1. Bennett JE, Dolin R, Blaser MJ, editors. Mandell, Douglas, and Bennett's principles and practice of infectious diseases. 9th ed. Philadelphia (PA): Elsevier; c2020. 3839 p.
2. Ziegler JL. Endemic Kaposi's sarcoma in Africa and local volcanic soils. Lancet. 1993 Nov 27;342(8883):1348–51.
3. Haffner SM. Coronary heart disease in patients with diabetes. N Engl J Med. 2000 Apr 6;342(14):1040–2.
4. Stein ME, Lachter J, Spencer D, Bezwoda WR. Chemotherapy for AIDS-related and endemic African Kaposi's sarcoma in southern Africa. Int J Dermatol. 1995 Oct;34(10):7–32.
5. Cioc AM, Allen C, Kalmar JR, Suster S, Baiocchi R, Nuovo GJ. Oral plasmablastic lymphomas in AIDS patients are associated with human herpesvirus 8. Am J Surg Pathol. 2004 Jan;28(1):41–6.

The Other Coinfection

Eugene M. Tan, MD, Jasmine R. Marcelin, MD, and Stacey A. Rizza, MD

24

Case Presentation

A 51-year-old man, an immigrant from South Sudan, presented to his primary care provider with recurrent, right-sided, upper-quadrant abdominal pain that was associated with meals and suggestive of biliary colic. His body mass index was approximately 25, and he denied alcohol use. An abdominal ultrasound showed a 3-mm gallbladder polyp but no signs of cholelithiasis or parenchymal liver disease. However, he had thrombocytopenia (49,000 platelets/mcL). Laboratory tests showed the following: alkaline phosphatase, 144 U/L; aspartate transaminase, 54 U/L; alanine transaminase, 32 U/L; total bilirubin, 1.5 mg/dL; and albumin, 3.0 g/dL.

The patient underwent a laparoscopic cholecystectomy because of concern for cholecystitis, but the cholangiogram showed normal findings intraoperatively. Postoperatively, he had persistent bleeding at the incision sites, and an evaluation for coagulopathy showed low fibrinogen levels (166 mg/dL [reference range, 200–375 mg/dL]). His hemoglobin level decreased from 11.9 g/dL preoperatively to 9.2 g/dL postoperatively. His international normalized ratio was 1.6, and he received fresh frozen plasma and vitamin K. Hemostasis was achieved with compressive dressings, blood transfusions, and albumin infusions.

Computed tomography of the abdomen showed moderate hemoperitoneum, blood in the abdominal wall musculature, splenomegaly, and a cirrhotic-appearing liver, which was the likely cause of his coagulopathy. He was generally somnolent and received a diagnosis of hepatic encephalopathy, which was treated with lactulose and rifaximin. Upper endoscopy showed large esophageal varices, which were banded.

To further evaluate the cause of his cirrhosis, hepatitis B virus (HBV) serology testing was performed, and total antibody tests were positive for HB core (HBc), HB envelope (HBe), and HB surface (HBs). HBc immunoglobulin (Ig) M, HBs antigen (HBsAg), and HBe antigen tests were negative, consistent with a resolved HBV infection. Given his prior residence in Africa, he was tested for hepatitis D virus (HDV) total antibodies, with positive results. HDV RNA testing could not be performed during his hospitalization, but 3 months later, tests for HDV RNA and HBV DNA were negative. Other tests were unrevealing with respect to the cause of cirrhosis; results were negative for anti–hepatitis A IgM, hepatitis C and E serologies, anti–smooth muscle antibodies, antimitochondrial antibodies, and α₁-antitrypsin. His ferritin level was normal, ruling out hemochromatosis.

The patient recovered quickly, and he was not treated with any antiviral medications. At a 1-year follow-up evaluation, his cirrhosis and hepatic encephalopathy were well controlled with lactulose and nadolol. Ultrasonographic screening for hepatocellular carcinoma was negative.

Discussion

Originally discovered in Italy in 1977, HDV is the smallest RNA virus (1,679 nucleotides) that infects humans. HDV infection is endemic in northeast and southeast Asia (genotypes 1, 2, and

4), the Amazon basin (genotypes 1 and 3), central Africa (genotypes 5-8), eastern Europe (genotype 1), and the Middle East (genotype 1). HDV is most often transmitted sexually or parenterally. Uncommonly, HDV can be transmitted perinatally or via blood transfusion or hemodialysis.

HDV has the same 3 envelope proteins as HBV, and HDV can replicate only in individuals who also have an active HBV infection (1,2). Patients may have an acute HBV and HDV coinfection from concurrent transmission, or they may have HDV superinfection of a chronic HBV infection. Of the 350 million chronic carriers of HBV worldwide in 2011, more than 15 million had antibodies against HDV (2). HBV vaccination has decreased the overall prevalence of HDV, but rates of HDV infection can still be as high as 70% for carriers of HBsAg in parts of Africa, Asia, and South America (2).

While HBV and HDV coinfection can present as a mild, self-limited infection, it may progress to fulminant hepatitis or cirrhosis in 20% of patients. Laboratory evaluations show 1) high HDV RNA levels; 2) positive test results for anti-HDV IgM, which later converts to anti-HDV IgG; and 3) positive test results for anti-HBc IgM (1). HBsAg levels should be positive for HDV to be infective. However, HBV DNA levels usually are below the assay's threshold of detection because HDV can suppress HBV replication (2).

Patients with an HDV superinfection of a chronic HBV infection can present with acute hepatitis or exacerbation of an existing liver disease. Laboratory tests can distinguish between acute HBV-HDV coinfection, acute HDV superinfection, and chronic HDV infection (Table 24.1). In HDV superinfection, test results may be positive for HDV antibodies, negative for anti-HBc IgM, and positive for anti-HBc IgG. Other laboratory test results that may suggest chronic HBV infection include positivity for HBsAg, HBe antigen, HBV DNA, and anti-HBs and anti-HBe antibodies (1). Acute HDV viremia can increase alanine transaminase levels and suppress HBV (2). In 90% of superinfections, progression to chronic HDV infection can occur (1), with HDV RNA levels decreasing as HBV resumes replication (2). Seventy percent of such patients can have cirrhosis developing within 5 to 10 years. The incidence of cirrhosis is 3 times higher for patients with HDV superinfection of a chronic HBV infection compared with patients with HBV monoinfection (1).

To diagnose HDV infection, all patients with positive test results for HBsAg should undergo testing for anti-HDV IgG or total antibodies. Our patient had a negative result for HBsAg, but he underwent HDV IgG testing because the cause of his cirrhosis was unclear. For patients with positive results for anti-HDV IgG or total antibody tests, further testing for HDV RNA, HDV antigen, or anti-HDV IgM is recommended, depending on the tests that are accessible in local laboratories. HDV RNA levels should be obtained by using real-time polymerase chain reaction, which is more sensitive than HDV IgM (2). HDV antigen is only transiently detectable in serum (1), but serum HDV RNA should typically be detectable until the patient responds to treatment. If HDV RNA is detected, a biopsy should be performed to assess the severity of liver disease. Although HDV genotyping is available only in major academic centers, it may be helpful because genotype 1 may be associated with a higher risk of cirrhosis (2). HDV may be associated with a 3-fold increased risk of hepatocellular carcinoma (1). Screening for hepatitis C virus and HIV should also be performed (2).

Treatment goals include suppressing replication of HDV and HBV, which can be shown by a sustained virologic response for HDV, 6 months after treatment and HBsAg clearance. Monotherapy with lamivudine, ribavirin, famciclovir, adefovir, or entecavir have shown little efficacy against HDV, and treatment decisions primarily should be focused on HBV. To tailor antimicrobial activity against HDV, an HBV treatment regimen could include weekly standard or pegylated interferon-alfa for 12 to 18 months (3). Fifty percent of patients who achieve a sustained virologic response at 6 months after treatment may still have detectable HDV RNA levels during the next 4 years of follow-up (4). Therefore, patients should ideally be monitored

Table 24.1.	Diagnosis of Hepatitis D Virus Infection in Different Clinical Settings		
Diagnostic Markers	Acute HBV/HDV Coinfection	Acute HDV Superinfection	Chronic HDV Infection
HBsAg	Positive	Positive	Positive
Anti-HBc, IgM	Positive	Negative	Negative
Serum HDAg (by EIA/RIA)	Early and short-lived, frequently missed	Early and transient, frequently missed	Not detectable
Serum HDV RNA (by RT-PCR)	Early and transient but lasts longer than HDAg	Early and persistent	Positive
Anti-HDV, total	Late, low titer	Rapidly increasing titers	High titers
Anti-HDV, IgM	Transient, may be the only marker	Rapidly increasing and persistent titers	Variable titers, usually high
Liver HDAg	Not indicated	Positive	Usually positive, may be negative in late stages

Abbreviations: Anti-HBc, hepatitis B core antigen; Anti-HDV, antibody to hepatitis D virus; EIA, enzyme immunoassay; HBsAg, hepatits B surface antigen; HBV, hepatitis B virus; HDAg, hepatitis D virus antigen; HDV, hepatitis D virus; IgM, immunoglobulin M; RIA, radioimmunoassay; RT-PCR, reverse transcription polymerase chain reaction.

From Diagnosis of hepatitis D virus infection. UpToDate [cited 2020 Sep 9]. Available from: https://www.uptodate.com/contents/diagnosis-of-hepatitis-d-virus-infection?search=diagnosis%20of%20hepatitis%20d%20virus%20infection%20in%20different%20clinical%20settings&source=search_result&selectedTitle=1~150&usage_type=default&display_rank=1; used with permission.

for several years. Patients who are also positive for HBV DNA should have an HBV polymerase inhibitor (eg, adefovir, tenofovir) as the mainstay of their treatment regimen (3).

Our patient's presentation is atypical because his laboratory test results (positive for total HBc antibody, negative for HBc IgM, positive for HDV total antibody, negative for HDV RNA) did not suggest acute HBV-HDV coinfection or HDV superinfection of a chronic HBV infection. HDV RNA, HDV antigen, and anti-HDV IgM tests were not performed during his hospitalization, but 3 months later, a follow-up test for HDV RNA was negative. We note that serum tests for HDV RNA are positive within a few weeks of infection, and positivity may be transient (5), which may explain his negative results at the 3-month follow-up evaluation. If HDV RNA levels were elevated during his hospitalization, that finding would be consistent with HDV superinfection. The patient denied any history of alcohol use, and his body mass index was approximately 25, so nonalcoholic fatty liver disease was less likely. An extensive autoimmune serology panel also was negative.

Cryptogenic cirrhosis may be the best description of his disease. Regardless of the exact cause, the patient has done well since his hospitalization, and after 1 year of follow-up, a screening test for hepatocellular carcinoma was negative.

References

1. Noureddin M, Gish R. Hepatitis delta: epidemiology, diagnosis and management 36 years after discovery. Curr Gastroenterol Rep. 2014 Jan;16(1):365.
2. Hughes SA, Wedemeyer H, Harrison PM. Hepatitis delta virus. Lancet. 2011 Jul 2;378(9785):73–85. Epub 2011 Apr 20.
3. Heidrich B, Manns MP, Wedemeyer H. Treatment options for hepatitis delta virus infection. Curr Infect Dis Rep. 2013 Feb;15(1):31–8.
4. Heidrich B, Yurdaydın C, Kabacam G, Zachou K, Bremer B, Dalekos GN, et al. Long-term follow-up after PEG-IFNa2a-based therapy of chronic hepatitis delta. [Oral Presentation 46]. J Hepatol. 2013 Apr;58(Suppl 1):S20.
5. Negro F. Hepatitis D virus coinfection and superinfection. Cold Spring Harb Perspect Med. 2014 Nov 3;4(11):a021550.

An Earache Too Far

25

Zerelda Esquer-Garrigos, MD, Jasmine R. Marcelin, MD, Alfonso Hernandez-Acosta, and Priya Sampathkumar, MD

Case Presentation

A 62-year-old woman with a history of uncontrolled type 2 diabetes mellitus had an episode of acute otitis media that was managed on an outpatient basis with amoxicillin (500 mg, oral, twice daily). Five days later, she presented to the emergency department with a fever, headache, and confusion. The initial evaluation showed that she was febrile (37.9°C) and tachycardic (heart rate, 115 beats/min). Nuchal rigidity was noted during the physical examination. An otoscopic examination showed erythema in the ear canal and purulence behind the tympanic membrane. A computed tomographic scan of the head showed no intracranial abnormalities. Two sets of peripheral blood cultures were obtained. Cerebrospinal fluid (CSF) analysis showed a glucose level of 10 mg/dL, a protein level of 130 mg/dL, and a white blood cell count of 1.5×10^9/L with 95% polymorphonuclear leukocytes. Gram-positive, lancet-shaped diplococci were observed in the CSF.

Bacterial meningitis was suspected, and the patient began receiving intravenous (IV) vancomycin (20 mg/kg, every 8-12 hours) plus ceftriaxone (2 g, every 12 hours). Because the patient also had a possible Streptococcus pneumoniae infection, she received dexamethasone (0.15 mg/kg, every 6 hours) with the first dose of antimicrobials plus rifampin (600 mg IV, once daily). On hospital day 3, the patient underwent myringotomy and tympanostomy tube placement for source control.

Tests for S pneumoniae antigen were positive in the CSF and urine, and a CSF culture also identified this microorganism. Susceptibility tests on the S pneumoniae isolate showed a minimum inhibitory concentration to penicillin of <1.0 but >0.12 mcg/mL. Ceftriaxone therapy was continued and vancomycin and rifampin were

withdrawn. She received antimicrobial therapy for 2 weeks from the date of source control.

A review of immunization records showed that she had received the pneumococcal polysaccharide vaccine (PPSV23) in 2008. She received a dose of the pneumococcal conjugate vaccine (PCV13) during her hospitalization, and a second dose of PPSV23 was scheduled to be administered 8 weeks later.

Discussion

Despite the development of effective systemic antibiotic therapy, bacterial meningitis continues to be a significant cause of morbidity and mortality in the United States (1). Numerous studies of different populations report that S pneumoniae is the species most commonly involved in bacterial meningitis cases (2,3). The prevalence of S pneumoniae in bacterial meningitis can range from 50% to 70%, and incidence rates increase with age (1,3). In recent years, pneumococcal vaccination has decreased the incidence of meningitis cases caused by the serotypes included in the vaccine (4).

For many years, the main therapy for pneumococcal meningitis was penicillin and other β-lactams such as cephalosporins. However, recent studies in the United States suggest that treatment with third-generation cephalosporins (eg, ceftriaxone, cefotaxime) can lead to clinical failure in 2% to 3% of cases because of emerging antibiotic resistance (5). Thus, the current recommendation is to treat suspected pneumococcal meningitis with vancomycin plus a third-generation cephalosporin until susceptibilities are determined.

Adjuvant corticosteroid therapy has been recommended for patients with suspected bacterial meningitis (6). Corticosteroids decrease inflammatory cytokines present in the CSF, and cytokines are thought to be implicated in the overall inflammatory response in meningitis (7). Adjunct therapy with dexamethasone, administered before or concomitant with the first dose of antimicrobial therapy, is associated with a decrease in overall mortality and the incidence of neurologic sequelae (8).

Although no clinical trials have assessed the use of rifampin in bacterial meningitis, guidelines from the Infectious Diseases Society of America suggest that rifampin may be indicated if the patient is concomitantly receiving dexamethasone and vancomycin. Additionally, it may be indicated if the infectious organism is susceptible to ceftriaxone, with a minimum inhibitory concentration >2 mg/mL (6).

References

1. Thigpen MC, Whitney CG, Messonnier NE, Zell ER, Lynfield R, Hadler JL, et al; Emerging Infections Programs Network. Bacterial meningitis in the United States, 1998–2007. N Engl J Med. 2011 May 26;364(21): 2016–25.

2. Durand ML, Calderwood SB, Weber DJ, Miller SI, Southwick FS, Caviness VS Jr, et al. Acute bacterial meningitis in adults: a review of 493 episodes. N Engl J Med. 1993 Jan 7;328(1):21–8.

3. Schuchat A, Robinson K, Wenger JD, Harrison LH, Farley M, Reingold AL, et al. Bacterial meningitis in the United States in 1995: Active Surveillance Team. N Engl J Med. 1997 Oct 2;337(14):970–6.

4. Whitney CG, Farley MM, Hadler J, Harrison LH, Bennett NM, Lynfield R, et al; Active Bacterial Core Surveillance of the Emerging Infections Program Network. Decline in invasive pneumococcal disease after the introduction of protein-polysaccharide conjugate vaccine. N Engl J Med. 2003 May 1;348(18):1737–46.

5. Weinstein MP, Klugman KP, Jones RN. Rationale for revised penicillin susceptibility breakpoints versus *Streptococcus pneumoniae*: coping with antimicrobial susceptibility in an era of resistance. Clin Infect Dis. 2009 Jun 1;48(11):1596–600.

6. Tunkel AR, Hartman BJ, Kaplan SL, Kaufman BA, Roos KL, Scheld WM, et al. Practice guidelines for the management of bacterial meningitis. Clin Infect Dis. 2004 Nov 1;39(9):1267–84. Epub 2004 Oct 6.

7. Scheld WM, Dacey RG, Winn HR, Welsh JE, Jane JA, Sande MA. Cerebrospinal fluid outflow resistance in rabbits with experimental meningitis: alterations with penicillin and methylprednisolone. J Clin Invest. 1980 Aug;66(2):243–53.

8. de Gans J, van de Beek D; European Dexamethasone in Adulthood Bacterial Meningitis Study Investigators. Dexamethasone in adults with bacterial meningitis. N Engl J Med. 2002 Nov 14;347(20):1549–56.

Not So Good **26**

Douglas W. Challener, MD, and Jasmine R. Marcelin, MD

Case Presentation

A 66-year-old man presented after a syncopal event. An anterior mediastinal tumor was identified, and pathologic findings from a tumor biopsy were consistent with T-cell lymphoblastic lymphoma. The lymphoma did not respond to 4 cycles of hyper-CVAD (cyclophosphamide, vincristine, doxorubicin, and dexamethasone). Another mediastinal biopsy after the chemotherapy was instead consistent with thymoma. Ultimately, the patient underwent thymectomy and did well with few complications, except for left hemidiaphragmatic paralysis.

Several years after the thymectomy, he began to have recurrent episodes of pneumonia, which led to 9 hospitalizations within 1 year. With each hospitalization, he was diagnosed with community-acquired pneumonia and treated with oral levofloxacin, after which he would show improvement and be dismissed from the hospital. However, shortly after completing each antibiotic treatment course, he would again become ill and require rehospitalization.

Most recently, the patient was hospitalized with a *Pseudomonas aeruginosa* bloodstream infection and pneumonia due to *Stenotrophomonas maltophilia*. During this hospitalization, additional immunologic testing showed a CD4$^+$ count of 14 cells/mcL (reference range, 365-1,437 cells/mcL), immunoglobulin (Ig) G of 11 mg/dL (reference range, 767-1,590 mg/dL), IgM of less than 5 mg/dL (reference range, 37-286 mg/dL), and IgA of 8 mg/dL (reference range, 61-356 mg/dL). He received a diagnosis of Good syndrome (GS). He recovered in the hospital with courses of meropenem and trimethoprim-sulfamethoxazole (TMP-SMX). He received 2 doses of intravenous immunoglobulin in the hospital and was ultimately dismissed with prescriptions for TMP-SMX for pneumocystis prophylaxis, azithromycin for *Mycobacterium avium* complex prophylaxis, and acyclovir for herpes simplex virus prophylaxis. He now presents for discussion of further prophylaxis and treatment.

Discussion

GS is a rare primary immunodeficiency that was first recognized by Dr Robert Good in 1954. Most simply, GS is a hypogammaglobulinemia associated with the presence of a thymoma, and approximately 10% of patients with an acquired hypogammaglobulinemia will have a thymoma (often the spindle-cell type). Patients with GS often are adults who present with recurrent upper respiratory tract infections and anterior mediastinal masses. The syndrome is most common in Europe, although few data suggest greater risk for any particular racial or ethnic population. In the United States, the incidence rate is 0.15 cases per 100,000 persons. GS affects men and women equally and typically presents in the sixth decade of life, much later than the age at presentation for other primary immunodeficiencies (1).

GS has no formal diagnostic criteria (2). The syndrome is defined most commonly as a thymoma plus humoral and cellular immune deficiency. T and B cells are depleted, and patients have recurrent infections caused by encapsulated organisms and opportunistic pathogens. GS can be considered a subset of common variable immunodeficiency, although peripheral B cells are reduced in GS. GS can be regarded as an adult-onset primary immunodeficiency with thymoma, hypogammaglobulinemia, diminished B and T cells, and an inverted CD4+/CD8 + ratio (1,3).

The cause of GS is not known. The lymphopenia and impaired maturation of myeloid and erythroid cells suggest a primary defect in the bone marrow; such a mechanism would be consistent with studies that report an absence of B-cell precursors in bone marrow samples (4). The pathogenesis and presentation of GS are heterogeneous and may vary widely among patients; further studies are needed to establish a common pattern of immunologic abnormalities (5).

The primary clinical manifestations of GS are caused by the immunodeficiency. Occasionally, autoimmune manifestations also are present and usually are observed within 6 years after the first symptoms. Most often, the thymoma diagnosis precedes the immunodeficient state by months to years. In these cases, spindle cells are the most common histologic finding (6).

Patients with GS are susceptible to a wide range of infections. Commonly, they have respiratory tract infections caused by bacterial pathogens such as *Haemophilus influenzae* or *Pseudomonas* species. In contrast to patients with AIDS, patients with GS uncommonly have *Mycobacterium* and *Toxoplasma* species infections (2). More than half the patients with GS have chronic diarrhea. In most cases, the diarrhea occurs without a definite infectious cause and instead is due to villous atrophy (1).

Autoimmune diseases such as myasthenia gravis and pure red cell aplasia are commonly associated with GS. Although patients have hypogammaglobulinemia overall, a considerable proportion of patients will have autoantibodies in their serum. The thymoma in GS may inhibit the thymus's production of self-tolerant T cells. The T lymphocytes may then attack B-cell precursors in the bone marrow, preventing their maturation and ultimately resulting in hypogammaglobulinemia (1).

Treatment of GS consists of thymectomy and immunoglobulin replacement with intravenous immunoglobulin. Immunodeficiency does not resolve after thymectomy. The autoimmune component of the disease may also persist, and immunosuppression is sometimes needed. It is often challenging to determine whether a patient's symptoms are due to an infection or are an autoimmune manifestation of the disease (2).

After diagnosis, patients should be tested for antibodies to toxoplasma and cytomegalovirus. Cytomegalovirus-negative blood should be used for transfusion for those with negative serologic test results. Live vaccines should be avoided. Appropriate immunizations should be provided, including pneumococcal, meningococcal, and *H influenzae* type B vaccinations.

Some have advocated prophylactic treatment with TMP-SMX for patients with GS who have CD4+ counts that are lower than 200 cells/mcL, as is done for patients with AIDS (7). However, TMP-SMX use in this setting is controversial; no studies have specifically addressed this management approach (1).

References

1. Kelesidis T, Yang O. Good's syndrome remains a mystery after 55 years: a systematic review of the scientific evidence. Clin Immunol. 2010 Jun;135(3):347–63. Epub 2010 Feb 10.
2. Kelleher P, Misbah SA. What is Good's syndrome? Immunological abnormalities in patients with thymoma. J Clin Pathol. 2003 Jan;56(1):12–6.
3. Miyakis S, Pefanis A, Passam FH, Christodulakis GR, Roussou PA, Mountokalakis TD. Thymoma with immunodeficiency (Good's syndrome): review of the literature apropos three cases. Scand J Infect Dis. 2006;38(4):314–9.
4. Tarr PE, Sneller MC, Mechanic LJ, Economides A, Eger CM, Strober W, et al. Infections in patients with immunodeficiency with thymoma (Good syndrome): report of 5 cases and review of the literature. Medicine (Baltimore). 2001 Mar;80(2):123–33.
5. Tarr PE, Lucey DR; Infectious Complications of Immunodeficiency with Thymoma (ICIT) Investigators. Good's syndrome: the association of thymoma with immunodeficiency. Clin Infect Dis. 2001 Aug 15;33(4):585–6.
6. Johnson SB, Eng TY, Giaccone G, Thomas CR Jr. Thymoma: update for the new millennium. Oncologist. 2001;6(3):239–46.
7. Multani A, Gomez CA, Montoya JG. Prevention of infectious diseases in patients with Good syndrome. Curr Opin Infect Dis. 2018 Aug;31(4):267–77.

A Little Atypical

27

Prakhar Vijayvargiya, MBBS, Jasmine R. Marcelin, MD,
Zerelda Esquer-Garrigos, MD, and Jennifer A. Whitaker, MD

Case Presentation

A 52-year-old man was admitted to the hospital with left buttock and low back pain. He was a former smoker with a history of HIV infection, osteoarthritis, and chronic back pain. His symptoms were attributed to degenerative joint disease, but the emergency department evaluation showed that he was febrile (temperature of 39.3°C) and required oxygen support to keep saturation above 90%. A chest radiograph showed a patchy consolidative opacity in the right midlung that was not present on a chest radiograph obtained 5 months before the current presentation. He was admitted to the hospital, and the infectious diseases service was consulted.

During an interview, he reported chills but denied fever (before coming to the hospital), and he also did not have chest pain, shortness of breath, or cough. His most recent CD4$^+$ T-cell count was 687 cells/mcL, and his viral load was below the detectable range; his antiretroviral therapy regimen included dolutegravir, abacavir, and lamivudine. Antibiotic therapy with vancomycin, piperacillin-tazobactam, and levofloxacin was started for presumed pneumonia in an immunocompromised patient. Urine tests for *Legionella* and streptococcal antigens were negative, as were bacterial blood cultures.

Further evaluation included a computed tomographic scan of the lungs that showed fairly extensive consolidation in the right lower lobe. Bronchoscopy was performed, and a *Legionella* polymerase chain reaction (PCR) test on the bronchoalveolar lavage was positive. Legionnaires disease (LD) was diagnosed, and antibiotics were de-escalated to levofloxacin monotherapy. Levofloxacin subsequently induced transaminitis, and his antibiotic therapy was changed to azithromycin. He completed 21 days of therapy and had a full clinical and radiographic recovery.

Discussion

LD is caused by an intracellular gram-negative bacillus of the genus *Legionella*. *Legionella pneumophila* is the species most associated with human infection. *Legionella* thrives in aquatic ecosystems, where it establishes a symbiotic relationship with free-living amoebae. This symbiotic relationship allows the bacteria to survive inside pulmonary macrophages.

Human infection occurs via inhalation of infectious aerosols. The major risk factors are exposure to warm water reservoirs such as cooling towers, whirlpool spas, water fountains, and air conditioning systems. Clinical syndromes resulting from *Legionella* infection include LD and Pontiac fever (Table 27.1).

Fever with pulse-temperature dissociation, diarrhea, nonproductive cough, and confusion can indicate LD, but these symptoms are not specific enough to allow differentiation from community-acquired pneumonia. Laboratory tests that are used to diagnose LD include *Legionella* urine antigen, sputum culture, PCR, and serology. The preferred method for diagnosis is to perform both a urine antigen test and a sputum culture (4). *Legionella* PCR assays can be performed, when available. Sensitivity of the *Legionella* urine antigen test ranges from 70% to 90% (4).

Table 27.1 Comparison of Legionnaires Disease and Pontiac Fever		
Disease Characteristic	Legionnaires Disease	Pontiac Fever
Clinical syndrome	Pneumonia	Flu-like illness
Pathogenesis	Replication of organism	Inflammatory response to endotoxin
Symptoms	Fever, rigors, dyspnea, cough, headache, diarrhea, confusion	Fever, headache, myalgia, asthenia
Incubation period	2-10 d (1)	23-92 h (2)
Epidemiology	Sporadic or epidemic	Epidemic
Outcome	Mortality rate is 10%-15% (3)	Self-resolves in <1 wk Hospitalization is uncommon

It is most sensitive for detecting *L pneumophila* serogroup 1. For immunocompromised patients and those with nosocomial LD, other *Legionella* species and serogroups are more likely to cause LD; therefore, the *Legionella* urine antigen test has lower sensitivity in these patient groups.

Sputum cultures require special growth media (buffered charcoal yeast extract), and the culture turnaround time is 3 to 7 days (4). Cultures are not sensitive for patients with mild disease but are very sensitive for those with severe, untreated disease. Neither bronchoscopy nor lung biopsy is required for a good culture yield, assuming a good-quality sputum specimen. Sputum cultures may be positive, despite the presence of epithelial cells and lack of leukocytes (4).

A *Legionella* PCR test can increase the diagnostic yield; however, it is not approved by the US Food and Drug Administration, and *Legionella* PCR testing may not be readily available at all centers. Not all patients with LD have seroconversion; therefore, antibody assays are neither sensitive nor specific. Other nonspecific laboratory clues include hyponatremia, hypophosphatemia, elevated transaminases, hyperbilirubinemia, myoglobinuria (a urine dipstick test is positive for blood, but with microscopy, the urine is negative for red blood cells), and elevated lactate dehydrogenase.

Levofloxacin and azithromycin are the antibiotics that are most active against LD. Tetracycline, other fluoroquinolones, and macrolides also can be used because these agents have intracellular bacteriocidal activity against *L pneumophila*. Therapy should begin with parenteral antibiotics, which can be changed to oral antibiotics as soon as clinical improvement is apparent. Addition of rifampin is not recommended because it has been associated with worse outcomes.

The usual antibiotic course lasts for 7 to 10 days, with up to 21 days of therapy recommended for immunocompromised patients. In 1 study, 500 mg of levofloxacin, administered orally for 7 to 14 days, was shown to be as effective as 750 mg of levofloxacin, administered orally for 5 days (5). Combination therapy with azithromycin and a fluoroquinolone is recommended only for severe cases. Most patients respond promptly to therapy, and symptom improvement is seen in 12 to 24 hours.

The proportion of LD in hospitalized cases of community-acquired pneumonia ranges from 2% to 15%. Population-based studies do not suggest any seasonal pattern. However, more cases are reported in the summer, likely because of increased testing.

LD is noncontagious and person-to-person transmission does not occur (1). Patient isolation is not necessary. However, every nosocomial outbreak of LD needs extensive investigation to identify the potential source and to prevent further spread.

References

1. Fraser DW, Tsai TR, Orenstein W, Parkin WE, Beecham HJ, Sharrar RG, et al. Legionnaires' disease: description of an epidemic of pneumonia. N Engl J Med. 1977 Dec 1;297(22):1189–97.

2. Luttichau HR, Vinther C, Uldum SA, Moller J, Faber M, Jensen JS. An outbreak of Pontiac fever among children following use of a whirlpool. Clin Infect Dis. 1998 Jun;26(6):1374–8.

3. Benin AL, Benson RF, Besser RE. Trends in Legionnaires disease, 1980-1998: declining mortality and new patterns of diagnosis. Clin Infect Dis. 2002 Nov 1;35(9):1039–46.

4. Murdoch DR. Diagnosis of Legionella infection. Clin Infect Dis. 2003 Jan 1;36(1):64–9.

5. Yu VL, Greenberg RN, Zadeikis N, Stout JE, Khashab MM, Olson WH, et al. Levofloxacin efficacy in the treatment of community-acquired legionellosis. Chest. 2004 Jun;125(6):2135–9.

The Initial Diagnosis Was Cholecystitis

28

Poornima Ramanan, MD

Case Presentation

A 64-year-old woman from Wisconsin presented with a 1-week history of fever, malaise, loss of appetite, and abdominal pain and was hospitalized with a presumptive diagnosis of acute cholecystitis. Around the time of symptom onset, the patient had noticed a painful lesion on the dorsal aspect of her left hand, which she attributed to an insect bite, and a painful swelling near the medial aspect of her left elbow. Her medical history was significant for severe rheumatoid arthritis, which was treated with adalimumab (40 mg, subcutaneous, every 2 weeks), hydroxychloroquine (200 mg, oral, twice daily), and prednisone (5 mg, oral, once daily). One week before symptom onset, the patient had been horseback riding and had camped overnight by the Mississippi River, where she was exposed to ticks and fleas. She had an indoor cat but did not have any recent cat scratches or bites. She denied any recent travel outside Wisconsin.

During the physical examination, the patient was not in acute distress, had stable vital signs, and was afebrile. The dorsal aspect of the left hand had a tender, nonpurulent, ulcerative lesion with central black eschar, surrounded by erythema (Figure 28.1). A tender, firm, mobile, left olecranon lymphadenopathy was also palpable. Fullness was noted in the left axillary region. The rest of the examination was unremarkable.

Laboratory data also were unremarkable, except for mild hepatic transaminitis (alanine aminotransferase, 69 U/L; aspartate aminotransferase, 61 U/L). Computed tomography of the chest showed numerous bilateral indeterminate pulmonary and pleural nodules and a lobulated, 3.9-cm mass in the left supraclavicular-infraclavicular space and left axilla (Figure 28.2).

Ultrasonographically guided aspiration of the left axillary mass yielded 6 mL of purulent material that showed many polymorphonuclear cells but no organisms with Gram stain. The fungal and

Figure 28.1 Erythematous, Nonpurulent, Ulcerative Lesion With Central Black Eschar on the Dorsal Aspect of the Patient's Left Hand

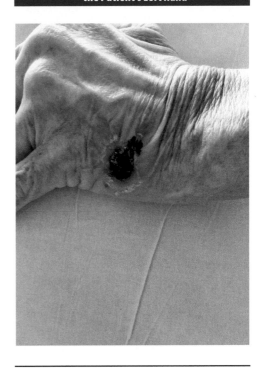

Figure 28.2   Computed Tomographic Image of the Chest With Intravenous Contrast

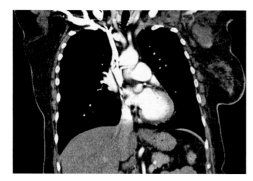

The image shows numerous bilateral indeterminate pulmonary and pleural nodules and a lobulated mass (measuring approximately 3.0×3.9 cm) in the left axilla and infraclavicular space.

acid-fast smears were negative. After 24 hours of culture, poor filmy growth was noted on chocolate and blood agar, but eosin methylene blue agar showed no growth. Gram stain of the culture isolate showed tiny, gram-negative coccobacilli that appeared like "grains of sand." The organism was oxidase negative and catalase positive. The axillary abscess specimen and culture isolate were sent to the Wisconsin Department of Health. Blood cultures remained negative. The state laboratory identified the organism as *Francisella tularensis* by using a *Francisella* polymerase chain reaction assay directly on the abscess specimen and by using matrix-assisted laser desorption/ionization–time of flight mass spectrometry (MALDI-TOF MS) to analyze the culture isolate.

A diagnosis of ulceroglandular and pneumonic tularemia was made. The patient showed clinical improvement after receiving 2 weeks of intravenous gentamicin and levofloxacin, followed by several weeks of oral ciprofloxacin and doxycycline. The microbiology laboratory received early notification of a clinical suspicion of tularemia, which helped the laboratory technicians avoid further exposure to this infectious organism.

Discussion

Tularemia is a rare but potentially fatal zoonotic infection that is most often caused by *F tularensis*, a fastidious, aerobic, gram-negative coccobacillus. The organism was first isolated in 1911 from ground squirrels in Tulare County, California, during an outbreak of plague-like illness in rodents (1). This facultative intracellular pathogen evades the host immune response by surviving in host macrophages (2). Tularemia has been reported from many countries in the Northern hemisphere and from 49 US states (all except Hawaii) (1-3). Most US cases are reported in Missouri, Arkansas, Oklahoma, Massachusetts, South Dakota, and Kansas (3).

The major reservoirs of *F tularensis* are various terrestrial and aquatic small mammals such as rabbits, hares, ground squirrels, muskrats, and water rats. In the United States, ticks and biting flies are the major vectors of transmission, whereas mosquitoes are additional vectors in Europe (1). The most common modes of transmission include arthropod bites, direct contact with infected animal tissue through hunting or butchering, ingestion of contaminated water or meat, inhalation of aerosols containing bacteria, or being bitten by animals (eg, cats) that recently ingested an infected small mammal (1). Occupations with high risk of acquiring tularemia include microbiology laboratory technicians, landscapers, veterinarians, hunters, and meat handlers. *F tularensis* is a bioterrorism tier 1 select agent because of its low infectious dose (as low as 10 bacteria), potential for airborne transmission, difficulty in making a rapid diagnosis, and history of being developed as a bioweapon (3).

The incubation period for tularemia is usually short (3-5 days) (1). In humans, *F tularensis* causes 6 distinct clinical syndromes that are dictated by its mode of transmission: ulceroglandular, glandular, oculoglandular, typhoidal, oropharyngeal, and pneumonic tularemia (2,3). Among these, ulceroglandular tularemia is the most common clinical presentation; it is characterized by fever, a single cutaneous ulcer with central eschar at the site of percutaneous inoculation (usually by arthropod bite), and tender regional lymphadenopathy. The differential diagnosis of ulceroglandular tularemia usually includes cat scratch disease, bubonic plague, mycobacterial infections, sporotrichosis, rat bite fever, and toxoplasmosis.

Complications include lymph node suppuration, hematogenous spread to other organs, secondary pneumonia, and sepsis. Oculoglandular tularemia occurs after conjunctival contamination and presents as painful, unilateral conjunctivitis with localized lymphadenopathy. Pneumonic tularemia occurs by inhalation of infected aerosols or through hematogenous spread; it may be misdiagnosed as slowly resolving community-acquired pneumonia because most patients respond to quinolones that are used for empiric treatment of community-acquired pneumonia. Oropharyngeal tularemia occurs after ingestion of contaminated meat or water and presents as pharyngitis and tonsillitis, with tender cervical lymphadenopathy. Typhoidal tularemia is a systemic illness presenting with high fever (typhoid-like illness) without localized skin lesions or lymphadenopathy (1,3).

Tularemia is most commonly diagnosed by serologic findings plus appropriate clinical findings and epidemiologic exposure. A 4-fold increase in antibody titers between acute and convalescent sera is essential for confirmation of the diagnosis. False-negative serologic results may be seen in early infection because clinically significant antibody titers are detected only 1 to 2 weeks after symptom onset (1). *F tularensis* has been isolated from cultures of blood, lymph nodes, skin lesions, conjunctiva, and oropharyngeal specimens. Despite its fastidious nature, *F tularensis* often grows aerobically in cysteine-enriched media such as chocolate agar, modified Thayer-Martin medium, and buffered charcoal yeast agar. Poor growth may also be seen from initial plating on blood agar; however, the organism does not grow on routine media used for isolation of gram-negative bacteria. *F tularensis*

should be suspected when a slow-growing, poorly staining, gram-negative coccobacillus is recovered from chocolate agar but shows no growth on eosin methylene blue or MacConkey agar. Reliable identification of the culture isolate may be obtained by MALDI-TOF MS or other molecular methods. *F tularensis* may be directly identified from clinical specimens with nucleic acid amplification tests, direct immunofluorescent antibody assays, and immunohistochemical staining (1). These tests are available only in specialized laboratories.

F tularensis is innately resistant to β-lactam antibiotics (1). Aminoglycosides are bactericidal to *F tularensis* and are the first-line treatments for tularemia in humans. Fluoroquinolones and tetracyclines are alternative agents that are effective against *F tularensis* (1). Routine antimicrobial susceptibility testing is not essential for patient care because acquired antimicrobial resistance has not been reported.

The main strategies for preventing tularemia include protection against arthropod bites, avoiding direct exposure to infected animal meat, and taking adequate safety precautions when working with suspected culture isolates in the microbiology laboratory (2). Standard isolation precautions are used for patients with tularemia because human-to-human transmission has not been documented. However, microbiology laboratory staff should be notified about any patients clinically suspected to have tularemia to avoid potential laboratory exposures and to initiate specific evaluations for the organism (1).

References

1. Maurin M, Gyuranecz M. Tularaemia: clinical aspects in Europe. Lancet Infect Dis. 2016 Jan;16(1):113-24.
2. Ellis J, Oyston PC, Green M, Titball RW. Tularemia. Clin Microbiol Rev. 2002 Oct;15(4):631–46.
3. Centers for Disease Control and Prevention (CDC). Tularemia: United States, 2001-2010. MMWR Morb Mortal Wkly Rep. 2013 Nov 29;62(47):963–6.

Complicated Urinary Tract Infection With a Multidrug- Resistant Organism

29

Prasanna P. Narayanan, PharmD, RPh,
Omar M. Abu Saleh, MBBS, and John C. O'Horo, MD

Case Presentation

An 88-year-old man who recently emigrated from India presented with fever, nausea, and back pain. His medical history was unremarkable, except for hypertension. He recently had a complicated urinary tract infection in the setting of left-sided obstructive uropathy due to a staghorn calculus (Figure 29.1). He was treated with ciprofloxacin at an outside hospital, but after discharge, his urine cultures grew *Klebsiella pneumoniae* (susceptibility pattern shown in Table 29.1).

Upon presentation at our institution, he had fevers up to 39°C and left-sided costovertebral angle tenderness that was elicited with percussion, consistent with pyelonephritis. Findings from a cardiopulmonary examination were unremarkable. The white blood cell count was 17×10^3 cells per high-power field, serum creatinine was 1 mg/dL, and estimated creatinine clearance was calculated to be 37 mL/min. An urgent consultation with a urologist was requested for consideration of nephrostomy tube placement to decompress the left renal collection system.

Because the patient had recently emigrated from India, concern was high for infection with an organism producing New Delhi metallo-β-lactamase (NDM). He began empiric therapy with colistin and tigecycline. The susceptibility profile of the isolate was consistent with a carbapenem-resistant *Enterobacteriaceae* (CRE).

NDM expression was later confirmed by molecular testing of the *K pneumoniae*. The isolate was susceptible to colistin and had intermediate susceptibility to tigecycline. The patient received an 8-day course of colistin after nephrostomy and decompression. His treatment was complicated by acute kidney injury (AKI), which was believed to have multifactorial causes, including colistin

Figure 29.1 Computed Tomographic Image of the Abdomen and Pelvis

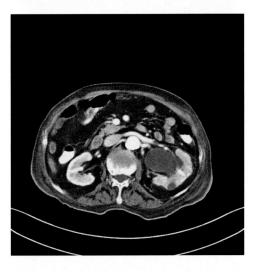

A large obstructing calculus in the mid left ureter was the cause of hydroureteronephrosis and pyelonephritis.

Table 29.1 *Klebsiella pneumoniae* Susceptibility Pattern, Initial Report[a]	
Antimicrobial Agent	**Minimum Inhibitory Concentration, mcg/mL[b]**
Amikacin	≥64
Ampicillin	≥32
Cefazolin	≥64
Cefepime	≥64
Cefoxitin	≥64
Ceftazidime	≥64
Ceftriaxone	≥64
Ciprofloxacin	≥4
Gentamicin	≥16
Levofloxacin	≥8
Meropenem	≥16
Nitrofurantoin	128
Piperacillin-tazobactam	≥128
Tobramycin	≥16
Trimethoprim-sulfamethoxazole	≥320

[a] Additional susceptibility tests were performed with colistin, chloramphenicol, tigecycline, and ceftazidime-avibactam.

[b] Minimum inhibitory concentration values indicate resistance to all antimicrobial agents shown in the table.

administration. Although the colistin dose was adjusted, it was stopped on day 8 after considering the negative findings from blood cultures, the progressive AKI, and the clinical improvement. His AKI eventually resolved upon discontinuation of colistin.

Discussion

The prevalence of antibiotic-resistant, gram-negative bacteria (GNB) has been increasing for the past 2 decades and continues to rise globally. Previously, the predominant mechanisms of GNB resistance included extended-spectrum β-lactamase and AmpC β-lactamase enzymes, decreased influx porin activity and expression, increased efflux pump activity, and alterations in the penicillin-binding proteins produced by many *Enterobacteriaceae* species (1). Although the GNB that produce extended-spectrum β-lactamase and AmpC β-lactamase are resistant to cephalosporins, they generally can be treated effectively with carbapenems. In the early 2000s, CRE emerged as a new public health threat, and CRE are now found in many regions of the United States, particularly the East Coast. The rapid and wide spread of these resistant GNB is likely due to inappropriate use and overuse of antimicrobial agents, transmission through medical tourism, and nontherapeutic use of antibiotics in livestock. The most common types of CRE include those that produce NDM, *K pneumoniae* carbapenemase (KPC), and OXA-48 carbapenemase; these CRE types often are resistant to carbapenems and multiple additional antibiotic classes. Organisms producing OXA-48 are the least prevalent and can be susceptible to cephalosporins, but because they often co-produce extended-spectrum β-lactamase, they may be resistant to all β-lactams (2).

CRE have been identified in inpatient and outpatient settings. Outcomes of these infections are poor, with mortality rates approaching 44% (2). These infections are also associated with markedly increased costs and longer hospitalizations. Carbapenemase-producing bacteria are generally identified through cultures and susceptibility testing. Carbapenemase production may be definitively confirmed with a phenotypic test (eg, modified Hodge test) or polymerase chain reaction (PCR) test to specifically identify genes encoding KPC, NDM, or OXA-48 carbapenemase. The sensitivity of PCR tests ranges from 97% to 100%. However, a limitation of molecular testing is that it will identify only currently recognized carbapenemase genes and may not include all genes involved in carbapenemase production (3).

Current antimicrobial options for CRE infections are limited, which increases the risk of patient mortality. Aminoglycosides, colistin, polymyxin B, and tigecycline are commonly used when in vitro testing shows susceptibility. Combination therapy may be used, although high-quality data about treatment outcomes are lacking.

Because of the limited antibiotic options available and the high expense of newer agents that target GNB, the polymyxin class of antibiotics has reemerged as a therapeutic option for CRE and other drug-resistant GNB. The 2 polymyxins that have been marketed for pharmacologic use are colistin (polymyxin E) and polymyxin B. They have a unique mechanism of action in that they act as "detergents" to destabilize the cell membrane; this destabilization leads to increased permeability and eventual cell lysis. Polymyxin antibiotics, along with tigecycline, maintain their activity against a range of CRE, but as use of these drugs against CRE and other drug-resistant GNB grows, reports of resistance are expected to increase. The mechanism underlying polymyxin resistance is not well understood, but it likely involves loss of the lipopolysaccharide target on the cell membrane. It is important to note that neither polymyxin is intrinsically active against *Proteus*, *Serratia*, *Morganella*, or *Providencia* species (4).

Despite the higher prevalence of colistin use in the past, recent research has indicated that polymyxin B has a more favorable pharmacokinetic profile (5). Administered as a prodrug, colistin subsequently is hydrolyzed to its active form, colistin methanesulfonate. However, for patients with normal renal function, only a small percentage is converted. Even when a loading dose is administered, therapeutic concentrations are not achieved quickly. Most of the active and inactive forms are eliminated renally, and dose adjustments are required for patients with renal dysfunction. Conversely, polymyxin B is administered in its active form and is not cleared through the kidneys; thus, it more reliably achieves prompt and adequate concentrations and does not require renal dose adjustments. A disadvantage to polymyxin B is that it cannot be used to treat urinary tract infections because its concentration in the urine is low (for urinary tract infections, colistin is the preferred polymyxin) (6).

Polymyxin B and colistin potentially can cause neurotoxicity and nephrotoxicity, but both are generally reversible upon discontinuation of the medication. Historically, polymyxin B was believed to be more nephrotoxic than colistin, which resulted in the predominant use of colistin, but the older studies had limitations such as different dosing strategies and formulations, varying definitions of nephrotoxicity, potentially confounding and noncontrolled risk factors, small sample sizes, and supportive care that was drastically different from today's standards. Newer studies with fewer limitations have shown that the risk of nephrotoxicity is either the same or lower with polymyxin B.

Fortunately, newer antibiotics are in development to combat CRE infections. For example, ceftazidime-avibactam is a recently approved β-lactam and β-lactamase inhibitor combination. Avibactam is effective against a wide range of β-lactamases, and when it is combined with ceftazidime, it can treat most CRE infections, except for those caused by NDMs. Uniquely, NDMs are not hydrolyzed by aztreonam. Aztreonam-avibactam is being developed as a new combination drug that is active against NDMs, with the avibactam component serving to inhibit other β-lactamases (7). New additions to the armamentarium include cefiderocol (a siderophore cephalosporin) (8) and the novel cefepime-zidebactam combination (9), both of which seem to have activity against CRE, including NDMs and other metallo-β-lactamase–producing GNBs.

References

1. Ruppe E, Woerther PL, Barbier F. Mechanisms of antimicrobial resistance in gram-negative bacilli. Ann Intensive Care. 2015 Dec;5(1):61. Epub 2015 Aug 12.
2. Vasoo S, Barreto JN, Tosh PK. Emerging issues in gram-negative bacterial resistance: an update for the practicing clinician. Mayo Clin Proc. 2015 Mar;90(3):395-403.
3. Lutgring JD, Limbago BM. The problem of carbapenemase-producing-carbapenem-resistant-*Enterobacteriaceae* detection. J Clin Microbiol. 2016 Mar;54(3):529–34. Epub 2016 Jan 6.
4. Falagas ME, Kasiakou SK. Colistin: the revival of polymyxins for the management of multidrug-resistant gram-negative bacterial infections. Clin Infect Dis. 2005 May 1;40(9):1333–41. Epub 2005 Mar 22. Erratum in: Clin Infect Dis. 2006 Jun 15;42(12):1819. Dosage error in article text.
5. Pogue JM, Ortwine JK, Kaye KS. Clinical considerations for optimal use of the polymyxins: a focus on agent selection and dosing. Clin Microbiol Infect. 2017 Apr;23(4):229–33. Epub 2017 Feb 24.
6. Nation RL, Velkov T, Li J. Colistin and polymyxin B: peas in a pod, or chalk and cheese? Clin Infect Dis. 2014 Jul 1;59(1):88–94. Epub 2014 Apr 3.
7. Doi Y, Paterson DL. Carbapenemase-producing *Enterobacteriaceae*. Semin Respir Crit Care Med. 2015 Feb;36(1):74–84. Epub 2015 Feb 2.
8. Kohira N, West J, Ito A, Ito-Horiyama T, Nakamura R, Sato T, et al. In vitro antimicrobial activity of a siderophore cephalosporin, S-649266, against *Enterobacteriaceae* clinical isolates, including carbapenem-resistant strains. Antimicrob Agents Chemother. 2015 Nov 16;60(2):729–34.
9. Sader HS, Rhomberg PR, Flamm RK, Jones RN, Castanheira M. WCK 5222 (cefepime/zidebactam) antimicrobial activity tested against gram-negative organisms producing clinically relevant β-lactamases. J Antimicrob Chemother. 2017 Jun 1;72(6):1696–703.

Thrombocytopenia

30

Jithma P. Abeykoon, MD, Omar M. Abu Saleh, MBBS, and Candido E. Rivera, MD

Case Presentation

A 71-year-old man with a history of chronic obstructive pulmonary disease (GOLD class II) and hypertension presented with a productive cough and colorless to yellow sputum production. He was feeling well about 11 months before the current presentation but underwent chest radiography for an episodic cough. The radiograph showed an indeterminate cavitated opacity in the left upper lobe. The patient denied fevers, chills, nausea, vomiting, chest pain, shortness of breath, hematemesis, epistaxis, and weight loss (his current weight was 70 kg). A computed tomographic (CT) image of the chest confirmed the cavitating lung mass on the left upper lobe and enabled a CT-guided biopsy. Histologically, the biopsy showed only necrotic material and was negative for malignancies.

The patient then underwent a bronchoscopy with biopsy. Histologic analysis of this biopsy specimen showed nonnecrotizing granulomatous inflammation. Multiple sputum cultures and bronchoalveolar lavage cultures were positive for *Mycobacterium avium* complex (MAC). He began treatment with azithromycin (250 mg, once daily), ethambutol (1,200 mg, once daily), and rifampin (600 mg, once daily) for a planned duration of 12 months after sputum culture conversion.

His long-term medications before the MAC infection included multivitamins, hydrochlorothiazide, fluticasone-salmeterol, tiotropium, and albuterol (inhaled). He had been taking hydrochlorothiazide for years without any known hematologic adverse effects, although this medication can cause thrombocytopenia. His complete blood count at baseline was normal, with a platelet count of $234,000\times10^6$/L. In addition, his liver enzymes, creatinine, and electrolyte levels were within normal limits.

After therapy for MAC was initiated, his platelet count decreased progressively to $61,000\times10^6$/L in a 10-month period, but his hemoglobin level and total white blood cell counts remained normal. A peripheral blood smear showed thrombocytopenia with well-granulated platelets and occasional large or giant forms, suggesting a consumptive process, but findings were equivocal for a specific diagnosis. The rest of his laboratory tests, which included an evaluation of electrolyte levels and liver function, showed results within normal limits. A physical examination did not reveal any rashes, petechiae, purpura, or hepatosplenomegaly.

With his worsening thrombocytopenia that was temporally associated with rifampin exposure, plus the lack of other identifiable causes, rifampin was replaced with rifabutin (azithromycin and ethambutol were continued). No changes were made to any of his long-term medications, including hydrochlorothiazide, given the stability of his platelet count for years before MAC therapy was initiated. Within a month after switching from rifampin to rifabutin, his platelet count improved to $93,000\times10^6$/L. Two months after rifampin discontinuation, his platelet count was $214,000\times10^6$/L and remained stable thereafter.

Discussion

Antimicrobial use, especially long-term use, can be associated with a myriad of adverse effects, including hematologic toxicities such as leukopenia, anemia, and drug-induced thrombocytopenia (DITP). The treating physician should be familiar with these toxicities so that an effective and individualized strategy of monitoring and treatment is implemented appropriately.

DITP is commonly attributed to antimicrobial agents. To determine whether DITP is the cause of thrombocytopenia, the following clinical criteria have been formulated (1):

  a. Drug exposure must precede the onset of thrombocytopenia
  b. The patient should completely recover from the thrombocytopenia and sustain recovery after discontinuing the suspected drug
  c. Other causes of thrombocytopenia must be excluded (including idiopathic thrombocytopenic purpura, thrombotic thrombocytopenic purpura, or bone marrow failure, if consistent clinical features are present)
  d. A drug rechallenge, if deemed safe and necessary, should give the same clinical presentation with thrombocytopenia (this criterion is not required for the diagnosis)

DITP can be either immune mediated or attributable to bone marrow suppression. A recent systematic review (covering reports published from 1940-2012) identified 153 drugs that are believed to have a high probability of causing immune-mediated thrombocytopenia (1). On the basis of clinical and laboratory (in vitro) evidence of DITP, the drugs were categorized into 2 groups, definite or probable. Rifampin had enough in vivo and in vitro evidence to support its categorization as a definite cause of DITP. Other antimicrobial agents in this category are penicillin, ceftriaxone, trimethoprim-sulfamethoxazole, and vancomycin. Non–immune-mediated thrombocytopenia, usually attributable to bone marrow suppression, is another well-described adverse effect of certain antimicrobial agents, including linezolid and valganciclovir.

Rifampin-induced thrombocytopenia was first reported in 1970 (2), and its incidence rate is estimated to be approximately 6% (3). The pathophysiology of rifampin-induced thrombocytopenia is associated with immunoglobulin (Ig) G and IgM antibodies that are directed against surface antigens in platelets (1-3). Rifampin can act like a hapten and can bind with plasma proteins, generating a hapten-molecule complex with specific IgM and IgG antibodies (2,4,5). These antibodies can induce complement fixation on the platelet surface (classic pathway), thus initiating platelet destruction (3,4). In addition to thrombocytopenia, rifampin is also an important cause of drug-induced leukopenia and neutropenia.

The median time to presentation with thrombocytopenia after rifampin exposure is 1 to 2 weeks, but this time can range from several hours to several years, depending on the history of rifampin exposure. The patient described above did not have a history of rifampin exposure and therefore may not have had any preformed antibodies. This possibility is supported by the somewhat long period (10 months) from rifampin initiation to severe thrombocytopenia because the rate of antibody-driven platelet destruction depends on the antibody titer.

The therapy for DITP is discontinuation of the offending agent. For this patient, rifampin was discontinued and replaced with rifabutin, which also is associated with a risk of thrombocytopenia. Although rifampin and rifabutin are in the same drug class, multiple small studies have shown that most patients who could not tolerate rifampin were successfully transitioned to rifabutin. Certain intolerances were more likely to recur after transitioning to rifabutin, including arthralgia, dermatologic concerns, and cholestasis. Other adverse events such as hepatitis and gastrointestinal intolerance recurred less frequently and may partly reflect the different immune-mediated response to rifabutin versus rifampin (5).

DITP in current medical practice largely remains a clinical diagnosis. One exception is heparin-induced thrombocytopenia, for which specific diagnostic tests are available. Although DITP is associated with a high incidence of morbidity and mortality, the possibility of completely reversing it by discontinuing the offending agent indicates that an accurate and timely diagnosis is vital.

References

1. Arnold DM, Kukaswadia S, Nazi I, Esmail A, Dewar L, Smith JW, et al. A systematic evaluation of laboratory testing for drug-induced immune thrombocytopenia. J Thromb Haemost. 2013 Jan;11(1):169–76.
2. Blajchman MA, Lowry RC, Pettit JE, Stradling P. Rifampicin-induced immune thrombocytopenia. Br Med J. 1970 Jul 4;3(5713):24–6.
3. Poole G, Stradling P, Worlledge S. Potentially serious side effects of high-dose twice-weekly rifampicin. Br Med J. 1971 Aug 7;3(5770):343–7.
4. Bansal R, Sharma PK, Sharma A. A case of thrombocytopenia caused by rifampicin and pyrazinamide. Indian J Pharmacol. 2013 Jul-Aug;45(4):405–7.
5. Chien JY, Chien ST, Huang SY, Yu CJ. Safety of rifabutin replacing rifampicin in the treatment of tuberculosis: a single-centre retrospective cohort study. J Antimicrob Chemother. 2014 Mar;69(3):790–6. Epub 2013 Nov 14.

When Transplant Goes Viral: The Perils of Overimmunosuppression

Cybele L. Abad, MD, and Raymund R. Razonable, MD

31

Case Presentation

The patient was a 57-year-old man with end-stage heart disease due to restrictive cardiomyopathy that was caused by prior radiotherapy for Hodgkin lymphoma. He underwent cardiac transplant 2 years before the current hospitalization.

At the time of cardiac transplant, he received induction with antithymocyte globulin and then had maintenance therapy with tacrolimus, mycophenolate mofetil, and prednisone. He had several episodes of acute rejection that were treated with augmented immunosuppression (eg, increased dose of tacrolimus or prednisone). He also had allograft dysfunction due to antibody-mediated rejection and was treated with rituximab and plasmapheresis.

The donor (D) was cytomegalovirus (CMV) seropositive, and the patient (recipient [R]) was CMV seronegative (CMV D⁺/R⁻ mismatch), and the patient therefore had prophylaxis with oral valganciclovir for 6 months. Nine months after transplant, he presented with nausea, vomiting, and diarrhea. Upper endoscopy (esophagogastroduodenoscopy) showed mucosal ulcers, and a biopsy was consistent with primary CMV gastrointestinal disease (Figure 31.1). He started receiving intravenous (IV) ganciclovir and showed improvement in his clinical symptoms. His viral load, which peaked at 3,340,000 IU/mL of plasma, subsequently declined (Figure 31.2) but was always detectable. The persistent CMV viremia (after 3 months of IV ganciclovir) prompted genotypic resistance testing, which showed a *UL97* L595S/L variant. Because his viral load remained low (<5,000 IU/mL of plasma), he had maintenance therapy with IV ganciclovir for another 4 months. Immunologic tests indicated the absence of global and CMV-specific CD8⁺ T-cell function. An attempt at reducing

Figure 31.1 Biopsy Specimen From a Patient With Cytomegalovirus Colitis

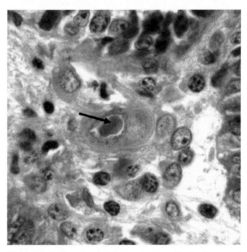

The classic "owl-eye" intranuclear inclusion and intracytoplasmic inclusions are shown. The dense intranuclear inclusion with surrounding halo is formed when the mass of viral particles shrinks away from the nuclear membrane during fixation (hematoxylin-eosin, original magnification ×1,000; oil immersion).

(From Dioverti MV, Razonable RR. Cytomegalovirus. Microbiol Spectr. 2016 Aug;4[4]; used with permission.)

Figure 31.2   Clinical Course and Treatment of a Patient With Cytomegalovirus Disease After Heart Transplant

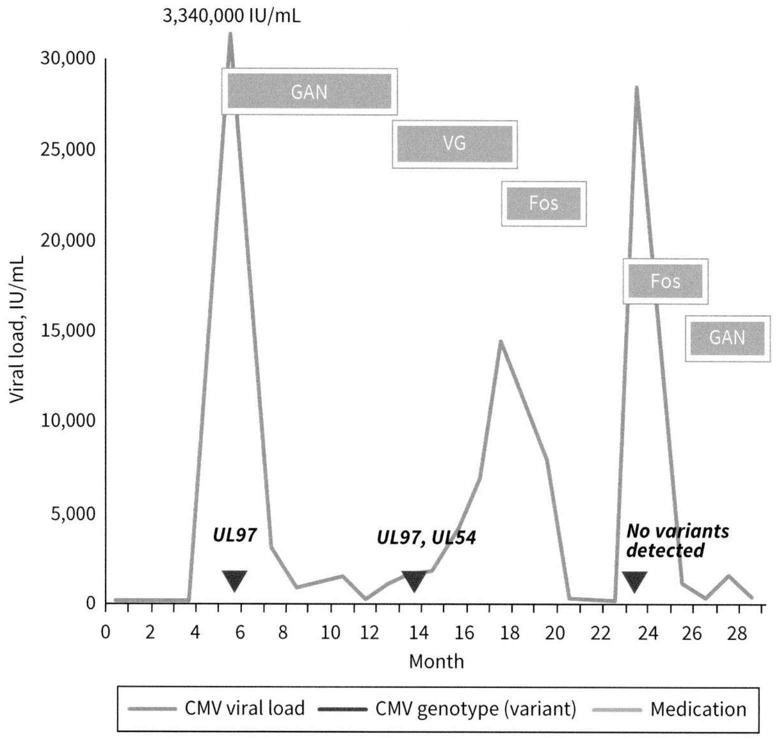

CMV indicates cytomegalovirus; Fos, foscarnet; GAN, ganciclovir; VG, valganciclovir.

the dose of immunosuppressive drugs was complicated by acute rejection. In an effort to relieve him of IV infusions, he was transitioned to oral valganciclovir 7 months later, when his viral load stabilized at 1,000 IU/mL of plasma.

Two weeks after transitioning to valganciclovir, his viral load increased to 14,500 IU/mL, and he had dyspnea, cough, and radiographic findings of pneumonitis. Genotypic testing showed *UL54* P522S, which conferred ganciclovir and cidofovir cross-resistance (Figure 31.2). The patient was hospitalized for initiation of IV foscarnet therapy.

After initiating IV foscarnet, the viral load declined rapidly to undetectable levels. However, he remained without CMV-specific CD8+ T cells. He was also nonresponsive to mitogen, suggesting a high degree of immunosuppression. He later had severe foscarnet-related

adverse effects, including renal failure requiring hemodialysis, severe mucositis, and mucosal ulcerations that impaired oral nutrition, resulting in severe generalized debility and failure to thrive. Foscarnet was discontinued after 2 months. A week later, his viral load increased to 28,300 IU/mL. Foscarnet was restarted, but the patient continued to have progressive adverse effects. After a thorough discussion about the goals of care, and considering his severe debility and failure to thrive, he was transitioned to palliative care.

Discussion

CMV D+/R− status and overimmunosuppression were interrelated factors that predisposed this patient to have CMV disease (1,2). The lack of preexisting cell-mediated and humoral immunity in this CMV D$^+$/R$^-$ solid-organ transplant recipient, coupled with the suppressed ability to mount an immune response because of augmented drug-induced immunosuppression, allowed uncontrolled replication of donor-transmitted CMV that caused severe, tissue-invasive CMV disease.

Antiviral prophylaxis is one of the recommended methods of preventing CMV disease in recipients of solid-organ transplants. The duration of therapy is usually 3 to 6 months, depending on the risk profile, with a longer duration for patients who are CMV D$^+$/R$^-$ and for patients with augmented immunosuppression. Therapy is extended for up to at least 12 months among CMV D$^+$/R$^-$ lung recipients, who have a higher risk of CMV disease compared with kidney, liver, and heart recipients. Despite the efficacy of antiviral prophylaxis in preventing CMV infection and disease during drug administration, about 25% of CMV D$^+$/R$^-$ solid-organ transplant recipients have subsequent development of CMV disease within 3 to 6 months after completing prophylaxis, termed *delayed* or *late-onset primary disease*. Recent literature suggests that individuals who persistently lack CMV-specific T-cell immunity are more likely to have delayed-onset CMV disease; hence, it often affects patients who receive intensified immunosuppression, usually for the treatment of rejection (3), as was seen in our patient.

The standard treatment recommendation for CMV disease is IV ganciclovir; for mild to moderate cases, oral valganciclovir is appropriate. Our patient was considered to have severe disease because of the high CMV viral load; hence, he was treated initially with IV ganciclovir. However, he remained viremic at low levels after prolonged therapy because he was unable to develop any CMV-specific cellular and humoral immunity. The persistent viremia in the setting of prolonged exposure to antiviral drugs, especially at suboptimal systemic drug levels, may lead to selection of drug-resistant viral variants. Indeed,

during the patient's illness, we noted the emergence of *UL97* and, subsequently, *UL54* variants, which limited the antiviral treatment options (4,5). *UL97* encodes the viral kinase that is required for initial phosphorylation of ganciclovir into its active, triphosphorylated form. Hence, sequence variants in the *UL97* gene can keep ganciclovir in its inactive, nonphosphorylated form that is unable to serve as a competitive substrate for the *UL54*-encoded CMV DNA polymerase. CMV DNA polymerase is the target for all 3 available anti-CMV drugs (ie, ganciclovir, foscarnet, and cidofovir), so a variant in the *UL54* gene may lead to cross-resistance among these 3 currently approved anti-CMV drugs.

Foscarnet is the main choice for treating CMV disease due to a *UL97*-variant virus. However, it has a high risk of numerous adverse effects, including nephrotoxicity, hyperkalemia, hypomagnesemia, and other electrolyte imbalances (all of these were experienced by our patient). In addition, mucositis and mucosal ulcerations are other known adverse effects (6); our patient was also affected severely by these issues. Cidofovir is another option for ganciclovir-resistant CMV, but it is associated with considerable renal toxicity. Cross-resistance is more common between ganciclovir and cidofovir, as was observed with this patient. Hence, foscarnet is the recommended regimen when ganciclovir resistance is suspected.

Treatment options for drug-resistant CMV are limited. Novel drugs such as maribavir and letermovir are currently under clinical investigation as possible alternatives because their mechanisms of action are different from that of standard antiviral drugs. Maribavir is in the benzimidazole drug class that directly inhibits *UL97* kinase and prevents encapsidation, whereas letermovir acts as a viral terminase complex inhibitor. Letermovir was recently approved for CMV prophylaxis for recipients of allogeneic hematopoietic stem cell transplants. However, letermovir has not been studied with active CMV disease and thus is not indicated for its treatment. Both novel drugs, if proven effective in therapeutic clinical trials, will be welcome additions to the existing armamentarium for CMV infections.

References

1. Eid AJ, Razonable RR. New developments in the management of cytomegalovirus infection after solid organ transplantation. Drugs. 2010 May 28;70(8):965-81.
2. Manuel O, Pang XL, Humar A, Kumar D, Doucette K, Preiksaitis JK. An assessment of donor-to-recipient transmission patterns of human cytomegalovirus by analysis of viral genomic variants. J Infect Dis. 2009 Jun 1;199(11):1621–8.
3. Kumar D, Chernenko S, Moussa G, Cobos I, Manuel O, Preiksaitis J, et al. Cell-mediated immunity to predict cytomegalovirus disease in high-risk solid organ transplant recipients. Am J Transplant. 2009 May;9(5):1214–22.
4. Limaye AP. Antiviral resistance in cytomegalovirus: an emerging problem in organ transplant recipients. Semin Respir Infect. 2002 Dec;17(4):265–73.
5. Razonable RR, Paya CV. Herpesvirus infections in transplant recipients: current challenges in the clinical management of cytomegalovirus and Epstein-Barr virus infections. Herpes. 2003 Dec;10(3):60–5.
6. Gilquin J, Weiss L, Kazatchkine MD. Genital and oral erosions induced by foscarnet. Lancet. 1990 Feb 3;335(8684):287.

Ulcerative Skin Lesions in a Returned Traveler

32

Madiha Fida, MBBS, Eugene M. Tan, MD, and Mark J. Enzler, MD

Case Presentation

A 69-year-old man with a history of hypertension and gout presented with a 3-month history of ulcerative lesions on the right lower extremity. He had vacationed in the Amazonian region of Ecuador 7 months earlier, and his activities included hiking in areas with volcanic sand, rain forests, and beaches. He did not recall any insect bites. He had received pretravel immunizations, including a vaccine for yellow fever, and took atovaquone-proguanil for malaria prophylaxis. He first noticed 3 tender lesions on the medial aspect of his right thigh, approximately 2 months after his return, which gradually increased in size and then developed central ulcerations (Figure 32.1). He also had myalgias, fatigue, and night sweats. He did not respond to two 10-day courses of oral doxycycline for a possible bacterial skin or soft tissue infection.

With the continued lack of improvement, a skin punch biopsy was performed and showed mixed acute and chronic dermal inflammation and intramonocytic amastigotes, consistent with cutaneous leishmaniasis (CL) (Figure 32.2). A biopsy sample was also sent to the Centers for Disease Control and Prevention (CDC) for culture, and *Leishmania* (*Viannia*) *braziliensis* was detected by culture and speciated by polymerase chain reaction (PCR) and isozyme electrophoresis.

The patient was treated with 6 infusions of liposomal amphotericin B (dose, 3 mg/kg of body weight) during a 2-week period. Although this therapy was briefly interrupted because of an acute kidney injury, he was able to complete the

Figure 32.2 Histopathology of the Skin Biopsy Specimen

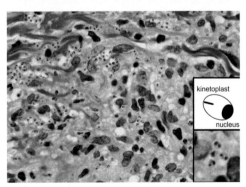

The amastigote form of *Leishmania* species is seen (hematoxylin-eosin; original magnification ×1,000 [inset, ×2,000]). The Jones silver method was used to highlight the kinetoplast.

(Courtesy of B.S. Pritt, MD, Mayo Clinic, Rochester, Minnesota; used with permission.)

Figure 32.1 Noduloulcerative Lesions on the Right Medial Thigh at the Initial Presentation

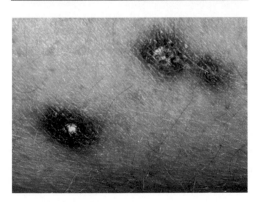

treatment regimen. The skin lesions completely healed within 4 weeks of initiating therapy. The patient had no relapse during 6 months of follow-up after completing treatment.

Discussion

In a study of returning overseas travelers who sought medical care, 8,227 of 42,173 patients (19.5%) presented with dermatologic problems; skin concerns were the third-most common reason to seek care (after travel-related gastrointestinal infections [34.0%] and fever [23.3%]) (1). Of these 8,227 cases, 264 (3.2%) had CL or mucosal leishmaniasis. In a prospective study of patients with travel-related dermatoses, 8 of 269 (3.0%) were CL cases (2).

Leishmaniasis may present as a disseminated infection (visceral) or with single or multiple lesions involving the skin or the oral or nasal mucosa. Leishmaniasis is transmitted by the bite of infected sand flies. The sand fly genus *Phlebotomus* is found in Asia, Africa, the Middle East, and southern Europe (associated with "Old World" CL), whereas the genus *Lutzomyia* is found in Mexico and South and Central America (associated with "New World" CL). In the Old World, CL is caused by *Leishmania aethiopica*, *Leishmania tropica*, and *Leishmania infantum*, whereas in the New World, it is caused by various species, including *Leishmania mexicana*, *Leishmania (Viannia) guyanensis*, *Leishmania (Viannia) panamensis*, and *L (V) braziliensis*. The incubation period of CL varies from weeks to months. Cutaneous lesions initially present as a papule, which ulcerates in 1 to 4 weeks (ulcers are painless and typically have rolled-up edges), followed by healing with atrophic scarring in 6 to 12 months. Certain CL species acquired in Central or South America may later spread to the mucosal surfaces of the nose or mouth.

The diagnosis of CL is made by histopathologic observation of the amastigote form of the parasite, by parasite cultures, or by molecular methods requiring the expertise of specialty laboratories such as the CDC. Histopathologically, typical amastigotes with kinetoplasts can be seen within the macrophages (Figure 32.2). Cultures require special liquid media, and the parasite can take up to 4 weeks to grow. PCR testing has a sensitivity of up to 97% and can be performed on the punch biopsy specimen, skin scrapings, or lesion aspirates (3). PCR can also be used for species identification, with high sensitivity and specificity. Because CL induces a poor antibody response, serology has no role in the diagnosis of CL.

The decision to treat CL is made after considering multiple factors, including the number and location of lesions, the host's immune status, and infection with a species associated with mucocutaneous disease, because for immunocompetent individuals, infection may resolve without treatment (4). The American Society of Tropical Medicine and Hygiene and the Infectious Diseases Society of America have published guidelines intended for American and Canadian practitioners for the management of all forms of leishmaniasis (4). They recommend determining whether the CL is simple or complex from the number, size, and location of lesions, whether the infecting species is prone to mucosal dissemination (eg, *L [V] braziliensis*), and other factors. Therapeutic options for simple CL include local therapies such as cryotherapy, thermotherapy, and photodynamic therapy or topical paromomycin, which is not readily available in North America. Complex CL can be treated with systemic therapies such as oral miltefosine (approved for CL caused by *L [V] braziliensis*, *L [V] guyanensis*, and *L [V] panamensis*) or parenteral agents such as liposomal amphotericin B, pentavalent antimonials (available only from the CDC on an Investigational New Drug protocol), and pentamidine (3).

Preventive strategies include individual protective measures such as minimizing exposed skin, using bed nets, applying insect repellents to bare skin, and wearing permethrin-treated clothing. Education regarding individual protective measures remains an integral part of pre-travel counseling to prevent arthropod-borne diseases. Public health measures for prevention include vector and reservoir control.

References

1. Leder K, Torresi J, Libman MD, Cramer JP, Castelli F, Schlagenhauf P, et al; GeoSentinel Surveillance Network. GeoSentinel surveillance of illness in returned travelers, 2007-2011. Ann Intern Med. 2013 Mar 19;158(6):456–68.
2. Caumes E, Carriere J, Guermonprez G, Bricaire F, Danis M, Gentilini M. Dermatoses associated with travel to tropical countries: a prospective study of the diagnosis and management of 269 patients presenting to a tropical disease unit. Clin Infect Dis. 1995 Mar;20(3):542–8.
3. Boggild AK, Ramos AP, Espinosa D, Valencia BM, Veland N, Miranda-Verastegui C, et al. Clinical and demographic stratification of test performance: a pooled analysis of five laboratory diagnostic methods for American cutaneous leishmaniasis. Am J Trop Med Hyg. 2010 Aug;83(2):345–50.
4. Aronson N, Herwaldt BL, Libman M, Pearson R, Lopez-Velez R, Weina P, et al. Diagnosis and treatment of leishmaniasis: Clinical practice guidelines by the Infectious Diseases Society of America (IDSA) and the American Society of Tropical Medicine and Hygiene (ASTMH). Am J Trop Med Hyg. 2017 Jan 11;96(1):24–45. Epub 2016 Dec 7.

HIV Prevention

33

Saira R. Ajmal, MD, and Mary J. Kasten, MD

Case Presentation

A 56-year-old transgender woman was referred to the HIV clinic for consideration of preexposure prophylaxis (PrEP). She reported coming out as transgender 8 years prior and identified as bisexual. She had 3 adult children from 2 prior marriages to women. She received weekly intramuscular estrogen and daily oral progesterone as hormone replacement therapy to synchronize her sexual characteristics with her gender identity. She was being seen at the Mayo Clinic Transgender and Intersex Specialty Care Clinic (Rochester, Minnesota), with the goals of undergoing surgery for breast augmentation and gender reassignment.

She was interested in learning about and potentially starting PrEP because she engaged in high-risk sexual practices. She stated that she was a sex worker, with 8 to 10 clients per month, most of whom were male truck drivers. She engaged in receptive-oral and receptive-anal sex, with appropriate protection 60% to 70% of the time. She denied a history of any sexually transmitted infections (STIs) and reported testing for STIs at Planned Parenthood every few months. Her medical history included elevated blood pressure, persistent depressive disorder, gender dysphoria, attention-deficit/hyperactivity disorder, and traumatic brain injury. She reported a history of nasal septal perforation, attributable to trauma, that required repairs. She denied use of illicit substances.

The patient had a strong indication for PrEP, given her risk factors. Baseline screening for HIV, gonorrhea, chlamydia, syphilis, and hepatitis C was performed, as was a urinalysis and serum creatinine test. Her vaccinations were updated. The baseline test results were normal, and she began PrEP with tenofovir disoproxil fumarate/emtricitabine (TDF/FTC) at her follow-up visit. A 90-day supply was provided, and a 1-month follow-up visit was scheduled to assess tolerance and to verify stable renal function.

Discussion

Approximately 2 million new HIV infections occur annually worldwide (1). Multiple studies have shown that PrEP with daily TDF/FTC can reduce the risk of HIV infection by more than 90% for patients who are highly adherent (2). PrEP, unlike treatment for prevention, allows individuals at risk of acquiring HIV to have control over decreasing their risk.

Two landmark trials showed the efficacy of PrEP in preventing HIV transmission in men who have sex with men (MSM) and heterosexual men and women. The iPrEx trial enrolled HIV-seronegative men or transgender women who had sex with men and randomized them to receive TDF/FTC or a placebo. TDF/FTC was associated with a 44% reduction in the incidence of HIV (1). In the Partners-PrEP trial, HIV-serodiscordant heterosexual couples were monitored after being randomly assigned to receive TDF/FTC, TDF, or placebo (3). Both active treatments reduced incidence of HIV in heterosexual men and women (TDF/FTC, 75%; TDF, 67%) (3). Of note, 2 trials from Africa (FEM-PrEP and VOICE) that enrolled HIV-negative women did not show a reduction in the acquisition of HIV with TDF or TDF/FTC, but adherence was low (4,5). The iPrEx trial also showed that the protective effect of TDF/FTC increased with higher adherence. Together, these studies highlight the importance of adherence for the efficacy of PrEP.

When considering PrEP, the first step is to determine the risk of HIV acquisition on the basis of sexual risk behaviors during the past 6 months. Higher risk is associated with condomless receptive penile-anal or penile-vaginal sex with nonmonogamous partners, a serodiscordant relationship, sex while using drugs, intravenous drug use, history of STI, or a higher frequency or number of sexual partners. If the patient is considered to have high risk of HIV acquisition, the risk of treatment needs to be evaluated and the patient's HIV-negative status needs to be confirmed. Evaluation should include a baseline HIV test, ideally with a fourth-generation antigen-antibody test; an HIV RNA test should be performed if the patient had signs of viral illness in the past 4 weeks, a screening test with indeterminate results, or a high-risk exposure within 4 weeks of starting PrEP. The baseline assessment also should include a renal function estimate because PrEP should be prescribed only if the estimated glomerular filtration rate (eGFR) is greater than 60 mL/min per 1.73 m^2; TDF/FTC has not been studied in HIV-uninfected patients with an eGFR less than 60 mL/min per 1.73 m^2, and TDF has been associated with nephrotoxicity in patients with HIV. A hepatitis B screen should be performed because of the potential for a hepatitis flare if TDF/FTC is discontinued because they have activity against hepatitis B.

Individuals should be counseled about symptoms of acute HIV infection, condom use, and safe drug use. An initial 1-month follow-up visit should be scheduled to evaluate for any adverse effects, with follow-up appointments every 3 months thereafter, at which patients should be screened for symptoms of HIV, counseled regarding safe sex and drug use, and assessed for adherence and adverse effects of therapy. HIV screening and pregnancy testing (for individuals who can become pregnant) should be performed at each 3-month follow-up visit, and STI screening should be performed every 3 months for the highest-risk patients and those with symptoms suggestive of infection. STI screening

tests can be performed every 6 months for asymptomatic individuals who are not in the highest-risk groups. Individuals with high risk of renal injury (eg, patients with hypertension, diabetes mellitus) should have a urinalysis performed every 3 to 6 months and creatinine levels should be assessed every 3 months. Individuals with average risk of renal injury should have their creatinine levels checked at least every 6 months. The need to continue PrEP should be reassessed at least on an annual basis, and PrEP should be continued for 1 month after the last high-risk exposure.

HIV infection is common among transgender persons; a 2013 meta-analysis of data from 15 countries reported a prevalence of 19.1% (6). No evidence-based prevention interventions are specific to this population. Because of the lack of data about PrEP outcomes for transgender women, an unplanned exploratory analysis of iPrEx trial data was recently performed to compare PrEP outcomes for transgender women and MSM (7). The subset analysis of the transgender population in the iPrEX trial showed that compared with MSM, transgender women generally had less education, more sexual partners, less condom use for receptive-anal intercourse, more STIs, and more substance use, and they more commonly had a history of transactional sex. When serum drug levels were measured, a lower proportion of transgender study participants had protective levels compared with MSM, but the difference was not significant. The analysis showed that MSM were more likely to use PrEP if they engaged in condomless receptive-anal intercourse, whereas transgender women were less likely to use PrEP with the same risk factor. The authors concluded that PrEP is protective in this group if they are adherent (none of the seroconverters had protective drug levels). Individuals with the highest risk of HIV were less likely to have protective drug levels, and TDF levels were lower in those who were receiving hormone therapy, which raised concerns about whether the patients' questions about potential drug interactions were not fully addressed. Prior research in HIV-positive transgender women showed that they prioritized hormone use over other health concerns and were hesitant to start antiretroviral therapy because they feared it would negatively interact with hormone therapy (8).

In conclusion, PrEP is an important health care need for individuals with increased risk of HIV infection. PrEP protects against acquisition of HIV infection when patients are highly adherent, and it appears to be protective for cisgender and transgender individuals. Transgender individuals may face health care disparities attributable to cultural biases and perceived stigma. Data suggest that this population may have concerns that health care providers may not be cognizant of, including the fear of drugs interacting with hormone therapy. Thus, this case emphasizes the importance of provider education and appropriate counseling when seeing patients for PrEP.

References

1. Grant RM, Lama JR, Anderson PL, McMahan V, Liu AY, Vargas L, et al; iPrEx Study Team. Preexposure chemoprophylaxis for HIV prevention in men who have sex with men. N Engl J Med. 2010 Dec 30;363(27):2587–99. Epub 2010 Nov 23.

2. Anderson PL, Glidden DV, Liu A, Buchbinder S, Lama JR, Guanira JV, et al; iPrEx Study Team. Emtricitabine-tenofovir concentrations and pre-exposure prophylaxis efficacy in men who have sex with men. Sci Transl Med. 2012 Sep 12;4(151):151ra125.

3. Baeten JM, Donnell D, Ndase P, Mugo NR, Campbell JD, Wangisi J, et al; Partners PrEP Study Team. Antiretroviral prophylaxis for HIV prevention in heterosexual men and women. N Engl J Med. 2012 Aug 2;367(5):399–410. Epub 2012 Jul 11.

4. Van Damme L, Corneli A, Ahmed K, Agot K, Lombaard J, Kapiga S, et al; FEM-PrEP Study Group. Preexposure prophylaxis for HIV infection among African women. N Engl J Med. 2012 Aug 2;367(5):411–22. Epub 2012 Jul 11.

5. Marrazzo JM, Ramjee G, Richardson BA, Gomez K, Mgodi N, Nair G, et al; VOICE Study Team. Tenofovir-based preexposure prophylaxis for HIV infection among African women. N Engl J Med. 2015 Feb 5;372(6):509–18.

6. Baral SD, Poteat T, Stromdahl S, Wirtz AL, Guadamuz TE, Beyrer C. Worldwide burden of HIV in transgender women: a systematic review and meta-analysis. Lancet Infect Dis. 2013 Mar;13(3):214–22. Epub 2012 Dec 21.

7. Deutsch MB, Glidden DV, Sevelius J, Keatley J, McMahan V, Guanira J, et al; iPrEx investigators. HIV pre-exposure prophylaxis in transgender women: a subgroup analysis of the iPrEx trial. Lancet HIV. 2015 Dec;2(12):e512-9. Epub 2015 Nov 6.

8. Sevelius JM, Patouhas E, Keatley JG, Johnson MO. Barriers and facilitators to engagement and retention in care among transgender women living with human immunodeficiency virus. Ann Behav Med. 2014 Feb;47(1):5–16.

Progressive, Cutaneous Nodules in an Immunocompromised Patient

34

Madiha Fida, MBBS, and Omar M. Abu Saleh, MBBS

Case Presentation

A 57-year-old woman presented with disseminated, painful skin lesions. Her medical history included granulomatosis with polyangiitis, for which she had been taking high-dose corticosteroids (prednisone, 80 mg/d) for about 1 year, and she had diabetes mellitus and Hashimoto disease. The skin lesions had started in the lower extremities about 5 months before her presentation and then spread to her torso, upper limbs, and face. Initially, the skin eruption was thought to have an autoimmune cause, and her immunosuppression therapy was modified to include methotrexate and rituximab. The skin lesions, however, continued to worsen.

A physical examination showed that she had a generalized cutaneous eruption with morphologically varied lesions, including crusted nodular lesions, erythematous macules, papular lesions with areas of ulceration, and violaceous lesions (Figure 34.1).

Laboratory tests included those for serum antineutrophil cytoplasmic antibodies, antinuclear antibodies, HIV, and fungal serologies. Tuberculin skin testing was negative, and a serum QuantiFERON-TB test showed indeterminate results. Chest radiography showed no pulmonary involvement. A skin biopsy was performed and showed gram-positive bacilli within the granulomas that also stained positive for bacilli with the Fite and Grocott-Gomori methenamine silver stains. Supplemental staining with periodic acid–Schiff–diastase was weakly positive (Figure 34.2).

Cultures from the skin biopsy grew *Mycobacterium chelonae* that was susceptible to tobramycin, clarithromycin, and tigecycline and resistant to moxifloxacin, trimethoprim-sulfamethoxazole, imipenem, doxycycline, and ciprofloxacin. She was started on combination therapy with tobramycin, azithromycin, and moxifloxacin, and after 6 weeks, she noted marked

Figure 34.1   Bilateral, Diffuse, Nodular, Ulcerative Skin Lesions

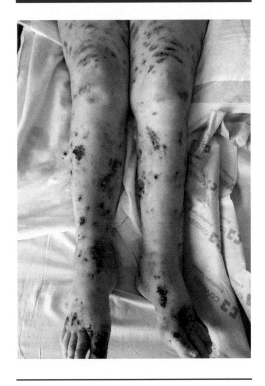

Figure 34.2   Histopathologic Evaluation of a Skin Biopsy Specimen

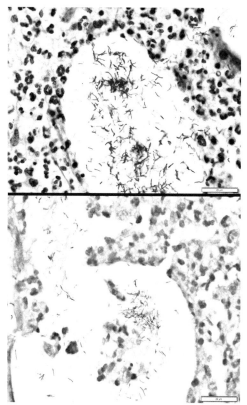

Upper panel, Gram-variable rods were seen in the biopsy specimen (original magnification, ×400). Lower panel, Rods were positive for Fite stain (original magnification, ×400).

improvement in the skin lesions. Moxifloxacin was used, despite in vitro evidence of resistance to ciprofloxacin, because of the possibility of in vivo activity. She was later switched to azithromycin monotherapy, to be continued indefinitely while receiving immunosuppression therapy.

Discussion

Chronic, progressive, subcutaneous nodules that begin on the acral areas of the body should always raise the concern for infection, especially in immunocompromised individuals. Impaired cell-mediated immunity that is attributable to long-term corticosteroid use should raise considerations for cutaneous nontuberculous mycobacteria, *Nocardia* species, and endemic fungal infections (eg, blastomycosis, sporotrichosis) in the appropriate settings. Cutaneous mold infection is more likely in the setting of profound, prolonged neutropenia and a more acute presentation. These pathogens must be included in the clinical considerations because they influence how the microbiology laboratory stains samples and incubates cultures. Routine Gram stain and bacteria cultures should be requested, but the laboratory should also be asked to perform stains and cultures for fungal, *Nocardia*, and mycobacterial organisms, and select pathogens should be specified, if possible. For example, laboratories typically use lower incubation temperatures when *Mycobacterium marinum* or *Mycobacterium haemophilum* are suspected, and growth media is supplemented with hemin when culturing for *M haemophilum*.

M chelonae is one of the rapidly growing nontuberculous mycobacteria (RGM), which is known for its growth in low temperature and hence the skin tropism. It is widely distributed in soil, dust, and water, and it can cause localized and disseminated cutaneous infections, especially in immunocompromised individuals. Other infections caused by *M chelonae* include keratitis associated with contact lens use and ocular surgery (1), catheter-related bloodstream infections, and pulmonary infections. Sporadic outbreaks have been associated with tattoos from parlors that used contaminated ink (2), facial infections after face lifts because of contaminated methylene blue dye, and localized infections from mesotherapy. Risk factors for infection include prolonged corticosteroid use, autoimmune disorders, leukemia, chemotherapy, and organ transplant (3). Cutaneous lesions are typically painful and nodular, and they present most commonly on the lower extremities.

Diagnosis of *M chelonae* infection is made by culturing the organism from the tissue biopsy specimen. *M chelonae* readily grows in Middlebrook and BACTEC culture media, as well as routine bacteriologic media. It typically grows within 7 days and hence is considered an RGM. Biochemical tests, drug susceptibility patterns, and polymerase chain reaction–based restriction fragment length polymorphism analysis can be performed to differentiate *M chelonae* from other RGMs, including *Mycobacterium fortuitum* complex and *Mycobacterium abscessus* complex. *M chelonae* is typically resistant to antituberculous agents, but it is susceptible to numerous other antimicrobial agents, including macrolides, tobramycin, fluoroquinolones, sulfonamides, imipenem, linezolid, and cefoxitin. *M chelonae* does not contain the *erm* gene, which can confer inducible macrolide drug resistance. Therefore, although macrolides are typically active against *M chelonae*, they should never be used as a monotherapy (4).

Treatment generally depends on the location and severity of the infection and the underlying immune status of the patient. Treatment typically is a course of combination therapy with 2 to 4 agents, followed by several months' therapy with 1 to 2 agents. For patients with limited cutaneous involvement, the recommended treatment is oral therapy with 2 agents, for a minimum of 4 months. For patients with more extensive disease (eg, severe skin and soft tissue involvement, disseminated infections), intravenous therapy plus oral therapy for 2 to 8 weeks is recommended, followed by oral therapy alone for 6 to 12 months. Tobramycin is the aminoglycoside of choice for *M chelonae* (5, 6).

For an immunocompromised patient with new skin lesions, infection with atypical organisms such as RGMs should be kept in the differential diagnosis. For our patient, diagnosis was delayed because the skin lesions initially were attributed to the underlying autoimmune disorder. This case underscores the important point that tissue biopsies should not be delayed for immunocompromised individuals with new skin lesions because they have risk of infection with atypical organisms.

References

1. Chang MA, Jain S, Azar DT. Infections following laser in situ keratomileusis: an integration of the published literature. Surv Ophthalmol. 2004 May-Jun;49(3):269–80.
2. Drage LA, Ecker PM, Orenstein R, Phillips PK, Edson RS. An outbreak of *Mycobacterium chelonae* infections in tattoos. J Am Acad Dermatol. 2010 Mar;62(3):501–6. Epub 2009 Sep 6.
3. Wallace RJ Jr, Brown BA, Onyi GO. Skin, soft tissue, and bone infections due to *Mycobacterium chelonae chelonae*: importance of prior corticosteroid therapy, frequency of disseminated infections, and resistance to oral antimicrobials other than clarithromycin. J Infect Dis. 1992 Aug;166(2):405–12.
4. Wallace RJ Jr, Tanner D, Brennan PJ, Brown BA. Clinical trial of clarithromycin for cutaneous (disseminated) infection due to *Mycobacterium chelonae*. Ann Intern Med. 1993 Sep 15;119(6):482–6.
5. Wallace RJ Jr, Swenson JM, Silcox VA, Bullen MG. Treatment of nonpulmonary infections due to *Mycobacterium fortuitum* and *Mycobacterium chelonei* on the basis of in vitro susceptibilities. J Infect Dis. 1985 Sep;152(3):500–14.
6. Uslan DZ, Kowalski TJ, Wengenack NL, Virk A, Wilson JW. Skin and soft tissue infections due to rapidly growing mycobacteria: comparison of clinical features, treatment, and susceptibility. Arch Dermatol. 2006 Oct;142(10):1287–92.

Two Problems

35

Anil C. Jagtiani, MD, and Zelalem Temesgen, MD

Case Presentation

A 65-year-old man had received a diagnosis of HIV 23 years before his current presentation. His HIV was well controlled with lamivudine, zidovudine, and tenofovir; his most recent CD4 count was 638 cells/mm³, and his HIV viral load was less than 20 copies/mL. He had no history of opportunistic infections but did recall methicillin-resistant *Staphylococcus aureus* pneumonia. He began antiretroviral therapy 16 years earlier and had received different combinations of agents because of intolerances. He had no documented history of resistance to antiretroviral drugs, including zidovudine, lamivudine, indinavir, and ritonavir. The patient was sexually active and monogamous with his long-time male partner, who also was HIV positive (the partner's infection was well controlled with emtricitabine, tenofovir, and efavirenz).

He had a hepatitis non-A, non-B coinfection for approximately 22 years that was later confirmed to be an infection with hepatitis C virus (HCV), genotype 1a. He was treated with a combination of interferon and ribavirin for 1 year, after which he had sustained virologic control. Unfortunately, his condition progressed to end-stage liver disease and cholangiocarcinoma that was complicated by recurrent ascending cholangitis. He required multiple hospitalizations, antibiotic courses, and biliary stents.

He began our standard institutional protocol for initial treatment of cholangiocarcinoma, which consisted of 5-fluorouracil and concurrent radiotherapy, followed by capecitabine and brachytherapy. Before the transplant, his antiretroviral regimen was adjusted to emtricitabine, tenofovir, and raltegravir to avoid interactions between tacrolimus and efavirenz. He subsequently underwent deceased-donor liver transplant; induction therapy consisted of thymoglobulin, which was followed by maintenance with mycophenolic acid, tacrolimus, and prednisone. After transplant, he received valganciclovir and trimethoprim-sulfamethoxazole for prophylaxis against cytomegalovirus and pneumocystis pneumonia, respectively. His posttransplant course was uncomplicated, and he was discharged home.

Discussion

HIV infection had been a contraindication for organ transplant because of concerns of increased risk of opportunistic infections and progression of HIV to AIDS; however, that has not proven to be the case, and solid-organ transplant is increasingly common in the management of end-organ disease for patients with HIV (1,2). In fact, after the HIV Organ Policy Equity Act (HOPE Act) was passed into law, organs from HIV-infected donors could be used for transplant into HIV-infected recipients in some centers.

With the marked improvements in HIV therapy, patients are now presenting with long-term complications from other comorbidities. The patient described above was coinfected with HIV and HCV, and the accelerated progression to cirrhosis and complication with cholangiocarcinoma necessitated a liver transplant. For liver transplant recipients, recurrence of HCV with progression to cirrhosis has a large impact on survival. Studies of liver transplant recipients with HIV and HCV coinfection consistently have shown lower survival rates, more aggressive HCV recurrence, and graft loss when compared with patients with HCV monoinfection. Predictors of poor outcomes include older age of the donor, low body mass index of the recipient, need for simultaneous kidney transplant, and use of HCV seropositive donors (1,3). However, patients with HIV monoinfection have outcomes similar to those of HIV-negative candidates.

Patients with HIV and HCV coinfection have a much higher rate of acute cellular rejection, and the higher rate is thought to be attributable to multiple factors, including drug-drug interactions (may affect levels of immunosuppressive drugs and possibly total body drug exposure), immune dysregulation inherent to HIV infection (may induce allosensitization), and more T cells with a memory phenotype (4,5). Of note, treatment of acute rejection has been associated with recurrent cirrhosis and graft loss, which can further worsen graft and patient survival (1). In addition, a higher risk of hepatitis C recurrence after transplant has been associated with worse patient and graft survival for patients with coinfections.

To improve transplant outcomes in patients with HIV, selection of donors and recipients is of utmost importance, as is aggressive and timely management of posttransplant complications. Recipients need to meet stringent criteria before transplant: 1) CD4 count greater than 200 cells/mcL for 3 months; 2) undetectable viral load or detectable due to intolerances but able to be suppressed after transplant; 3) documented medication adherence; 4) absence of malignancy, opportunistic infections, or malnutrition (wasting); 5) acceptance of lifelong *Pneumocystis* prophylaxis; and 6) availability of follow-up with experienced providers and access to immunosuppressive drugs and laboratory monitoring (6). Each transplant center also may have other specific inclusion criteria.

Of note, clinically significant drug interactions must be considered when taking care of these patients. The most important interactions affect patients receiving a protease inhibitor–based

regimen because calcineurin inhibitors and mTOR inhibitors will need dose adjustment, typically to low doses (eg, once or twice weekly tacrolimus doses may be sufficient). In addition, nonnucleoside reverse transcriptase inhibitors (eg, efavirenz) may induce rapid clearance of calcineurin inhibitors, and therefore, dose adjustments and frequent monitoring are required (6). For this reason, HIV integrase inhibitors are the preferred agents in highly active antiretroviral regimens because of their lack of drug interactions and their minimal adverse effects.

In terms of preventive measures, patients with HIV who are transplant recipients should remain on lifelong *Pneumocystis* prophylaxis and azithromycin for *Mycobacterium avium* complex if CD4 counts are less than 75 cells/mcL. All patients should be screened for cytomegalovirus, hepatitis A virus, hepatitis B virus, and *Toxoplasma*, in addition to routine pretransplant serologic screening and other screening tests as needed, depending on exposure history and prophylaxis recommendations.

Although patients with coinfections consistently have poorer outcomes, such as accelerated cirrhosis and high mortality rates, patients with HIV infection do benefit from organ transplant (3). In addition, the wait-list mortality rate is higher for transplant candidates with coinfection compared with monoinfection, suggesting that the Model for End-Stage Liver Disease score may not be a good predictor of mortality in this population. More data are needed to quantify the survival benefit of liver transplant for this patient population. Most outcome data and experience in transplant for patients with HIV and HCV are from the era before direct-acting antiviral therapies for HCV were available. Presumably, treatment and high cure rates of HCV infection, before and after transplant, will likely change the outlook for patients with HIV-HCV coinfection in the near future.

References

1. Terrault NA, Roland ME, Schiano T, Dove L, Wong MT, Poordad F, et al; Solid Organ Transplantation in HIV: Multi-Site Study Investigators. Outcomes of liver transplant recipients with hepatitis C and human immunodeficiency virus coinfection. Liver Transpl. 2012 Jun;18(6):716-26.

2. Miro JM, Montejo M, Castells L, Rafecas A, Moreno S, Aguero F, et al; Spanish OLT in HIV-Infected Patients Working Group investigators. Outcome of HCV/HIV-coinfected liver transplant recipients: a prospective and multicenter cohort study. Am J Transplant. 2012 Jul;12(7):1866–76. Epub 2012 Apr 4.

3. Locke JE, Durand C, Reed RD, MacLennan PA, Mehta S, Massie A, et al. Long-term outcomes after liver transplantation among human immunodeficiency virus-infected recipients. Transplantation. 2016 Jan;100(1):141–6.

4. Stock PG, Barin B, Murphy B, Hanto D, Diego JM, Light J, et al. Outcomes of kidney transplantation in HIV-infected recipients. N Engl J Med. 2010 Nov 18;363(21):2004–14. Erratum in: N Engl J Med. 2011 Mar 17;364(11):1082.

5. Haidar G, Singh N. Improving the outcomes of human immunodeficiency virus/hepatitis C virus-coinfected transplant recipients: the answer is blowin' in the wind. Liver Transpl. 2017 Jun;23(6):727–9.

6. Blumberg EA, Rogers CC; AST Infectious Diseases Community of Practice. Human immunodeficiency virus in solid organ transplantation. Am J Transplant. 2013 Mar;13 Suppl 4:169–78.

36

Patient With Diplopia and Thoracic Pain

Alexandra S. Higgins, MD, Patrick S. Hoversten, MD, and Mark J. Enzler, MD

Case Presentation

A 61-year-old man presented to his primary care physician in early July with a large erythematous rash on his left buttock. He was a campground caretaker from northern Minnesota and had a history of hypertension, coronary artery disease, and treated prostate cancer. He was treated for 1 week with an unknown antibiotic and the rash resolved. A Lyme serology test was negative. Additionally, the patient fell from a ladder, landing on his back, in mid-July. Soon after the fall, he had a severe headache, with pain localizing to his left ear, occiput, and eye, plus 8 weeks of diplopia. He was seen by a neuro-ophthalmologist who diagnosed idiopathic isolated sixth nerve palsy. Magnetic resonance imaging (MRI) of the head was unrevealing. The patient subsequently had lancinating pain that localized to his thoracic and upper lumbar spinal and paraspinal region, plus severe lower abdominal pain and intermittent paresthesias of his bilateral arms. He was later hospitalized 3 times in his home area, and he required narcotics for pain control. An MRI of the cervical and thoracic spine showed spondylosis at the C6 level and a slight disk protrusion at T7 without cord compression. Computed tomographic images of the abdomen and pelvis were normal. He received multiple courses of low-dose prednisone and gabapentin but showed no meaningful improvement.

He pursued a second opinion at our institution in September and reported severe truncal and abdominal pain with numbness and a tingly sensation with a belt-like distribution. He noted intermittent pain in his arms, particularly the upper back of his arms, that was associated with tingling and numbness. He denied any weakness. A neurologic examination showed slight sensory loss over the left anterior abdomen (just above the umbilicus) and no motor deficits. An electromyographic examination showed no electrophysiologic evidence of a large-fiber peripheral neuropathic disorder or myopathy. A thermoregulatory sweat test showed evidence of clear anhidrosis of the left side of the abdomen at T10 and right side at T5, with bilateral patches of anhidrosis over the shoulders and left thigh (Figure 36.1). This finding was consistent with a patchy polyradiculopathy or small-fiber neuropathy.

A Lyme serology test was repeated at our institution and showed evidence of seroconversion, with positive results for an immunoglobulin (Ig) G qualitative enzyme immunoassay (EIA) and an IgG Western blot (WB) (8 bands present, with 5 bands required for positivity). The IgM EIA was positive, with 2 bands detected. A cerebrospinal fluid (CSF) analysis showed an elevated IgG level, with 12 oligoclonal bands that were not present in the serum, elevated protein level (122 mg/dL), normal glucose level (54 mg/dL), and mild lymphocytic pleocytosis (34 total nucleated cells; 94% lymphocytes and 6% monocytes). A CSF Lyme qualitative EIA was positive, with an immunoblot showing 7 IgG bands and 2 IgM bands. No CSF WB diagnostic criteria have been established for neuroborreliosis.

Figure 36.1   Thermoregulatory Sweat Test

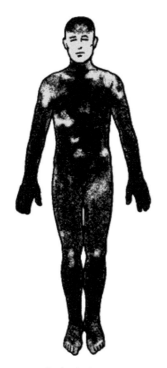

Sweating in purple shaded area. Pretest temperature was 35.7°C. Posttest temperature was 37.6°C.

The final diagnosis was Bannwarth syndrome or Lyme neuroborreliosis involving the central nervous system (cranial neuropathies and lymphocytic pleocytosis) and peripheral nervous system (inflammatory thoracic radiculopathies). The patient was treated with a 28-day course of intravenous ceftriaxone, which resulted in near-complete resolution of his pain.

Discussion

Lyme disease is the most common tick-borne infection in North America and Europe. It is caused most frequently by *Borrelia burgdorferi* in the United States and by *Borrelia garinii* and *Borrelia afzelii* in Europe (1,2). The nervous system is the third most common site of involvement for *Borrelia* infections (after skin and joints), and 10% to 15% of patients with Lyme disease have neurologic involvement. Acute neurologic Lyme disease that is associated with the triad of lymphocytic meningitis, cranial neuropathy (most commonly the seventh cranial nerve [2]), and radiculoneuritis is termed *Bannwarth syndrome* (1). Although Bannwarth syndrome is more likely to be associated with European Lyme disease, a cluster of 5 cases of neuroinvasive Lyme disease presenting with Bannwarth syndrome was reported in the United States in 2017 (3). Acute neurologic manifestations of Lyme disease have a broad differential diagnosis that includes other causes of facial palsy (herpes zoster, Guillain-Barré syndrome, HIV, sarcoidosis, Sjögren syndrome, tumor, stroke, basilar meningitides), viral meningitis, mechanical radiculopathy, and multiple sclerosis (4).

Lyme disease serologic testing consists of 2-tiered antibody testing that starts with an EIA and, if positive or indeterminate, is followed by a confirmatory IgM and IgG WB for antibodies against *B burgdorferi* to increase the specificity of initial testing (5). This approach is reasonably sensitive (>87%) and specific (99%) for disseminated Lyme disease (5). Neuroinvasive Lyme infection should be considered for patients with exposure to ticks in a Lyme-endemic region and present with the following constellation of findings: cranial motor neuropathy, painful radiculoneuritis (classic finding), and lymphocytic meningitis that, taken together, constitute Bannwarth syndrome. Diagnostic testing for neuroborreliosis consists of CSF analysis showing lymphocytic pleocytosis, elevated protein level, and normal glucose level, keeping in mind that neurologic Lyme disease limited to the peripheral nervous system may have normal CSF findings (1). Serologic testing, as previously described, is typically positive (4). Presence of intrathecal antibodies to *B burgdorferi* is the most useful laboratory finding for the diagnosis of neuroborreliosis, and it is performed by comparing CSF and serum Lyme quantitative EIAs that are corrected for breakdown of the blood-brain barrier (1). If the CSF screening test for Lyme disease with a qualitative EIA is positive, then quantitative serum and CSF Lyme EIAs should be performed simultaneously and a Lyme antibody index calculated. An antibody index greater than 1.5 indicates the presence of intrathecal antibodies against the *Borrelia* species associated with Lyme disease, ie, it is suggestive of neuroinvasive Lyme disease (6). In the United States, treatment of neuroborreliosis with meningitis or radiculopathy consists of 2 to 4 weeks of intravenous ceftriaxone (2 g, once daily); if the patient is unable to tolerate β-lactam antibiotics, then doxycycline may be used (2).

The patient described above had a history of a rash, followed by sixth cranial nerve palsy and painful polyradiculitis. An early Lyme serology test was negative, which is often the case during the first 2 weeks of infection. The patient's initial symptoms were attributed to a mechanical injury after a fall. The rash most likely was erythema chronicum migrans, a skin manifestation of early Lyme infection. The presence of 12 CSF oligoclonal bands and the patient's clinical response to ceftriaxone therapy supported the diagnosis of Bannwarth syndrome. The patient's multiple inflammatory radiculopathies were confirmed with

a thermoregulatory sweat test. Neuroborreliosis should be considered in the differential diagnosis of patients presenting with polyradiculitis who reside in Lyme-endemic regions.

References

1. Halperin JJ. Neuroborreliosis. J Neurol. 2017 Jun;264(6):1292-7. Epub 2016 Nov 24.
2. Wormser GP, Dattwyler RJ, Shapiro ED, Halperin JJ, Steere AC, Klempner MS, et al. The clinical assessment, treatment, and prevention of Lyme disease, human granulocytic anaplasmosis, and babesiosis: clinical practice guidelines by the Infectious Diseases Society of America. Clin Infect Dis. 2006 Nov 1;43(9):1089–134. Epub 2006 Oct 2. Erratum in: Clin Infect Dis. 2007 Oct 1;45(7):941.
3. Shah A, O'Horo JC, Wilson JW, Granger D, Theel ES. An unusual cluster of neuroinvasive Lyme disease cases presenting with Bannwarth syndrome in the Midwest United States. Open Forum Infect Dis. 2017 Dec 23;5(1):ofx276.
4. Stanek G, Wormser GP, Gray J, Strle F. Lyme borreliosis. Lancet. 2012 Feb 4;379(9814):461–73. Epub 2011 Sep 6.
5. Hinckley AF, Connally NP, Meek JI, Johnson BJ, Kemperman MM, Feldman KA, et al. Lyme disease testing by large commercial laboratories in the United States. Clin Infect Dis. 2014 Sep 1;59(5):676–81. Epub 2014 May 30.
6. Halperin JJ. Nervous system Lyme disease. Clin Lab Med. 2015 Dec;35(4):779–95. Epub 2015 Sep 18.

Case Presentation

A 43-year-old man with HIV presents to the clinic with ongoing viremia (HIV viral load, 13,480 copies/mL) and a CD4 count of 142 cells/mcL. He is intermittently nonadherent with his medication regimen of coformulated darunavir (800 mg) and cobicistat (150 mg) plus coformulated tenofovir disoproxil fumarate (300 mg) and emtricitabine (200 mg), once daily. He has gastrointestinal disturbances (nausea, diarrhea, and vomiting) that he associates with the coformulated darunavir-cobicistat. He also has intermittent nonadherence with the boosted protease inhibitor (darunavir-cobicistat) because it interacts with his psychiatric medications. The fluctuant levels of his psychiatric medications make titration difficult; consequently, his major depression and schizophrenia are poorly controlled.

History of Antiretroviral Therapy and Identified Genotype Mutations

In 2004, the patient began receiving efavirenz plus zidovudine-lamivudine. This treatment was discontinued in 2005 because of worsening psychiatric issues, nightmares, and nonadherence. He did not receive antiretroviral therapy again until 2010. For 3 months in 2010, the patient was treated with atazanavir plus tenofovir disoproxil fumarate–emtricitabine. This treatment was discontinued because of severe scleral icterus, elevated bilirubin, and cutaneous bile salt deposition. He left care and was lost to follow-up from 2010 to 2014. He did not receive any antiretroviral therapy during this period. From 2014 to 2018, the patient received raltegravir (RAL) plus tenofovir disoproxil fumarate–emtricitabine. This treatment was discontinued because of virologic failure and integrase strand transfer inhibitor (INSTI) resistance that developed in the setting of substance abuse–related nonadherence in 2017 and 2018. Since 2018, the patient has received darunavir-cobicistat plus tenofovir disoproxil fumarate–emtricitabine.

The patient's historical HIV genotypes showed a K103N mutation in the reverse transcriptase gene. The protease inhibitor gene had an M36L mutation. Two INSTI mutations also were identified, N155H and Q148H. His current regimen (darunavir-cobicistat plus tenofovir disoproxil fumarate–emtricitabine) poses problematic drug interactions with other desired medication therapy for comorbid illness, and adverse effects are contributing to nonadherence. The medical team is revisiting an integrase inhibitor–based antiretroviral program, but the team is concerned about his prior integrase inhibitor resistance.

Discussion

Development of Resistance to Antiviral Drugs

The HIV virus has among the highest rates of genetic mutation of any biological entity, and it can develop considerable genetic diversity while replicating within a host. Ongoing viral replication in the setting of selective pressure from antiviral drugs facilitates the outgrowth of resistant quasispecies as dominant clones. Further replication leads to additional (secondary) mutations that enhance resistance and viral fitness.

When a single point mutation develops easily and conveys a high level of resistance to a drug, that drug is said to have a low genetic barrier to resistance. Drugs with a high genetic barrier to resistance often require multiple mutations before a notable effect on drug susceptibility is observed. Antiviral drugs with a high genetic barrier to resistance, in which mutations convey a large cost to viral fitness, are desirable for treatment.

Development of Resistance to RAL

RAL has a relatively low genetic barrier to resistance. Resistance typically occurs via 3 mutually exclusive primary pathways that evolve on separate viral genomes within quasispecies (Table 37.1) (1).

Development of a primary mutation can reduce the effectiveness of INSTIs, but it can also negatively affect viral fitness by reducing replicative capacity of variants carrying the mutation. Secondary mutations develop with ongoing viral replication under drug pressure, and these mutations usually enhance fitness of viral variants while further increasing the resistance (measured as fold change in the concentration of the drug that will provide 50% inhibition in vitro). The addition of G140S to Q148H provides a powerful example that shows how replication ability is notably enhanced with a potent increase in resistance to RAL (Table 37.2) (1,2).

In vivo evaluation of the progression of resistance to RAL shows that clones with the N155H

Table 37.1 Primary and Associated Secondary Mutations Conferring Resistance to Raltegravir

Primary Mutation	Associated Secondary Mutations
N155H	L74M, E92Q, T97A, G136R, V151I
Q148R/H/K	E138A/K, G140A/S
Y143R/C	L74A/I, E92Q, T97A, I203M, S230R

Data from Clavel (1).

Table 37.2 Characteristics of Select Mutations With Resistance to Raltegravir

Mutation	Fold Change in IC_{50}	Percentage of Wild-Type RC
N155H	31.5	59.9
Q148H	78.0	28.0
Q148H + G140S	1,436.0	90.5

Abbreviations: IC_{50}, concentration of drug that will provide 50% inhibition in vitro; RC, replicative capacity.

Data from Quercia et al (2).

mutation are more prevalent during the early development of resistance, but they are often replaced by the Q148 and Y143 mutations. Thus, the comparative viral fitness of N155H might enhance the initial development of resistance and virologic escape, but ongoing replication seems to lead to dominance of clones with Q148 and Y143 because these secondary mutations enhance resistance and virologic fitness relative to the N155H mutation (3).

Development of Resistance to Elvitegravir

Like RAL, elvitegravir (EVG) has a relatively low genetic barrier to resistance. Single primary mutations T66I and E92Q often develop early during EVG therapy, although Q148H and N155H also occur. Ongoing replication under EVG selection pressure increases diversity of viral genomes and secondary mutations, and the clones with T66I or E92Q can be replaced by others such as those with Q148R/K/H (4).

Cross-Resistance Between EVG and RAL

Viral variants with amino acid substitutions at positions 66, 92, 148, and 155 all affect the active site of the integrase enzyme by disrupting appropriate binding of the drug moiety and the ability to inhibit replication. These mutations confer a large degree of cross-resistance between EVG and RAL (Table 37.3). Thus, virologic failure from RAL or EVG resistance precludes use of the other drug in a salvage program.

Table 37.3   FC in IC$_{50}$ for Select Integrase Strand Transfer Inhibitor Mutations Conferring Resistance to RAL and EVG

Mutation	RAL[a]	EVG[a]
N155H	++	++
N155H + L74M	++	++
N155H + E92Q	+++	+++
Q148H	+	+
Q148H + E138K	++	++
Q148H + G140S	+++	+++
Y143H + N155H	++	++
Y143R	++	+
Y143R + T97A	+++	++
T66I + E92Q	++	+++
T66K + L74M	++	+++
T66I + Q148R	++	+++
E92Q + Q148R	+++	+++

Abbreviations: EVG, elvitegravir; FC, fold change; IC$_{50}$, concentration of drug that will provide 50% inhibition in vitro; RAL, raltegravir.

[a] + indicates low FC; ++, moderate FC; +++, high FC.

Data from Anstett et al (4).

Second-Generation INSTIs

Second-generation INSTIs include dolutegravir (DTG), bictegravir (BIC), and cabotegravir (CAB). Oral DTG was approved by the US Food and Drug Administration in 2013, and oral BIC was approved in 2018 as part of a coformulated single-tablet regimen (containing BIC, emtricitabine, and tenofovir alafenamide). CAB was approved in 2021 as a long-acting injectable formulation in combination with injectable rilpivirine.

Second-generation INSTIs have shown a high genetic barrier to resistance and have activity in the setting of many mutations that confer resistance to first-generation INSTIs (5). In vitro experiments indicate that second-generation INSTIs maintain their efficacy in the presence of multiple first-generation INSTI mutations and combinations (generated by site-directed

mutagenesis) (Table 37.4). BIC and DTG show similar activity, whereas CAB is less active for some double- and triple-mutation combinations. Fold-change values can be compared with ranges of expected activity, noting cutoffs above which the drug is considered resistant. The following fold-change values or ranges have been reported for currently approved INSTIs: RAL, 1.5; EVG, 2.5; DTG, 4 to 13; and BIC, 2.5 to 10 (5-7).

For patients whose RAL or EVG regimens have failed, in vitro assessments of their viral isolates reinforce the cross-resistance profile for first-generation INSTIs (EVG and RAL) and show continued activity of BIC, CAB, and DTG in the setting of single, first-generation INSTI mutations. Further, they show comparable fold change with continued activity of DTG and BIC in the presence of many mutation combinations that eliminate activity of first-generation INSTIs. Certain mutation combinations cause more dramatic loss of CAB activity (relative to BIC and DTG), whereas others cause resistance to all second-generation INSTIs (5-7).

Although in vitro assessments have value, little clinical data have been published for BIC or CAB activity in patients with strong antiretroviral drug resistance, prior INSTI failure, or first-generation INSTI resistance. However, clinical data for DTG have been published. The SAILING study (8) assessed treatment-experienced (but INSTI-naive) patients with resistance to at least 2 classes of antiretroviral agents and reported that 71% of patients had virologic suppression after 48 weeks of DTG treatment (50 mg, once daily, in combination with an optimized background regimen).

The VIKING-3 study assessed patients with prior INSTI treatment failure and first-generation INSTI resistance, and they showed that 116 of 183 patients (63%) attained viral loads of less than 50 copies/mL at 48 weeks after receiving DTG (50 mg, twice daily, in combination with an optimized background regimen) (3). Notably, treatment success rates decreased with increasing baseline integrase resistance. At 48 weeks, 71% of patients with no documented Q148H/K/R mutations (having

Table 37.4   IC$_{50}$ and FC in IC$_{50}$ for Select Second-Generation Integrase Strand Transfer Inhibitor Mutations

Mutation	DTG		CAB		BIC	
	IC$_{50}$, mean, nM	FC	IC$_{50}$, mean, nM	FC	IC$_{50}$, mean, nM	FC
Wild type (reference)	1.6	NA	2.4	NA	1.9	NA
N155H	3.6	2.3	2.2	0.9	2.7	1.4
Q148H	0.6	0.4	6.8	2.8	0.9	0.5
T66I	0.9	0.6	0.9	0.4	0.2	0.1
E92Q	2.3	1.4	4.2	1.8	2.0	1.1
R263K	11.3	7.0	13.4	5.6	4.1	2.2
Y143R	4.3	2.7	2.7	1.1	2.6	1.4
Q148H + G140S	5.8	3.6	36.3	15.1	5.5	2.9
Q148K + E138K	25.0	17.7	772.1	321.7	59.3	31.2
Y143H + N155H	1.7	1.1	1.2	0.5	2.7	1.4
N155H + E92Q	1.8	1.1	4.6	1.9	3.3	1.7
Y143H + N155H	2.5	1.6	3.7	1.5	4.0	2.1
Q148K + G140A + E138K	212.1	132.6	610.3	254.3	223.0	117.3
Q148R + G140A + L74M	12.0	7.5	53.2	22.1	11.7	6.2
Q148R + G140C + E138K	5.3	3.3	134.2	55.9	8.2	4.3
Q148H + G140S + T97A	55.9	35.0	43.7	18.2	29.5	15.5
Q148H + G140S + E138A	13.8	8.6	70.2	29.2	5.1	2.7
Q148H + G140S + Y143R	7.7	4.8	113.8	47.4	9.4	4.9

Abbreviations: BIC, bictegravir; CAB, cabotegravir; DTG, dolutegravir; FC, fold change; IC$_{50}$, concentration of drug that will provide 50% inhibition in vitro; NA, not applicable.

Data from Smith et al (5).

Y143, N155, T66, or E92) had a viral load of less than 50 copies/mL, whereas success rates decreased to 56% for patients with Q148 plus 1 mutation and to 29% for patients with Q148 and more than 2 secondary mutations (notably G140A/C/S, L74I, or E138A/K/T). The VIKING-3 study also showed that the higher dose was generally well tolerated, with very few withdrawals attributed to drug-related adverse effects. Thus, DTG (50 mg, administered twice daily) has a favorable adverse effect profile at an increased dose and has in vitro and clinical data to support its use in the setting of INSTI resistance with prior INSTI failure. However, caution should be exercised when INSTI resistance is present with a Q148 mutation and greater than 2 concerning secondary mutations, given

the lower response rates in VIKING-3 for this subgroup of patients. DTG at a dose of 100 mg, twice daily, has shown virologic success (viral load, <50 copies/mL) after 48 weeks in 4 of 5 heavily treatment-experienced patients with dual Q148 and G140 mutations. Although data are limited, this dosing scheme is a potential option for patients with multiple INSTI mutations.

Summary

First-generation INSTIs (EVG, RAL) have a lower genetic barrier to resistance than second-generation INSTIs (DTG, BIC, CAB). Primary resistance against RAL usually develops via

3 mutually exclusive pathways (N155, Q148, Y143). EVG often develops primary resistance via T66, E92, N155, or Q148 mutation development. First-generation INSTIs share a high level of cross-resistance. Second-generation INSTIs have in vitro activity against many first-generation INSTI mutations, with BIC and DTG showing comparable activities and CAB having less activity for some combinations. DTG at an increased dose has clinical data to support its use in a combination regimen for patients with first-generation INSTI failure and resistance.

References

1. Clavel F. HIV resistance to raltegravir. Eur J Med Res. 2009 Nov 24;14 Suppl 3(Suppl 3):47–54.
2. Quercia R, Dam E, Perez-Bercoff D, Clavel F. Selective-advantage profile of human immunodeficiency virus type 1 integrase mutants explains in vivo evolution of raltegravir resistance genotypes. J Virol. 2009 Oct;83(19):10245–9.
3. Castagna A, Maggiolo F, Penco G, Wright D, Mills A, Grossberg R, et al; VIKING-3 Study Group. Dolutegravir in antiretroviral-experienced patients with raltegravir- and/or elvitegravir-resistant HIV-1: 24-week results of the phase III VIKING-3 study. J Infect Dis. 2014 Aug 1;210(3):354-62. Epub 2014 Jan 19.
4. Anstett K, Brenner B, Mesplede T, Wainberg MA. HIV drug resistance against strand transfer integrase inhibitors. Retrovirology. 2017 Jun 5;14(1):36.
5. Smith SJ, Zhao XZ, Burke TR Jr, Hughes SH. Efficacies of cabotegravir and bictegravir against drug-resistant HIV-1 integrase mutants. Retrovirology. 2018 May 16;15(1):37.
6. Santoro MM, Fornabaio C, Malena M, Galli L, Poli A, Marcotullio S, et al; PRESTIGIO Study Group. Susceptibility to bictegravir in highly arv-experienced patients after inSTI failure. CROI Conference on retroviruses and opportunistic infections. CROI Foundation/IAS-USA; c2019; p. 206.
7. Saladini F, Giannini A, Boccuto A, Dragoni F, Appendino A, Albanesia E, et al. In vitro activity of DTG/BIC/E/CAB on first-generation InSTI-resistant HIV-1 [abstract]. CROI Conference on retroviruses and opportunistic infections. CROI Foundation/IAS-USA; c2019; p. 206.
8. Cahn P, Pozniak AL, Mingrone H, Shuldyakov A, Brites C, Andrade-Villanueva JF, et al; extended SAILING Study Team. Dolutegravir versus raltegravir in antiretroviral-experienced, integrase-inhibitor-naive adults with HIV: week 48 results from the randomised, double-blind, non-inferiority SAILING study. Lancet. 2013 Aug 24;382(9893):700–8. Epub 2013 Jul 3. Erratum in: Lancet. 2014 Jan 4;383(9911):30.

Bilateral Tinnitus

Christina G. O'Connor, PharmD, RPh

Case Presentation

A 43-year-old woman presented with left shoulder pain, nausea, and vomiting. Her medical history included congenital tetralogy of Fallot and a complex cardiac surgical history, including placement of an implantable cardioverter-defibrillator (ICD). She was hospitalized, and blood cultures showed branching, gram-positive cocci with a beaded appearance, initially suspected to be *Nocardia*. The patient began treatment with imipenem and trimethoprim-sulfamethoxazole (TMP-SMX). A transesophageal echocardiogram showed linear strands attached to the ICD leads.

The organism was identified as *Mycobacterium fortuitum*, and multiple blood cultures were subsequently positive. The patient began treatment with a macrolide-containing regimen and underwent ICD device removal. Cultures from the ICD pocket also were identified as *M fortuitum* complex. The isolate was susceptible to amikacin, ciprofloxacin, and moxifloxacin, intermediately sensitive to cefoxitin and imipenem, and resistant to clarithromycin, doxycycline, linezolid, minocycline, tobramycin, and TMP-SMX. Additional testing from an outside facility showed a minimum inhibitory concentration (MIC) of 0.12 mcg/mL for tigecycline, an MIC of 0.25 mcg/mL for clofazimine, and an MIC of 0.03 mcg/mL for bedaquiline.

After susceptibilities were determined, the patient was changed from a macrolide-containing regimen to imipenem-cilastatin (1,000 mg, intravenous [IV], every 12 hours), amikacin (500 mg, IV, every 24 hours), and moxifloxacin (400 mg, oral, once daily). The amikacin dosage was calculated to target a peak of 35 to 45 mcg/mL; the target dose was extrapolated backward from serum levels measured 2 and 6 hours after the end of an amikacin infusion. Monthly audiology testing and routine laboratory monitoring were recommended. At baseline, audiology testing showed normal findings for both ears. Her medical team planned to replace the cardiac device 1 month after blood culture results were negative.

The patient had a follow-up appointment with an infectious diseases clinician 2 months later. She was tolerating the antimycobacterial agents and was clinically stable overall. Weekly amikacin serum troughs were consistently undetectable. However, she reported symptoms of an upper respiratory tract infection with sinus congestion, plus bilateral tinnitus and left-sided hearing loss, which were attributed to her respiratory infection. Additionally, she indicated having otalgia at the tragus. No changes were made to the *M fortuitum* treatment plan at that time.

An audiology evaluation was completed several weeks later. Results were notable for mild to moderately severe sensorineural hearing loss (SNHL) at 6 to 8 kHz in the left ear. The audiologist graded the hearing loss as a grade 2 adverse event according to the National Cancer Institute Common Terminology Criteria for Adverse Events, version 4.03. Evaluation of the right ear and cochlear hair function showed normal findings. The patient continued to report bilateral intermittent tinnitus (lasting 2-3 seconds) occurring 2 to 3 times per week. She reported a new concern of dizziness, which she described as a sensation of the room spinning while she was standing or sitting.

Because of concerns about potential aminoglycoside toxicity, the IV amikacin was replaced with tigecycline (50 mg, IV, daily). Imipenem-cilastatin and moxifloxacin were continued. Several weeks after discontinuation of amikacin, her tinnitus and dizziness re-solved but the mild hearing loss remained. The patient successfully completed a prolonged course of tigecycline, imipenem-cilastatin, and moxifloxacin for the *M fortuitum* infection.

Discussion

This case is an example of an insidious presentation of likely antimycobacterial-related oto-toxicity in a patient with a serious and rare infectious syndrome and limited treatment options. Ototoxicity is a well-known complication of aminoglycosides, although it also has been reported with macrolides, another commonly used antimycobacterial agent.

Derived from soil actinomycetes, amino-glycosides are highly water soluble, positively charged protein synthesis inhibitors that share a common 6-membered cyclitol or hexose ring linked by glycosidic bonds (1). As a drug class, aminoglycosides are highly effective against most gram-negative bacteria and *Mycobacterium*, but they are associated with a risk of clinically significant adverse effects. Aminoglycosides exist in a naturally benign state as soft Lewis bases, but interaction with a Lewis acid (metal ion) will produce toxic, oxidatively active metal complexes (1). Hallmark toxicities of aminoglycosides are nephrotoxicity, neuromuscular blockade, and ototoxicity. Ototoxicity can be permanent, may be difficult to detect, and can manifest after the aminoglycoside has been stopped. Generally, hearing disturbances tend to arise after 72 hours of aminoglycoside exposure. Among patients receiving aminoglycoside courses of 5 to 7 days, up to 20% of patients have hearing loss and 15% have balance disturbances (1). Ototoxicity risk is considered highest with gentamicin, then tobra-mycin, and then amikacin. Amikacin tends to cause more cochlear toxicity, and gentamicin causes more vestibular toxicity. Several studies that investigated a potential link between aminoglycoside-induced renal dysfunction and

ototoxicity determined that these toxicities are independent. Patient-specific risk factors are not well established, aside from the mitochondrial sequence variant A1555G in the 12S ribosomal RNA gene (1,2). Pretreatment screening for this variant is not currently part of routine clinical practice.

A sign of aminoglycoside cochlear toxicity is bilateral SNHL, beginning at high frequencies. Vestibular toxicity can present with any combination of vertigo, nausea, vomiting, nystagmus, and ataxia (1). Vestibular damage is caused by the loss of hair cells in cristae ampullares and can involve type I and type II hair cells. Injury begins with the outer hair cells and progresses to inner hair cells in severe cases. Damage to sensory epi-thelia in the utricle and saccule may also occur (1,2). Gentamicin has been identified in hair cells months after systemic drug exposure (2).

The mechanism of ototoxicity with macrolides is not as well understood. Ion transport im-pairment at the level of the stria vascularis and central involvement in the auditory pathways have been proposed (3). Initially described with erythromycin in the 1970s, ototoxicity has sub-sequently been reported (although rarely) with azithromycin and clarithromycin. Erythromycin-related ototoxicity is characterized as temporary, pan-frequency SNHL and tinnitus that usually occur within the first 72 hours after drug initiation. Reversible, azithromycin-induced ototoxicity was described in the 1990s with the treatment of dis-seminated *Mycobacterium avium* in persons living with HIV or AIDS, although at least 1 case of ir-reversible, azithromycin-related SNHL has been reported. Patients with the highest risk are female, have advanced age, have renal or hepatic impair-ment, and receive high doses of macrolides (3,4).

The American Academy of Audiology (5) provides guidance on monitoring for drug-induced ototoxicity and includes specific recommendations for aminoglycosides. These guidelines stress the importance of obtaining audiology measurements at baseline, when-ever possible, noting that an examination often is not practical for patients who require urgent treatment with aminoglycosides. In such acute situations, the recommendation is to test within 2 days of aminoglycoside initiation. The primary methods for monitoring drug-induced ototoxicity are the basic audiologic assessment, high-frequency audiometry, and otoacoustic emission measurement. These may be used separately or in combination, depending on patient-specific considerations. The guidelines recommend monitoring on a weekly or biweekly basis, ideally, and follow-up testing should be conducted a few months after drug discontinuation because of the risk of delayed hearing loss. Access to frequent audiology testing may be challenging; thus, many specialists obtain measurements at baseline and once monthly thereafter, paired with patient self-monitoring and immediate testing if patient concerns arise. Patients and their caregivers should be educated about the risks and signs of various types of drug-induced ototoxicity.

In conclusion, aminoglycoside- and macrolide-related ototoxicity is a treatment-related adverse effect that is serious, difficult to detect, and potentially irreversible. Patients must be vigilantly monitored for signs of drug-induced ototoxicity by health care professionals. A multidisciplinary team that includes infectious diseases physicians, audiologists, and pharmacists is critical for early detection and prevention of harm.

References

1. Xie J, Talaska AE, Schacht J. New developments in aminoglycoside therapy and ototoxicity. Hear Res. 2011 Nov;281(1-2):28-37. Epub 2011 May 27.
2. Guthrie OW. Aminoglycoside induced ototoxicity. Toxicology. 2008 Jul 30;249(2-3):91–6. Epub 2008 Apr 29.
3. Schellack N, Naude A. An overview of pharmacotherapy-induced ototoxicity. South African Family Practice. 2013;55(4):357–65.
4. Ress BD, Gross EM. Irreversible sensorineural hearing loss as a result of azithromycin ototoxicity: a case report. Ann Otol Rhinol Laryngol. 2000 Apr;109(4):435–7.
5. American Academy of Audiology. Position statement and clinical practice guidelines: ototoxicity monitoring. 2009 [cited 2021 Feb 5]. Available from: https://audiology-web.s3.amazonaws.com/migrated/OtoMonGuidelines.pdf_539974c40999c1.58842217.pdf.

Fever in a Returning Traveler 39

Madiha Fida, MBBS, Lina I. Elbadawi, MD, and Mark J. Enzler, MD

Case Presentation

A 30-year-old female Somali immigrant with a history of treated latent tuberculosis presented to our travel clinic in late May with a 3-month history of intermittent fevers, severe fatigue, joint pain, epigastric pain, and an 8-kg weight loss. Her symptoms started 1 week after a 3-month trip to visit family in Somalia. She did not receive any pretravel vaccinations, nor did she take antimalarial chemoprophylaxis. She had never been sexually active. She reported frequent ingestion of unpasteurized camel milk during her trip.

The patient initially noted fevers at the end of her trip that were associated with frontal headaches. She managed these symptoms with over-the-counter nonsteroidal anti-inflammatory drugs (NSAIDs). She then had epigastric pain. Two months into her illness, she had asymmetric, painful swelling in both ankles and the proximal interphalangeal joints of her right hand.

The physical examination at presentation showed that her heart rate was 92 beats/min, blood pressure was 101/72 mm Hg, and temperature was 37.7°C. She had an antalgic gait because of ankle pain. She had mild epigastric tenderness with deep palpation and swelling of her right hand (third proximal interphalangeal joint) and proximal right foot. Findings from chest radiography and abdominal ultrasonography were unremarkable. Laboratory testing showed microcytic anemia, with a hemoglobin level of 11 g/dL that was managed with oral iron replacement therapy. Results of a blood malaria multiplex polymerase chain reaction (PCR) test and an HIV screening test were negative. Bacterial blood cultures were obtained. An esophagogastroduodenoscopy examination showed mild gastritis that was believed to be

caused by NSAID use. An empiric 14-day course of oral cefdinir, started 2 weeks before presentation, was unsuccessful.

The patient was hospitalized 3 days after her presentation to the travel clinic, when aerobic blood cultures grew tiny, coccobacillus-shaped, gram-negative organisms in multiple samples. The organism dimensions were approximately 1×0.5 µm (compared with 0.25-1×2 µm for *Escherichia coli*) (Figure 39.1).

The patient was empirically treated with intravenous (IV) piperacillin-tazobactam, without a clinical response. She was febrile on a daily basis during the hospitalization. On hospital day 4, her blood culture isolate was identified as *Brucella melitensis*, and the antimicrobial regimen was switched to oral doxycycline plus rifampin. Clues suggesting that the patient's blood isolate was a *Brucella* species were the organism's tiny size and the patient's past ingestion of unpasteurized

Figure 39.1   Gram Stain of Blood Culture

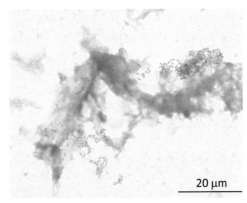

20 µm

Clumps of tiny, gram-negative coccobacilli (*Brucella melitensis*) are visible.

camel milk. A computed tomographic scan of the abdomen and pelvis showed normal findings, and a transthoracic echocardiogram did not show any signs of infective endocarditis. Repeat blood cultures remained positive on days 10 and 17 after initiation of doxycycline and rifampin, so oral ciprofloxacin (750 mg, twice daily) was added to her regimen. Her bacteremia cleared 24 days after initiation of *Brucella*-active antibiotic therapy.

At a follow-up appointment, she reported resolution of the joint pain and fever. Because she had a prolonged bloodstream infection, she was treated for 12 weeks, and repeat blood cultures were negative after completion of therapy.

Discussion

A common patient presentation in our travel clinic is fever in the returning traveler. In a study of 42,173 returning travelers who presented to a clinic or hospital, fever was the chief reason for seeking care for 23.3% of ill travelers (the cohort included 33 cases of brucellosis) (1). Globalization has had a large impact on exposure to infectious diseases, and world travel poses a challenge to local physicians who must consider unusual infections in the context of the traveler's itinerary, travel-related activities, and local infection epidemiology. Diagnostic considerations for a febrile traveler returning from Somalia should include falciparum malaria, typhoid fever, leptospirosis, brucellosis, viral infection (measles, HIV, chikungunya, and dengue), and tuberculosis.

Brucellosis is an uncommon reportable disease in the United States, with approximately 100 to 200 cases reported to the Centers for Disease Control and Prevention each year since 1990. Domestically acquired cases are typically associated with ingestion of unpasteurized dairy products (2). Previously, swine-associated brucellosis (*Brucella suis*) was acquired domestically by workers in slaughterhouses, but this

source has been eliminated as a result of the US Department of Agriculture National Brucellosis Eradication Program, which was expanded to cover swine herds in 1972. Brucellosis remains endemic in the Mediterranean basin, Persian Gulf, Indian subcontinent, and parts of Mexico and Central and South America, where ingestion of unpasteurized dairy products is common (3,4). Clinical presentation varies from asymptomatic infection to severe and fatal illness. Acute infection may be associated with nonspecific symptoms such as fever, night sweats, anorexia, myalgia, arthralgia, fatigue, and abdominal pain.

Brucellosis is a zoonotic infection that may be transmitted through direct inoculation (by handling infected animal tissues), inhalation of infected aerosols, or ingestion of food products derived from infected animals. Our patient likely acquired her infection by ingesting unpasteurized camel milk while traveling in Somalia. Brucellosis may present as a generalized infection, or it may be localized in 30% of patients. Affected systems are outlined in Table 39.1.

Brucella are facultative, intracellular bacteria that are classified into biovars on the basis of biologic and serologic criteria (4,5). Species that are pathogenic in humans include *B melitensis* (goats and sheep), *B suis* (pigs, including feral pigs), *Brucella abortus* (cattle), and *Brucella canis* (dogs). Although speciation may be performed by evaluating results of biochemical reactions, matrix-assisted laser desorption/ionization

Table 39.1	Clinical Presentation of Brucellosis
System	**Presentation**
Musculoskeletal	Arthritis, vertebral osteomyelitis or diskitis (spondylitis), sacral ileitis
Central nervous system	Neurobrucellosis
Pulmonary	Bronchitis, pneumonitis
Gastrointestinal	Hepatitis, splenic abscess, colitis
Cardiac	Endocarditis
Genitourinary	Orchitis, epididymitis

time-of-flight mass spectrometry is often used for identification in modern reference laboratories (4). Microscopically, *Brucella* appear as extremely small (0.6-1.5×0.5-0.7 μm), gram-negative coccobacilli. The incubation period of *Brucella* species is typically between 1 and 4 weeks, although it may be as long as several months. The microbiologic diagnosis is established by culture, serology, or PCR. Although cultures can be obtained from blood, bone marrow, or other body fluids, bone marrow specimens are the most sensitive source for culture. The laboratory should be warned when *Brucella* is suspected, to avoid infecting laboratory personnel. Several *Brucella* serologic tests are available, with the serum agglutination test and enzyme-linked immunosorbent assay being the most common. It may be difficult to interpret serologic test results of patients who reside in *Brucella*-endemic regions and patients who are recovering from infection because results may remain positive long after recovery in treated individuals.

Because *Brucella* is a predominantly intracellular bacterial pathogen, treatment of brucellosis requires combination antibiotic therapy with agents that are active intracellularly (4,5). The combination of oral doxycycline (100 mg, twice daily, for 6 weeks) plus streptomycin (1 g daily, intramuscular [IM] or IV, for the first 2-3 weeks) remains the treatment of choice for uncomplicated brucellosis, provided that the patient has normal renal function and no focal disease such as spondylitis, neurobrucellosis, or endocarditis; with this therapy, cure rates are up to 92% (4,6). Gentamicin (5 mg/kg once daily, IM or IV, for the first 5-7 days) may be substituted for streptomycin if streptomycin is unavailable and the patient has normal renal function. Spondylitis should be treated with 12 or more weeks of doxycycline plus 2 to 3 weeks of streptomycin. Nonaminoglycoside oral treatment regimens (eg, with gentamicin or streptomycin) may include 6 weeks of oral doxycycline (100 mg, twice daily) plus rifampin (600-900 mg, once daily), which is more convenient than administering parenteral aminoglycosides. However, a 2012 meta-analysis that included 9 studies and 930 patients showed that oral doxycycline plus rifampin had a higher combined rate of treatment failure and relapse compared with oral doxycycline plus parenteral streptomycin (18.2% vs 6.7%; odds ratio, 3.17 [95% CI, 2.05-4.91]) (6). Our patient's treatment providers elected not to prescribe streptomycin or gentamicin. Second-line agents with anti-*Brucella* activity include fluoroquinolones (ciprofloxacin and ofloxacin), which may be considered as part of a multidrug treatment regimen (as in this case) (4). For patients with neurobrucellosis, therapy should include ceftriaxone (2 g, IV, twice daily) for 1 month plus oral doxycycline and rifampin for 4 to 5 months. Optimal treatment of *Brucella* spondylitis and infective endocarditis is uncertain.

Travel-related infections may pose a diagnostic challenge. It is important to have a broad differential diagnosis that includes common and exotic infections.

References

1. Leder K, Torresi J, Libman MD, Cramer JP, Castelli F, Schlagenhauf P, et al; GeoSentinel Surveillance Network. GeoSentinel surveillance of illness in returned travelers, 2007-2011. Ann Intern Med. 2013 Mar 19;158(6):456–68.
2. McNabb SJ, Jajosky RA, Hall-Baker PA, Adams DA, Sharp P, Worshams C, et al; Centers for Disease Control and Prevention (CDC). Summary of notifiable diseases: United States, 2006. MMWR Morb Mortal Wkly Rep. 2008 Mar 21;55(53):1–92. Erratum in: MMWR Morb Mortal Wkly Rep. 2008 May 2;57(17):466.
3. Pappas G, Papadimitriou P, Akritidis N, Christou L, Tsianos EV. The new global map of human brucellosis. Lancet Infect Dis. 2006 Feb;6(2):91–9.
4. Gul HC, Erdem H. Brucellosis (*Brucella* species). In: Bennett JE, Dolin R, Blaser MJ, editors. Mandell, Douglas, and Bennett's principles and practice of infectious diseases. 9th ed. Philadelphia (PA): Elsevier; c2020. p. 2453–8.
5. Pappas G, Akritidis N, Bosilkovski M, Tsianos E. Brucellosis. N Engl J Med. 2005 Jun 2;352(22):2325–36.
6. Solis Garcia del Pozo J, Solera J. Systematic review and meta-analysis of randomized clinical trials in the treatment of human brucellosis. PLoS One. 2012;7(2):e32090. Epub 2012 Feb 29.

Dermatology Crisis

Sarwat Khalil, MBBS, and Omar M. Abu Saleh, MBBS

40

Case Presentation

A 67-year-old man from Minnesota with a history of nonalcoholic fatty liver disease and diabetes mellitus presented with an abdominal wall abscess that was treated with incision and drainage. He was prescribed a 2-week course of amoxicillin-clavulanate. Forty-eight hours later, he presented to the hospital with a 24-hour history of fever, chills, and a diffuse rash. He reported some skin discomfort and pruritus. He also had associated confusion, nausea, vomiting, and diarrhea. A physical examination showed that the patient was in distress, with a temperature of 39.4°C, heart rate of 127 beats/min, blood pressure of 84/54 mm Hg, and respiratory rate of 25 breaths/min. His oxygen saturation was 95% on ambient (room) air. His rash was diffuse and erythematous, with pustules, vesicles, and considerable dermal edema (Figures 40.1 and 40.2). The Nikolsky sign was negative. A chest radiograph was clear, and ultrasonography of the abdomen did not show any abnormalities. Initial laboratory test findings are shown in Table 40.1.

Amoxicillin-clavulanate was discontinued, and the patient began treatment with intravenous vancomycin and cefepime. A skin biopsy showed findings consistent with acute generalized exanthematous pustulosis (AGEP). The intravenous antibiotics were discontinued, and he began treatment with doxycycline. Gradually, his symptoms improved, and the rash resolved within 2 weeks after discontinuing the amoxicillin-clavulanate.

Discussion

Cutaneous reactions after antibiotic use most commonly present as exanthematous drug eruptions (80% of cases) or urticarial reactions (5%-10%) (1,2). These reactions are often mild and resolve quickly with discontinuation of the

Figure 40.1   Small, Pustular, Nonfollicular, and Erythematous Lesions of Acute Generalized Exanthematous Pustulosis

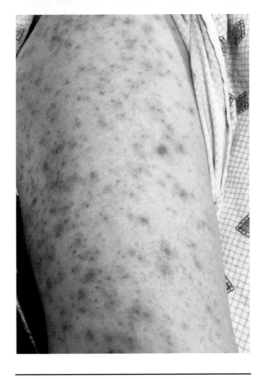

Figure 40.2   Close-up Image of Characteristic Pustular Lesions

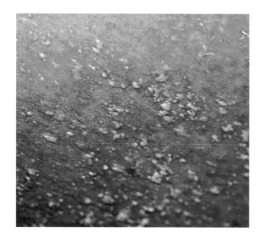

Table 40.1   Laboratory Test Results

Test	Value
White blood cell count, per mcL	32,000
Polymorphonuclear cells, %	94
Eosinophils, %	5
Aspartate aminotransferase, U/L	120
Alanine aminotransferase, U/L	240
Lactic acid, mmol/L	5

culprit drug. However, they can also rarely manifest as severe cutaneous reactions (<1 per 1,000 new cases) that are associated with severe, diffuse mucocutaneous involvement and severe systemic symptoms (2).

The type of drug reaction must be accurately established because some reactions are associated with a high risk of morbidity and mortality. The 3 most important drug reactions to consider are drug rash with eosinophilia and systemic symptoms (DRESS), Stevens-Johnson syndrome and toxic epidermal necrolysis (SJS-TEN), and AGEP. Several factors can be considered when determining the specific diagnosis, as summarized in Table 40.2, although the diagnosis is confirmed histopathologically.

Most AGEP cases are associated with antimicrobial agents, and aminopenicillins and macrolides are the more common culprits (2-4). AGEP and other skin reactions are T cell–mediated, delayed hypersensitivity reactions and can have varying severity. The AGEP rash usually appears within 24 to 48 hours of starting the offending drug, but the reaction can be delayed by up to a week (4). DRESS and SJS-TEN have a longer latency period of several days to weeks. The characteristic rash of AGEP consists of sterile, nonfollicular pustules on a background of erythematous and edematous dermis. It is more pronounced in skin folds, and facial edema is common. Lesions are mostly limited to the skin, and mucosal involvement is rare.

Although fever is present in AGEP, DRESS, and SJS-TEN, it is less pronounced in DRESS and SJS-TEN. Similarly, systemic signs are more severe and organ involvement is greater in DRESS and SJS-TEN. However, it is important to note that a small number of patients can have severe symptoms and organ involvement with AGEP, especially if patients are older or immunocompromised.

Common laboratory test findings include leukocytosis, with a markedly elevated neutrophil count. Peripheral eosinophilia is sometimes present. Classic histopathologic findings include considerable edema of the dermis and dermal infiltrates of neutrophils in the absence of bacteria (5). Tissue cultures are negative (3,5).

Symptoms resolve rapidly within 1 to 2 weeks after discontinuation of the offending agent, and patients rarely require any treatment. Desquamation occurs during the convalescence period. Death is rare (estimated at 2%) (3).

Table 40.2	Severe Cutaneous Drug Reactions			
Clinical Feature	Exanthematous Drug Eruption	Acute Generalized Exanthematous Pustulosis	Drug Rash With Eosinophilia and Systemic Symptoms	Stevens-Johnson Syndrome and Toxic Epidermal Necrolysis
Rash characteristics	Onset in 4-21 d after starting antibiotics (may be sooner in previously sensitized patients) Symmetric, maculopapular lesions Rapid spread, may coalesce	Onset in a few hours to ~3 d after the first dose of antibiotics Rapid evolution (within hours) Nonfollicular, sterile pustules on a background of edematous erythema More prominent in body folds	Onset in 2-8 wks (longer latency period) Severe, widespread rash involving >50% of body surface area Often a morbilliform eruption that rapidly progresses to diffuse erythema with follicular accentuation Associated with ≥2 of the following findings: facial edema, infiltrated lesions, scaling, or purpura	Onset in 1-4 wks, often starting on the face or thorax Ill-defined, coalescing, erythematous macules, with purpuric centers Markedly tender Positive Nikolsky sign
Systemic signs	Fever and other systemic symptoms are generally absent	Temperature >38°C	Temperature >38°C Malaise Lymphadenopathy (30%-60% of cases) ≥1 organ involved (90% of cases)	Often has a prodrome with influenza-like symptoms Temperature >38°C Oral mucosal involvement, with painful hemorrhagic erosions Severe conjunctivitis, corneal ulceration, uveitis (80% of cases) Urogenital involvement (67% of cases)
Laboratory test findings	Normal white blood cell count ± Eosinophilia	Leukocytosis Neutrophilia (>7,000×10^6/L) ± Mild eosinophilia	Leukocytosis Marked eosinophilia Atypical lymphocytes ± Elevated liver enzymes	Hematologic abnormalities (lymphopenia, anemia) Neutropenia (33% of cases) Eosinophilia is unusual Mildly elevated liver enzymes
Mucosal involvement	Absent	Rare	Infrequent	Common (>90% of cases)
Histopathologic findings	Superficial perivascular inflammatory infiltrate Subtle vacuolar interface dermatitis	Intracorneal or subcorneal spongiform pustules Dermal infiltrates rich in neutrophils Necrotic keratinocytes Marked edema of the dermis	Mild spongiosis with lymphocytic infiltrate, as well as eosinophils in the superficial dermis	Partial to full thickness epidermal necrosis with sparse inflammatory dermal infiltrate ± Subepidermal bullae Scant perivascular inflammatory cells with variable infiltrate

Abbreviation: ±, may be present or absent.

References

1. Stern RS. Clinical practice: exanthematous drug eruptions. N Engl J Med. 2012 Jun 28;366(26):2492–501.
2. Thong BY, Tan TC. Epidemiology and risk factors for drug allergy. Br J Clin Pharmacol. 2011 May;71(5): 684–700.
3. Saissi EH, Beau-Salinas F, Jonville-Bera AP, Lorette G, Autret-Leca E; Centres Regionaux de Pharmacovigilance. [Drugs associated with acute generalized exanthematic pustulosis]. Ann Dermatol Venereol. 2003 Jun-Jul;130(6-7):612–8. French.
4. Sidoroff A, Dunant A, Viboud C, Halevy S, Bavinck JN, Naldi L, et al. Risk factors for acute generalized exanthematous pustulosis (AGEP)-results of a multinational case-control study (EuroSCAR). Br J Dermatol. 2007 Nov;157(5):989–96. Epub 2007 Sep 13.
5. Halevy S, Kardaun SH, Davidovici B, Wechsler J; EuroSCAR and RegiSCAR study group. The spectrum of histopathological features in acute generalized exanthematous pustulosis: a study of 102 cases. Br J Dermatol. 2010 Dec;163(6):1245–52.

A 60-Year-Old Man With Multiple Falls

41

Madiha Fida, MBBS, Sara L. Cook, MD, PhD, and Omar M. Abu Saleh, MBBS

Case Presentation

A 60-year-old, previously healthy man presented with visual changes and an unsteady gait that had started 7 to 8 weeks ago. He first presented to the hospital 6 weeks earlier (2 weeks after symptom onset) and was admitted for further evaluation. Magnetic resonance imaging (MRI) of the cervical spine showed C6 to C7 disk bulging without any stenosis. A lumbar puncture was performed, but findings from a cerebrospinal fluid (CSF) analysis were essentially normal. He was discharged without a clear diagnosis. He continued to have frequent falls and had progressive confusion, tremors, worsening memory, and dysarthria in the subsequent weeks.

He did not have a history of fever, chills, neck stiffness, hallucinations, focal neurologic signs, or changes in bowel or bladder function. His medical history was significant only for a pituitary tumor, which was resected 2 years before his current presentation. He was born in the United States and had spent most of his life in the Midwest.

During the physical examination, he was somnolent and hypokinetic, with normal vital signs. He was able to open his eyes to voice but was able to make only incomprehensible sounds. His strength was reduced in all extremities, although his muscle tone and all deep tendon reflexes were normal. Plantar reflexes were intact bilaterally, and he had no neck stiffness. Laboratory tests, including complete blood counts and liver and kidney function, were within reference ranges. Tests for serum ceruloplasmin, antinuclear antibody, syphilis, and HIV were negative.

Computed tomography of the head without contrast did not show any intracranial abnormality. An MRI of the brain was obtained and showed uniform, symmetric signal abnormality in the caudate and putamen on T2 and fluid-attenuated inversion recovery (FLAIR)–weighted images (Figure 41.1). An electroencephalogram showed diffuse, nonspecific slowing of the background activity, consistent with moderately severe, diffuse cerebral dysfunction. The patient's neurologic status continued to decline, and he began to have startle myoclonus in the upper extremities and then the lower extremities. He eventually had akinetic mutism. A lumbar puncture was again performed, and the CSF analysis showed 3 nucleated cells, 11 erythrocytes, glucose level of 94 mg/dL (serum glucose was 123 mg/dL), and total protein level of 55 mg/dL (reference range, 0-35 mg/dL). Polymerase chain reaction tests for herpes simplex virus, varicella-zoster virus, cytomegalovirus, and Epstein-Barr virus in the CSF showed negative results. The CSF showed elevated 14-3-3 protein (3.9 ng/mL; reference range, <1.5 ng/mL), with elevated neuron-specific enolase (273 ng/mL; reference range, <15 ng/mL).

Given the imaging and CSF findings, a preliminary diagnosis of Creutzfeldt-Jakob disease (CJD) was made. After an extensive discussion with the family, the patient was transitioned to comfort care and died 1 week after the change

Figure 41.1   Magnetic Resonance Images of the Brain

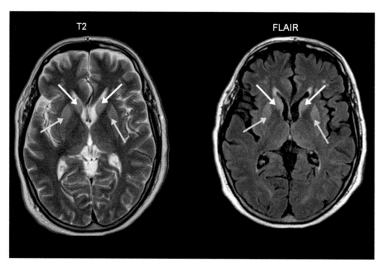

Uniform, symmetric signal abnormalities are seen in the caudate (white arrows) and putamen (yellow arrows) on T2 diffusion and fluid-attenuated inversion recovery (FLAIR)–weighted images.

in care status. An autopsy showed widespread, spongiform change in the neocortex and subcortical gray matter (Figure 41.2). Abnormal, protease-resistant prion protein was detected by Western blot analysis. Immunostaining with 3F4, the monoclonal antibody to prion protein, showed granular deposits that confirmed the diagnosis of CJD.

Figure 41.2   Photomicrograph of Brain Tissue Showing Creutzfeldt-Jakob Disease

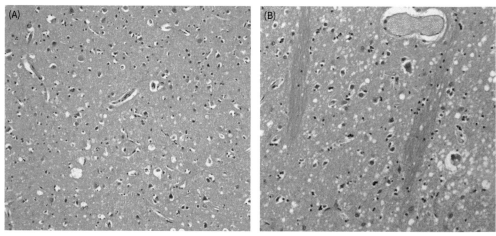

Tissue samples are stained with hematoxylin-eosin; original magnification, ×100. Prominent spongiotic changes are visible in the cortex (A) and basal ganglia (B).

Discussion

CJD, one of the most common forms of human prion disease, may be sporadic, familial, variant, or iatrogenic. The major pathologic finding of CJD is the abnormal prion protein that is highly resistant to digestion with protease. The abnormal protein subsequently accumulates and leads to progressive neurodegeneration.

More than 80% of CJD cases are caused by sporadic CJD, which typically affects people aged 57 to 62 years (1). Variant CJD has been associated with consumption of meat from cattle with bovine spongiform encephalopathy; it has predominantly psychiatric symptoms at presentation, with MRI showing symmetric FLAIR hyperintensities on the pulvinar (posterior) thalamic nuclei (termed the *pulvinar sign*). Iatrogenic CJD can occur after neurosurgical procedures with contaminated instruments, after corneal transplants and dural grafts, and with use of pituitary hormones extracted from patients with CJD (2-4).

Prions may remain infectious for several years in the dried form, so instruments should be kept moist until cleaned and decontaminated. Infectivity varies among different tissues and is highest for the brain, spinal cord, and eye; low-infectivity tissues include the CSF, lymph nodes, spleen, liver, kidneys, olfactory epithelium, and placenta (5). Valuable infection control guidelines for the prevention of iatrogenic and nosocomial transmission of transmissible spongiform encephalopathy have been developed by the World Health Organization (WHO). Disposable instruments should be incinerated if they come in contact with high- or low-infectivity tissues from patients with suspected or confirmed CJD. For reusable instruments that are heat sensitive, chemical sterilization agents such as sodium hypochlorite can be used; for heat-resistant instruments, chemical and autoclave sterilization are recommended. Instrument quarantine is often used when a patient is suspected of having CJD; instruments are subsequently processed according to the pathology results. The patient described above did have a pituitary tumor resected 2 years before disease development, but a definitive association is difficult to establish.

Clinical symptoms are characterized by rapidly progressive mental deterioration that may include dementia, behavioral changes, and impairment of memory and judgment. Myoclonus is a cardinal manifestation of CJD and is especially provoked by startling the patient. The diagnosis is made by considering a combination of clinical features, imaging findings, and CSF analysis, but the definitive diagnosis requires histopathologic analysis of brain tissue. Typical MRI findings include increased T2 and FLAIR signal intensity in the head of the caudate and putamen, which was seen in the patient described above, but different clinical syndromes and molecular subtypes may show different findings on MRI. Detection of 14-3-3 protein has 92% sensitivity and up to 80% specificity for diagnosing prion disease (6). Accumulation of the abnormal prion protein may be detected by immunohistochemical techniques. No effective treatment for CJD exists, and most individuals die within a year of diagnosis.

References

1. Ladogana A, Puopolo M, Croes EA, Budka H, Jarius C, Collins S, et al. Mortality from Creutzfeldt-Jakob disease and related disorders in Europe, Australia, and Canada. Neurology. 2005 May 10;64(9):1586–91.
2. Creange A, Gray F, Cesaro P, Adle-Biassette H, Duvoux C, Cherqui D, et al. Creutzfeldt-Jakob disease after liver transplantation. Ann Neurol. 1995 Aug;38(2):269–72.
3. Heckmann JG, Lang CJ, Petruch F, Druschky A, Erb C, Brown P, et al. Transmission of Creutzfeldt-Jakob disease via a corneal transplant. J Neurol Neurosurg Psychiatry. 1997 Sep;63(3):388–90.
4. Johnson RT, Gibbs CJ Jr. Creutzfeldt-Jakob disease and related transmissible spongiform encephalopathies. N Engl J Med. 1998 Dec 31;339(27):1994–2004.
5. WHO Infection Control Guidelines for Transmissible Spongiform Encephalopathies: report of a WHO consultation; Geneva, Switzerland, 23-26 March 1999. World Health Organization [cited 2021 Jan 29]. Available from: https://www.who.int/csr/resources/publications/bse/whocdscsraph2003.pdf?ua=1.
6. Muayqil T, Gronseth G, Camicioli R. Evidence-based guideline: diagnostic accuracy of CSF 14-3-3 protein in sporadic Creutzfeldt-Jakob disease: report of the guideline development subcommittee of the American Academy of Neurology. Neurology. 2012 Oct 2;79(14):1499–506. Epub 2012 Sep 19.

Flexor Tenosynovitis and Septic Arthritis After a Dog Bite

42

Talha Riaz, MBBS, and Omar M. Abu Saleh, MBBS

Case Presentation

A 52-year-old, right hand–dominant man was bitten by his brother's dog. The patient was trying to pet the dog when the dog bit his right middle finger. Forty-eight hours after the injury, he had marked swelling, redness, and pain in his right middle finger. The patient did not have a notable medical, surgical, or epidemiologic history. He had received a tetanus vaccine 1 month before the incident. The dog was also up to date with all its immunizations.

At presentation, the patient's vital signs were unremarkable. He had fusiform swelling of his right third finger, with puncture wounds on the dorsal and volar aspects of the proximal interphalangeal (PIP) joint, along with a small abscess on the dorsal aspect of the PIP joint (Figure 42.1).

The patient was able to actively extend and flex his right middle finger to 70 degrees. He had tenderness to palpation along the right long finger flexor tendon. A neurovascular examination had normal findings. An orthopedic hand surgeon evaluated the patient and, with regional

---

Figure 42.1   Images of the Dog Bite on the Patient's Right Middle Finger

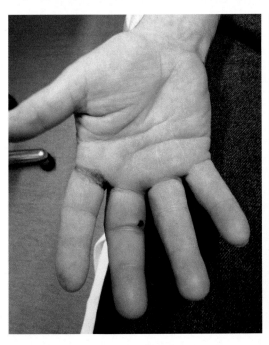
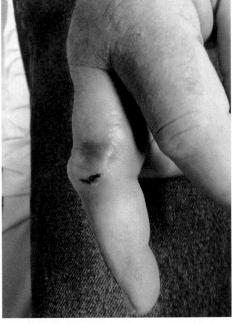

anesthesia, performed a bedside irrigation and débridement of the abscess. Scant purulence was noted, and specimens were obtained for Gram stain and cultures. The patient began treatment with intravenous ampicillin-sulbactam, and consultation with an infectious diseases physician was sought.

Pertinent laboratory test findings included elevated C-reactive protein (63.4 mg/L) and normal white blood cell and platelet counts. A radiograph of his hand did not show any fractures or retained foreign bodies. However, during the next 2 days, the patient had increased purulence and increased tenderness along the flexor and extensor tendons of his right middle finger. Wound cultures grew a gram-negative organism, *Pasteurella dagmatis*, that was sensitive to penicillin and ceftriaxone. Two days after the bedside procedure, he was taken to the operating room for irrigation and débridement of the flexor and extensor tendon sheaths and the PIP joint of the right long finger. Cloudy fluid was found along the flexor tendon sheath and around the PIP joint, and the joint capsule was punctured. His wounds were débrided and left to heal by primary intention. Intraoperative cultures grew oxacillin-sensitive, coagulase-negative *Staphylococcus*. Histopathologic evaluation of the flexor tenosynovium showed acute inflammation. His final diagnosis was flexor tenosynovitis and septic arthritis of the PIP joint of the right middle finger.

The patient was discharged home with a 3-week course of ceftriaxone (2 g, intravenous, once daily) and metronidazole (500 mg, oral, 3 times daily). At the end of therapy, his wounds had fully healed, and he had no signs of residual infection.

Discussion

Animal bites are a common health issue in the United States (1). According to 1 report, nearly 4.7 million Americans are bitten by animals annually (2). Dog bites are the most common type

of bite and typically involve those who own dogs as pets (3). In the United States, the reported incidence of emergency department–evaluated dog bite injuries ranges from 0.3% to 1.1% (4). Because dogs have rounded teeth and strong jaws, they can cause deep musculoskeletal injuries. Bites can cause puncture wounds and crush injuries (commonly on the right hand), and they can tear away body parts. Neurovascular structures can be damaged as well, depending on the depth of the bite.

Initial management of a dog bite warrants close inspection to ascertain the extent of injury, including identification of any devitalized tissues. Irrigation of the wound is critical for preventing infection. Microbiologic assessment is needed, and typically, aerobic and anaerobic cultures should be obtained, especially if the patient presents with an abscess. Radiographic imaging should be obtained to rule out fractures and foreign bodies. Patients should be assessed for the need for vaccination against rabies and tetanus. Patients require hospitalization if they have a late presentation, like the patient described above (who presented 48 hours after injury), and have an established infection that manifests as an abscess, cellulitis, and purulent discharge.

The bacteria that cause infection in bite wounds may originate from the dog's mouth, the patient's own skin, and the environment. Infection with *Streptococcus* species, *Staphylococcus* species, and oral anaerobes (eg, *Fusobacterium* and *Prevotella* species, *Capnocytophaga canimorsus*, *Pasteurella* species) warrant special attention. Of the bacteria from the Pasteurellaceae family that cause zoonotic infections in humans, *Pasteurella multocida* and *Pasteurella canis* are most commonly reported (5). *P dagmatis* is rather uncommon, although concurrent isolation of *P dagmatis* with another *Pasteurella* species has been reported (6). *Pasteurella* species are not susceptible to first-generation cephalosporins but are susceptible to penicillins.

For patients with a deep musculoskeletal injury, such as a puncture wound, it is important to ascertain whether bones, tendons, and joints have been infected. The choice of antibiotics and duration of therapy differ for cellulitis, tenosynovitis, and septic arthritis. For patients with a limited range of motion and chronic pain involving a joint, osteomyelitis also should be considered.

For dog bites, first-line oral therapy is amoxicillin-clavulanate. Other combinations of oral therapy include clindamycin or metronidazole plus either ciprofloxacin, levofloxacin, or trimethoprim-sulfamethoxazole. For higher-risk infections, as determined by the depth and extent of injury incurred plus the immune status of the patient, intravenous therapy is necessary. Intravenous options include ampicillin-sulbactam, cefoxitin, ertapenem, or moxifloxacin. No consensus has been reached about whether primary or secondary closure is more effective. Historically, primary closure has been linked with an increased risk of wound infection.

In conclusion, this case illustrates the importance of determining deeper bone and joint damage from a dog bite because the duration and choice of antibiotics differ for cellulitis versus tenosynovitis and septic arthritis.

References

1. DiPiro JT, Yee GC, Posey LM, Haines ST, Nolin TD, Ellingrod VL. Pharmacotherapy: a pathophysiologic approach, 11th ed. New York (NY): McGraw Hill Medical; 2020.

2. Sacks JJ, Kresnow M, Houston B. Dog bites: how big a problem? Inj Prev. 1996 Mar;2(1):52–4.

3. Presutti RJ. Prevention and treatment of dog bites. Am Fam Physician. 2001 Apr 15;63(8):1567–72.

4. Skurka J, Willert C, Yogev R. Wound infection following dog bite despite prophylactic penicillin. Infection. 1986 May-Jun;14(3):134–5.

5. Abrahamian FM, Goldstein EJ. Microbiology of animal bite wound infections. Clin Microbiol Rev. 2011 Apr;24(2):231–46.

6. Zbinden R, Sommerhalder P, von Wartburg U. Co-isolation of *Pasteurella dagmatis* and *Pasteurella multocida* from cat-bite wounds. Eur J Clin Microbiol Infect Dis. 1988 Apr;7(2):203–4.

Healthy Young Woman With Fever and Jaundice

43

FNU Shweta, MBBS, Eric C. Stone, MD, and Abinash Virk, MD

Case Presentation

A healthy, 22-year-old woman received vaccines for tetanus-diphtheria, hepatitis A, typhoid, and yellow fever (YF) before a trip to Bolivia. Five days after vaccination, she presented to an emergency department with myalgias, a fever of 39.7°C, and vomiting. She had tachycardia, tachypnea, and hypotension. A physical examination showed unremarkable findings, except for an enlarged and tender axillary lymph node ipsilateral to the vaccination site. She had mild leukocytosis with neutrophilic predominance and mildly elevated aspartate aminotransferase and international normalized ratio (INR) (Table 43.1).

Table 43.1.	Results of Hematologic Studies and Serum Levels of Yellow Fever Vaccine Viremia and Antibodies[a]							
Laboratory Test	**Reference Range**	**Postvaccine Day**						
		5	**6**	**7**	**8**	**9**	**10**	**11**
White blood cells, ×10⁹/L	3.5-10.5	11.5	9.0	2.0	4.0	2.0	5.2	0.8
Hemoglobin, g/dL	12.0-15.5	13.5	13.0	11.0	9.3	7.7	10.0	10.4
Platelets, ×10⁹/L	150-450	230	198	43	35	18	16	14
Bicarbonate (serum), mmol/L	22-29	25	24	16	8	18	20	19
Creatinine, mg/dL	0.6-1.1	1.1	0.9	2.7	5.3	3.7	1.9	1.8
AST, U/L	12-31	57	67	418	987	616	459	353
ALT, U/L	9-29	27	28	178	322	223	160	103
INR	0.9-1.1	1.3	1.1	1.4	1.5	1.4	1.3	1.5
Bilirubin, total, mg/dL	0.1-1.0	0.9	NA	4.0	7.4	6.7	7.0	7.3
Alkaline phosphatase, U/L	55-142	84	NA	414	157	111	NA	125
pH	7.35-7.45	NA	NA	7.31	7.15	7.24	7.20	7.16
Lactate, mmol/L	0.6-2.3	NA	NA	4.0	3.9	6.2	6.4	NA
PaO₂, mm Hg	70-100	NA	NA	35	59	49	34	39
PaCO₂, mm Hg	35-45	NA	NA	32	40	48	48	56
Viremia, PFU/mL	NA	61,000	106,500	46,500	329	89	47	67
Neutralizing antibodies, GMT	NA	<10	<10	<10	40	640	2,560	ND
Immunoglobulin M	NA	Neg	Neg	Neg	Pos	Pos	Pos	ND

Abbreviations: ALT, alanine aminotransferase; AST, aspartate aminotransferase; GMT, geometric mean titer; INR, international normalized ratio; NA, not available; ND, not determined; Neg, Negative; PFU, plaque-forming unit; pH, arterial blood pH; Pos, positive.

[a] The values shown are the most abnormal values reported during each 24-hour period.

Twenty-four hours later, she had abdominal pain, loose stools, and recurrent fever. Pancytopenia developed while her aspartate aminotransferase and total bilirubin levels and INR increased. She was transferred to the intensive care unit 7 days after the YF vaccination, and a chest radiograph showed new pleural effusions (Figure 43.1), leading to a tamponade-like physiology. An HIV serologic test was negative. The patient's condition worsened, despite hemodialysis and administration of vasopressors, intravenous (IV) immunoglobulin, and IV hydrocortisone (50 mg, every 6 hours). She required mechanical ventilation, nitric oxide therapy, high-frequency oscillatory ventilation, and extracorporeal membrane oxygenation. A repeat transthoracic echocardiogram showed an

Figure 43.1   Chest Radiograph

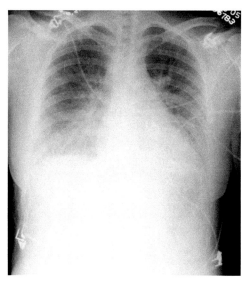

Image was obtained after admission to the intensive care unit.

(From Belsher JL, Gay P, Brinton M, DellaValla J, Ridenour R, Lanciotti R, et al. Fatal multiorgan failure due to yellow fever vaccine-associated viscerotropic disease. Vaccine. 2007 Dec 5;25[50]:8480-5. Epub 2007 Sep 18; used with permission.)

ejection fraction of 15%. Broad-spectrum antibiotic therapy was started.

Eleven days after YF vaccination, the patient died. Blood cultures grew group C β-hemolytic *Streptococcus*. Cultures of pleural fluid grew the same organism plus *Staphylococcus aureus*. An autopsy showed multiorgan failure and findings consistent with disseminated intravascular coagulation (Figure 43.2). The lungs showed diffuse alveolar hemorrhage and acute necrotizing bronchopneumonia. Postmortem blood cultures grew *S aureus*.

Tissue samples were sent to the Centers for Disease Control and Prevention for immuno-histochemical and histopathologic evaluation. Yellow fever vaccine (YFV) antigens were detected in the kidney but not in the liver, spleen, heart, or lungs. Histopathologic findings from the liver included microvesicular steatosis and Councilman bodies, which are seen in wild-type YF. Plasma and serum samples were tested with reverse-transcriptase polymerase chain reaction assays for 17D vaccine RNA. Estimated viral titers are shown in Table 43.1. Viremia decreased with the development of YF virus–specific neutralizing and immunoglobulin M antibodies but remained detectable. The consensus sequence of the patient's viral RNA showed 100% nucleotide identity to the virus from the vaccine lot.

Discussion

YFV is a live, attenuated viral vaccine that generates highly protective antibodies within 7 to 10 days after vaccination. Travelers to high-risk areas are advised to undergo vaccination; however, YFV can have rare but severe adverse events, including YFV-associated neurologic disease (YEL-AND; 0.8 events per 100,000 doses) and YFV-associated viscerotropic disease

Figure 43.2   Autopsy Specimens

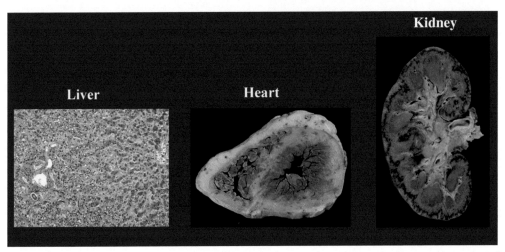

The liver shows midzonal necrosis, with sparing of hepatocytes around the central vein and portal triad (hematoxylin-eosin; original magnification, ×100). The heart shows circumferential subendocardial hemorrhage involving both ventricles, with petechial hemorrhages present over the epicardium. The kidney shows diffuse cortical hemorrhages with subcapsular infarction.

(From Belsher JL, Gay P, Brinton M, DellaValla J, Ridenour R, Lanciotti R, et al. Fatal multiorgan failure due to yellow fever vaccine-associated viscerotropic disease. Vaccine. 2007 Dec 5;25[50]:8480-5. Epub 2007 Sep 18; used with permission.)

(YEL-AVD; 0.3 events per 100,000 doses). Other severe adverse events include hypersensitivity reactions such as anaphylaxis, which affects about 1.3 per 100,000 doses, according to US national surveillance data. Therefore, a risk-benefit assessment and patient counseling should occur before vaccination.

The risks of YEL-AND and YEL-AVD increase with age and are up to 3 to 4 times higher for vaccine recipients aged 60 years and older. YEL-AND is characterized by encephalitis, meningitis, Guillain-Barré syndrome, or acute disseminated encephalomyelitis within 28 days after vaccination. Meningoencephalitis is the most common manifestation. Diagnosis can be aided by polymerase chain reaction testing of cerebrospinal fluid for YF virus or for antibodies specific to the YF virus. Most patients with YEL-AND recover without residual deficits. Treatment should be chosen on the basis of the presenting syndrome and a neurologic consultation is warranted. The patient described above had YEL-AVD, which is the most severe adverse reaction to YFV. It is characterized by acute multiorgan dysfunction after primary vaccination and causes death in up to 60% of cases. The average time to symptom onset is 3 to 14 days (1). YEL-AVD signs and symptoms mirror those of wild-type YF, and findings may include fever, nausea, vomiting, headache, diarrhea, myalgias, arthralgias, and malaise. Later stages may include hepatic failure, elevated liver enzyme and bilirubin levels, renal failure, hypotension, thrombocytopenia, respiratory failure, and bleeding diathesis. Less commonly, disseminated intravascular coagulation and rhabdomyolysis are observed. Dissemination of the live, attenuated virus is believed to cause YEL-AND and YEL-AVD. Treatment of YEL-AND and YEL-AVD is supportive (2).

References

1. Lindsey NP, Rabe IB, Miller ER, Fischer M, Staples JE. Adverse event reports following yellow fever vaccination, 2007-13. J Travel Med. 2016 Jul 4;23(5).

2. Gershman MD, Staples JE, Bentsi-Enchill AD, Breugelmans JG, Brito GS, Camacho LA, et al; Brighton Collaboration Viscerotropic Disease Working Group. Viscerotropic disease: case definition and guidelines for collection, analysis, and presentation of immunization safety data. Vaccine. 2012 Jul 13;30(33):5038–58. Epub 2012 May 4.

Does It Always Have to Be a Burning Sensation?

44

Aditya S. Shah, MBBS, and John W. Wilson, MD

Case Presentation

A 33-year-old man presented for discussion of preexposure prophylaxis for HIV. He reported sexual activity with men, including insertive and receptive anal intercourse and oral intercourse. He had no past medical problems and had no symptoms consistent with sexually transmitted infections (STIs), such as dysuria, rectal pain, skin lesions, fevers, chills, urethral discharge, lymphadenopathy, or oropharyngeal exudates.

At presentation, he received screening tests for HIV, syphilis, gonorrhea, and chlamydia. The HIV test was a fourth-generation antibody-antigen assay, and the syphilis test was a serologic immunoglobulin G assay. The patient's urine was tested for gonorrhea and chlamydia infection with ligase chain reaction (LCR) assays. The patient also had serologic tests for hepatitis A, B, and C viral infections. All baseline test results were negative for infection. However, because of his high-risk behavior, we additionally submitted an oropharyngeal swab for gonorrheal and chlamydial testing by LCR. Despite the absence of adverse throat symptoms, his test results were positive for *Neisseria gonorrhoeae* infection. The patient was treated with a single 250-mg dose of intramuscular ceftriaxone plus a single 1-g dose of oral azithromycin.

Discussion

Gonorrhea is caused by the gram-negative coccobacilli *N gonorrhoeae* (1). This infection can cause a wide spectrum of symptoms in men and women. Men with gonococcal urethritis often present with the more recognizable and frequent symptoms of urethral discharge and dysuria compared with women with cervicitis. In women, classic manifestations are cervicitis, infertility, ectopic pregnancy, chronic pelvic pain, and pelvic inflammatory disease, but women commonly may be asymptomatic. Thus, women must be tested for infection, regardless of symptoms, when their partner has a suspected or confirmed STI (1).

For men, classic manifestations of gonorrhea include urethritis (when limited to the urogenital region) and oropharyngeal exudates with lymphadenopathy (when limited to the oropharyngeal region) (1), although men may also have asymptomatic infections. Extragenital infections (eg, in the rectal and oropharyngeal regions [1]) are common in certain high-risk groups, namely men who have sex with men (MSM), but they are common and known complications in women as well. Thus, gonococcal infection should be considered for various genital and extragenital clinical presentations among sexually active individuals. The Centers for Disease Control and Prevention (CDC) also recommends annual screening for gonorrhea in all sexually active women younger than 25 years and older women with increased risk (eg, due to new or multiple sex partners or a sex partner with a sexually transmitted disease) (1).

With regard to diagnostic tests, a nucleic acid amplification test (NAAT) such as LCR is preferred for diagnosing genital and extragenital gonococcal infections (1,2). Compared with culture, NAATs have a faster turnaround time and improved sensitivity, although NAATs cannot provide antimicrobial susceptibility information (1,2). Another advantage of NAAT is that it can also be used with swabs from different anatomical locations, including the cervix, rectum, and throat (1,2).

Gram stains of urethral secretions showing neutrophils and intracellular, gram-negative diplococci have good sensitivity and specificity for diagnosing gonorrhea in symptomatic men. However, a negative Gram stain does not rule out infection. For symptomatic men, the main role of Gram stain is to diagnose the cause of urethritis (3). For men with urethritis due to gonorrhea, Gram stain of a urethral sample often shows gram-negative diplococci (3). Gram stain is less diagnostically useful in samples taken from the urogenital tract of women and from extragenital regions of men and women because of the presence of other commensal *Neisseria* species and other gram-negative bacteria (3).

For men, more than 50% of *N gonorrhoeae* infections are asymptomatic or mild (1). Symptoms may include epididymitis and urethritis (4). Classic symptoms of urethritis are urethral discharge and dysuria (1). Men with epididymitis usually have concerns about testicular pain and swelling, with concomitant urethritis. Laboratory tests such as a urinalysis often show more than 2 white blood cells per high-power field or more than 10 white blood cells per mcL on microscopic examination (2). NAATs are the most sensitive and specific diagnostic tests for gonorrhea and chlamydia infections that are limited to the urogenital tract (1,2).

The rectal and oropharyngeal regions are extragenital sites that can be infected with gonorrhea. For men (typically MSM), rectal manifestations include proctitis (4). Interestingly, for women, anal or rectal canal gonococcal infection can occur even in the absence of receptive anal intercourse, possibly because of contiguous spread of infection from the vagina to the anal region (4). Most cases of anorectal gonococcal infection are asymptomatic. Symptoms, if present, include constipation, anorectal discharge, bleeding, pain, and tenesmus (4).

Symptoms of oropharyngeal infection include oropharyngeal exudate, pain, and lymphadenopathy. The mode of infection is usually oral sexual exposure. However, most cases of oropharyngeal infection are asymptomatic, like the patient described above, so it is therefore important to test patients on the basis of high-risk behavior (3).

Several universal preexposure prophylaxis guidelines (from Canada [5] and from the CDC [2]) recommend screening for gonorrhea and chlamydia at 3-month intervals and at 3 sites: the pharynx, urethra, and rectum. This approach aims to screen all high-risk individuals and treat them and their contacts to prevent further linear transmission of infection. STIs are increasingly common in the United States, and providers should have a low threshold for testing and treating patients.

Ceftriaxone cures about 98% to 99% of uncomplicated gonorrhea infections (6), but dual treatment with ceftriaxone and azithromycin is recommended. The 2 main reasons for dual treatment of gonorrhea infection are the rising rates of drug-resistant gonorrhea and coinfection with chlamydia. Ceftriaxone and azithromycin have different mechanisms of action, which improve efficacy and possibly slow the emergence of ceftriaxone resistance. If patients have treatment failure, defined as symptoms that persist despite adhering to the recommended regimen of ceftriaxone and azithromycin, the CDC currently recommends culturing for *Neisseria* (1).

The classic treatment regimen for gonorrhea infection is intramuscular ceftriaxone (a single 250-mg dose) and oral azithromycin (a single 1-g dose). This regimen is used for uncomplicated genital gonorrhea infection and for extragenital infections in the pharyngeal and conjunctival regions (6). Patients with proctitis and epididymitis should receive intramuscular ceftriaxone (a single 250-mg intramuscular injection) plus doxycycline (100 mg, oral, twice daily for 10 days) (6). Retesting is recommended 3 months after the infection is treated because patients with gonorrhea constitute a high-risk group with potential for reinfection (6).

References

1. Centers for Disease Control and Prevention. Sexually transmitted disease surveillance: 2017 [Internet]. Atlanta (GA); US Department of Health and Human Services; 2018 [cited 2021 Mar 17]. Available from: https://www.cdc.gov/std/stats17/2017-STD-Surveillance-Report_CDC-clearance-9.10.18.pdf.

2. Centers for Disease Control and Prevention. Recommendations for the laboratory-based detection of *Chlamydia trachomatis* and *Neisseria gonorrhoeae*: 2014. MMWR Recomm Rep. 2014 Mar 14;63(RR-02):1–19.

3. Sherrard J, Barlow D. Gonorrhoea in men: clinical and diagnostic aspects. Genitourin Med. 1996 Dec;72(6):422–6.

4. Chan PA, Robinette A, Montgomery M, Almonte A, Cu-Uvin S, Lonks JR, et al. Extragenital infections caused by *Chlamydia trachomatis* and *Neisseria gonorrhoeae*: a review of the literature. Infect Dis Obstet Gynecol. 2016;2016:5758387. Epub 2016 Jun 5.

5. Canadian Guideline on HIV Pre-exposure Prophylaxis and Nonoccupational Postexposure Prophylaxis [Internet]. Toronto (Ontario) [cited 2021 Mar 18]. CATIE: Canada's source for HIV and hepatitis C information. Available from: https://www.catie.ca/en/canadian-guideline-prep-npep.

6. Workowski KA, Bolan GA; Centers for Disease Control and Prevention. Sexually transmitted diseases treatment guidelines, 2015. MMWR Recomm Rep. 2015 Jun 5;64(RR-03):1–137. Erratum in: MMWR Recomm Rep. 2015 Aug 28;64(33):924.

The Furuncle Keeps Getting Worse

45

Edison J. Cano Cevallos, MD, and Daniel C. DeSimone, MD

Case Presentation

A 52-year-old woman presented to the emergency department with concerns about chest pain and erythema circumscribing her left inframammary fold that started 3 days earlier as a small furuncle. She reported manipulating the lesion but was unable to extrude it successfully. Afterward, she noted local symptoms and generalized weakness, fever, nausea, and vomiting. Her medical history was remarkable for obesity (body mass index, 51 kg/m²), uncontrolled type 2 diabetes mellitus (a recent hemoglobin A_{1c} level was 9.8%), and severe chronic periodontitis that was diagnosed when she was 15 years old and required full-mouth extraction. She denied any previous similar episodes and had no history of recent antibiotic use or contact with people who were ill. A physical examination showed erythema and tenderness in the midsternal area, extending to the inframammary fold, with no fluctuance. Laboratory studies showed leukocytosis, with 13.5×10^9 cells/L and 79.3% neutrophils. She received 1 dose of piperacillin-tazobactam, and at discharge, she was prescribed amoxicillin-clavulanate for a week.

She did not improve, and 2 days later, she presented to the emergency department with worsening pain and progression of the chest wall erythema. A computed tomographic (CT) image with intravenous contrast showed cellulitis on the left side of her chest with phlegmonous changes, but no subcutaneous emphysema or pleural effusions were identified (Figure 45.1). She started treatment with oral trimethoprim-sulfamethoxazole because of concerns about methicillin-resistant *Staphylococcus aureus* and was discharged.

Despite the change in antimicrobial therapy, her condition progressively worsened and she presented again 4 days later, a total of 8 days after the furuncle was initially noted. She reported chest pain that was disproportionately high, with worsening erythema and tense skin induration. A repeat CT image of the chest showed interval progression of edematous changes and new multiloculated, emphysematous collections in the subcutaneous tissues that extended to the anterior margin of the pectoralis muscle and suggested a necrotizing infection (Figure 45.2).

Figure 45.1　Computed Tomographic Image

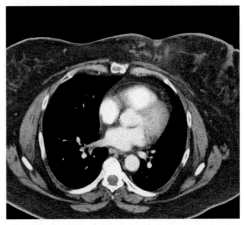

The image shows subcutaneous edema consistent with cellulitis of the left inframammary fold and a possible initial furuncle.

Figure 45.2   Computed Tomographic Image

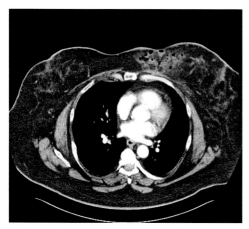

Emphysematous changes are seen 8 days after initial symptoms were noted.

The patient was transferred to our institution. At admission, she received piperacillin-tazobactam and vancomycin and underwent extensive débridement of skin and subcutaneous tissue (Figure 45.3). Multiple loculations and a large amount of purulence were noted with the incision, but the pectoralis muscle fascia

Figure 45.3   Site of Surgical Excision

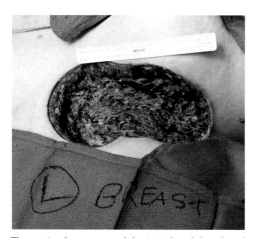

The excised area around the initial multiloculated abscess was 15×5×5 cm.

was intact and there was no evidence of muscle involvement.

Initial assessment of the purulent sample obtained intraoperatively showed non–spore-forming, gram-positive anaerobic bacillus (more than 2 species in semiquantitative cultures). *Actinomyces europaeus* was identified from anaerobic cultures. Other associated bacteria (termed *companion pathogens*) were identified by cultures, including *Corynebacterium simulans*, *Ralstonia pickettii*, *Dialister micraerophilus*, *Prevotella bergensis*, and *Porphyromonas levii* or *Porphyromonas somerae*. Other anaerobic flora that were susceptible to piperacillin-tazobactam were present, but specific species were not further identified.

The patient showed marked improvement after surgical débridement. The erythema that extended beyond the resection resolved in 2 days, and the wound was treated with negative pressure. The pathologic assessment confirmed abscesses with acute inflammation. At discharge, the patient began treatment with intravenous ertapenem for 4 weeks and then amoxicillin (875 mg, oral, twice daily for 6 months). She had a favorable response and no evidence of recurrence.

Discussion

The initial presentation was consistent with a chest wall cellulitis that started as a furuncle in a patient with diabetes mellitus. Nonetheless, the infection progressed deeper into the tissue, despite treatment with antibiotics that targeted common skin pathogens. Further deterioration after 8 days, with emphysematous changes on a chest CT image, raised concerns about the possibilities of antibiotic failure, uncommon pathogens, or need for surgical intervention. Her associated symptoms, clinical course, and imaging and laboratory findings were suggestive of a severe infection, even early in the course, and the surgical intervention was critical for providing a diagnosis and markedly improving her clinical status.

The genus *Actinomyces* comprises filamentous, gram-positive, non–spore-forming, anaerobic bacteria that are found ubiquitously in the soil and are also a commensal organism in the human mouth, gastrointestinal tract, and urogenital tract (1). Actinomycosis represents an invasive infection by an *Actinomyces* organism that is characterized by continuous and progressive spread, often across tissue planes. Sometimes, sinus tracts can form, and sulfur granules can be present in up to 75% of cases (2,3). *Actinomyces israelii* is the most prevalent species, but other clinically relevant species include *Actinomyces viscosus, Actinomyces meyeri, Actinomyces naeslundii, Actinomyces odontolyticus, Actinomyces gerencseriae, Actinomyces turicensis,* and *Actinomyces europaeus* (4).

The classic and most common presentation (~60% of reported cases) is cervicofacial actinomycosis. It is characterized by slow progression of a painless, indurated abscess that forms deep sinus tracts and most commonly originates from odontogenic infections (5). Actinomycosis also can arise from colonized sites, where a disruption of the tissues facilitates infection (eg, genitourinary tract infection due to an intrauterine device, invasion of the gastrointestinal tract after mucosal injury or surgery). Respiratory tract actinomycosis can present as a mass-like pulmonary consolidation, and its risk factors include alcohol abuse and poor dentition (2). A well-known phenomenon of actinomycosis is the presence of companion pathogens that facilitate virulence, as reported in the case description above.

Actinomycosis of the skin and soft tissues is rare and mostly occurs after direct inoculation. It presents as a superficial skin infection that progresses slowly to involve multiple tissue planes and form multiple sinus tracts. It responds poorly to oral antibiotics. Several cases of breast infections caused by *Actinomyces* species have been reported (6), with recent literature describing the emergence of *A europaeus* (7-12).

Surgical intervention is paramount in the management of patients with actinomycosis (13). Fortunately, *Actinomyces* species have good susceptibility to penicillin, ceftriaxone, vancomycin, linezolid, and ertapenem, despite small differences among species (14,15). A combination of surgical débridement plus intravenous antibiotics is widely recommended, followed by 3 to 6 months of treatment with oral antimicrobial agents, provided that the patient has improvement after surgical intervention and no evidence of recurrence (4).

References

1. Bennett JE, Dolin R, Blaser MJ, editors. Mandell, Douglas, and Bennett's principles and practice of infectious diseases. 9th ed. Philadelphia (PA): Elsevier; c2020. 3839 p.
2. Valour F, Senechal A, Dupieux C, Karsenty J, Lustig S, Breton P, et al. Actinomycosis: etiology, clinical features, diagnosis, treatment, and management. Infect Drug Resist. 2014 Jul 5;7:183–97.
3. Holm P. Studies on the aetiology of human actinomycosis. II. Do the other microbes of actinomycosis possess virulence? Acta Pathol Microbiol Scand. 1951;28(4):391–406.
4. Wong VK, Turmezei TD, Weston VC. Actinomycosis. BMJ. 2011 Oct 11;343:d6099.
5. Pulverer G, Schutt-Gerowitt H, Schaal KP. Human cervicofacial actinomycoses: microbiological data for 1997 cases. Clin Infect Dis. 2003 Aug 15;37(4):490–7. Epub 2003 Jul 30.
6. Bing AU, Loh SF, Morris T, Hughes H, Dixon JM, Helgason KO. *Actinomyces* species isolated from breast infections. J Clin Microbiol. 2015 Oct;53(10):3247–55. Epub 2015 Jul 29.
7. Nielsen HL. First report of *Actinomyces europaeus* bacteraemia result from a breast abscess in a 53-year-old man. New Microbes New Infect. 2015 May 14;7:21–2.
8. Silva WA, Pinheiro AM, Jahns B, Bogli-Stuber K, Droz S, Zimmerli S. Breast abscess due to *Actinomyces europaeus*. Infection. 2011 Jun;39(3):255–8. Epub 2011 Apr 21.
9. Zautner AE, Schmitz S, Aepinus C, Schmialek A, Podbielski A. Subcutaneous fistulae in a patient with femoral hypoplasia due to *Actinomyces europaeus* and *Actinomyces turicensis*. Infection. 2009 Jun;37(3):289–91. Epub 2008 Oct 14.
10. Funke G, Alvarez N, Pascual C, Falsen E, Akervall E, Sabbe L, et al. *Actinomyces europaeus* sp. nov., isolated

from human clinical specimens. Int J Syst Bacteriol. 1997 Jul;47(3):687–92.

11. Zarrif-Nabbali H, Bolanos-Rivero M, Navarro-Navarro R, Martin-Sanchez AM. [A sebaceous cyst infection by *Actinomyces europaeus*]. Enferm Infecc Microbiol Clin. 2016 May;34(5):324–5. Epub 2015 Sep 7. Spanish.

12. White SE, Woolley SD. *Actinomyces europaeus* isolated from a breast abscess in a penicillin-allergic patient. Case Rep Infect Dis. 2018 Jun 20;2018:6708614.

13. Cope VZ. Surgery in actinomycosis. In: Human actinomycosis: what the general practitioner ought to know about. London (Eng): William Heinemann Medical Books LTD; 2013. p. 69–70.

14. Barberis C, Budia M, Palombarani S, Rodriguez CH, Ramirez MS, Arias B, et al. Antimicrobial susceptibility of clinical isolates of *Actinomyces* and related genera reveals an unusual clindamycin resistance among *Actinomyces urogenitalis* strains. J Glob Antimicrob Resist. 2017 Mar;8:115–20. Epub 2017 Jan 18.

15. Goldstein EJ, Citron DM, Merriam CV, Warren YA, Tyrrell KL, Fernandez H. Comparative in vitro activities of ertapenem (MK-0826) against 469 less frequently identified anaerobes isolated from human infections. Antimicrob Agents Chemother. 2002 Apr;46(4):1136–40.

Oral Ulcers in an Immunocompromised Patient

46

Tariq Azam, MD, and Mark J. Enzler, MD

Case Presentation

A cachectic, 81-year-old man from rural southern Minnesota presented with concerns about progressive pain on the left lateral side of his tongue, a hard palate, and right upper gingival ulcerations. These lesions had been worsening for 6 months and were associated with odynophagia, an unintentional weight loss of 35 kg, severe fatigue, anorexia, dry cough, and intermittent diarrhea. The lesions appeared a few months after completing salvage therapy for non-Hodgkin lymphoma with bendamustine and rituximab. The salvage treatment was followed by rituximab maintenance therapy, but this therapy had been paused for the past 4 months because of the painful ulcers. A physical examination showed that the patient had normal vital signs, a normal heart and lungs, no palpable adenopathy, abdominal mass, or organomegaly, and no abdominal pain. An oral examination showed a large, deep ulceration on the left lateral aspect of the tongue (Figure 46.1), a large upper-gingival ulcer, and a soft-palate ulcer.

Lingual and gingival biopsies showed squamous mucosa with granulation tissue and acute and chronic inflammation. No direct immunofluorescence was performed and a polymerase chain reaction test for herpes simplex virus was negative. Histoplasma serology test results were negative in the setting of absent B cells. Laboratory tests showed a low level of T cells (197 cells/mcL; reference range, 500-1,600 cells/mcL) and immunoglobulin G (535 mg/dL; reference range, >766 mg/dL). Alanine aminotransferase was mildly elevated (55 U/L; reference range, ≤55 U/L),

as was alkaline phosphatase (216 U/L; reference range, ≤115 U/L). His white blood cell and platelet counts were normal, and he had mild normocytic, normochromic anemia (hemoglobin, 11.6 g/dL; reference range, 13.5-17.5 g/dL).

One week later, fungal cultures from a lingual ulcer swab grew *Histoplasma capsulatum*, and a test for *Histoplasma* urine antigen was markedly positive (12.5 IU/L; reference range, <0.5 IU/L). A subsequent hard-palate biopsy showed benign squamous mucosa with ulceration and granulomatous inflammation. Fungal staining with Grocott methenamine silver (GMS) showed small, budding yeast consistent with *Histoplasma* (Figure 46.2). He was diagnosed with disseminated histoplasmosis (DH) that manifested as oral histoplasmosis. He was hospitalized for initiation of induction antifungal therapy with intravenous amphotericin B, which he received for 2 weeks, and initiation of oral itraconazole. A

Figure 46.1   Left Lingual Ulceration

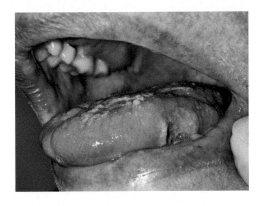

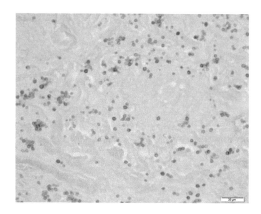

Figure 46.2   Grocott Methenamine Silver Stain of the Palate Ulcer Biopsy Specimen Shows Small Yeast Forms

colonoscopy showed colonic mucosa with active inflammation; focal ulcerations also were noted, with rare yeast forms that were identified with GMS staining. Cytomegalovirus was not identified by immunostaining.

One month after starting antifungal therapy, he had marked clinical improvement, with smaller ulcerations on his tongue, palate, and gingiva that were now pain free, and his anorexia resolved. A urine test for *Histoplasma* antigen showed negative results after 9 months of therapy, and the patient completed 12 months of itraconazole therapy.

Discussion

H capsulatum is the most common cause of endemic dimorphic fungal infection in the United States, and it is endemic in the Ohio and Mississippi River Valleys and parts of Central and South America. Infections are acquired by inhaling spores that are present in the environment, and the disease often is associated with bird or bat guano or farm exposures. Although most *H capsulatum* infections (>90%) are asymptomatic and self-limited, 1 in 2,000 acute

infections may result in severe, progressive DH (1). Immunocompromised patients are at increased risk for more severe forms of histoplasmosis in the setting of either acute or recrudescent infections (2,3). DH is associated with the spread of infection to extrapulmonary organs such as lymph nodes, skin, adrenal glands, brain, wrist tendons or synovium, gastrointestinal tract, liver, bone marrow, oral mucosa, and heart valves (rare). Our patient presented with classic findings of DH that included weight loss, liver enzyme abnormalities, diarrhea associated with colonic involvement, anemia, and multiple painful oral cavity ulcerations.

Diagnosis of DH requires a clinical suspicion of histoplasmosis for patients residing in *Histoplasma*-endemic regions and patients who have been exposed to birds or bird guano. DH is confirmed by *H capsulatum* cultured from bodily fluids or tissue biopsies. The presence of *Histoplasma* antigen in the blood or urine is highly suggestive of infection. *Histoplasma* complement fixation or immunodiffusion serologic tests may suggest histoplasmosis, but they do not confirm active *Histoplasma* infection (1,4). If histoplasmosis is suspected and the patient presents with oral manifestations, a biopsy of the lesion should be performed. The specimen will typically show granulomatous inflammation, and small yeast forms may be seen with fungal-specific staining. The biopsy specimen from the oral mucosa can be cultured, and identification of *H capsulatum* will confirm the diagnosis.

The frequency of severe DH cases has increased during the past 10 years. Patients often are immunocompromised and have been receiving tumor necrosis factor−α inhibitor therapies or other therapies that decrease immune function (5). Oral histoplasmosis has been a relatively uncommon manifestation of disseminated histoplasmosis, with only scattered single case reports published in the past 10 years, although surprisingly, a 1980 study by Goodwin et al (2) reported oral histoplasmosis in 28 (27%) of 102 patients with DH. More recently, our practice has seen an increase in patients with oropharyngeal histoplasmosis involving the tongue, gingiva, palate, or larynx as a manifestation of DH. Of the 9 patients in our practice with oral histoplasmosis–associated DH seen from 1995 through 2016, 5 were seen after 2012 (6).

Patients with DH-associated oral histoplasmosis present with severe pain from oral mucosal lesions that may involve the tongue, gingiva, or palate, and patients typically present with other manifestations of DH such as weight loss, anemia, and elevated liver enzymes (6). Laryngeal histoplasmosis may present with odynophagia, hoarse voice, and aspiration. Primary care physicians, dentists, and oral surgeons may not recognize the clinical significance of oral lesions in patients living in *Histoplasma*-endemic regions if DH is undiagnosed. In our case series (6), we noted a median delay in oral histoplasmosis diagnosis of 5 months (range, 1-12 months). Because painful oral lesions may be the only clinical manifestation of DH, clinicians should arrange for biopsy of oral or laryngeal lesions and have samples assessed histopathologically and with fungal-specific culture and stains.

References

1. Deepe GS. *Histoplasma capsulatum* (histoplasmosis). In: Bennett JE, Dolin R, Blaser MJ, editors Mandell, Douglas, and Bennett's principals and practice of infectious diseases. 9th ed. Philadelphia (PA): Elsevier. c2020. p. 3162–76.
2. Goodwin RA Jr, Shapiro JL, Thurman GH, Thurman SS, Des Prez RM. Disseminated histoplasmosis: clinical and pathologic correlations. Medicine (Baltimore). 1980 Jan;59(1):1–33.
3. Wheat LJ, Connolly-Stringfield PA, Baker RL, Curfman MF, Eads ME, Israel KS, et al. Disseminated histoplasmosis in the acquired immune deficiency syndrome: clinical findings, diagnosis and treatment, and review of the literature. Medicine (Baltimore). 1990 Nov;69(6):361–74.
4. Kauffman CA. Diagnosis of histoplasmosis in immunosuppressed patients. Curr Opin Infect Dis. 2008 Aug;21(4):421–5.
5. Vergidis P, Avery RK, Wheat LJ, Dotson JL, Assi MA, Antoun SA, et al. Histoplasmosis complicating tumor necrosis factor-α blocker therapy: a retrospective analysis of 98 cases. Clin Infect Dis. 2015 Aug 1;61(3):409–17. Epub 2015 Apr 13.
6. Pincelli T, Enzler M, Davis M, Tande AJ, Comfere N, Bruce A. Oropharyngeal histoplasmosis: a report of 10 cases. Clin Exp Dermatol. 2019 Jul;44(5):e181-8. Epub 2019 Feb 1.

It Must Be Something in the Water: A Hand Infection After Fishing

47

Kathryn T. del Valle, MD, and Aaron J. Tande, MD

Case Presentation

A 65-year-old man with a history of hypertension and seasonal allergies presented with pain and swelling in his left thumb and wrist that had been progressing for the past 3 months. His symptoms began while he was fishing in Texas, after his thumb was pierced by a saltwater catfish spine. A portion of the spine had broken off and remained in the pad of his thumb. Shortly after the injury, he received a 5-day course of amoxicillin. Although he had temporary relief of his symptoms, they returned and he was subsequently prescribed a 10-day course of doxycycline. After completing the antibiotic course, he had persistent pain and swelling that extended from his thumb into his entire hand and wrist.

Magnetic resonance imaging and radiography of the left upper extremity identified a foreign body in the pad of his left thumb, which was surgically excised. Antibiotics were not administered after surgery. Aerobic and anaerobic bacterial cultures from surgery were negative. Postoperatively, he had persistent pain and swelling and later had nodules develop on his fingers. The patient did not have systemic symptoms such as fever, chills, or sweating, nor did he report headache, shortness of breath, abdominal pain, nausea, vomiting, or diarrhea. He presented to our facility for further evaluation and management.

The initial physical examination at our hospital showed soft tissue swelling and thickening of the left dorsal hand and volar wrist, plus 2 nodular lesions on his third and fourth digits, without any purulent discharge (Figure 47.1). He also had mildly reduced wrist flexion.

He subsequently underwent irrigation and débridement of the left dorsal hand nodules and flexor tenosynovectomy of the left forearm. Purulence was encountered intraoperatively, and

Figure 47.1   *Mycobacterium marinum* Infection

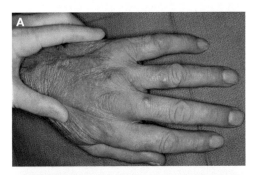

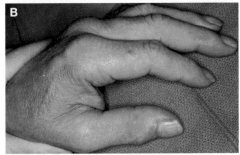

Photographs were taken before irrigation, débridement, and tenosynovectomy. A, Nodules on the third and fourth digits. B, Swelling of the first digit.

histopathologic analysis showed nonnecrotizing granulomatous and chronic lymphohistiocytic inflammation. Acid-fast and fungal stains were negative. Tissue cultures grew acid-fast bacilli (AFB) that were ultimately identified as *Mycobacterium marinum*. Bacterial cultures remained negative.

While histopathology and culture results were pending, he was treated with ertapenem, doxycycline, and levofloxacin; the latter 2 were prescribed for mycobacterial coverage. After final culture confirmation of *M marinum*, his antimicrobial therapy was transitioned to clarithromycin (500 mg, twice daily) and rifampin (600 mg, once daily). Ethambutol (15 mg/kg, once daily) was added several days later, given his tolerance of the initial regimen. Nearly 2 weeks later, final susceptibility tests showed that the *M marinum* isolate was susceptible to each of the 3 drugs in his regimen, as well as to doxycycline, amikacin, and rifabutin, but it was resistant to ciprofloxacin, moxifloxacin, and trimethoprim-sulfamethoxazole. He completed a 5-month treatment course with clarithromycin, ethambutol, and rifampin and had remarkable clinical improvement (Figure 47.2). At the time of treatment completion, his left hand, wrist swelling, and nodules had fully resolved.

Discussion

M marinum infections initially can mimic more common skin and soft tissue infections. However, a few crucial clues from this patient's clinical presentation raised suspicion for *M marinum* infection. First, the specific mechanism of injury was trauma in an aquatic setting (ie, direct injury from a saltwater fish). Although *M marinum* infections are associated with aquatic creatures, they can also occur after injuries from inanimate objects such as fishhooks and propeller blades; as such, aquarium hobbyists have markedly increased infection risk. Second, the patient's lack of response to standard antibiotic

Figure 47.2   After Treatment

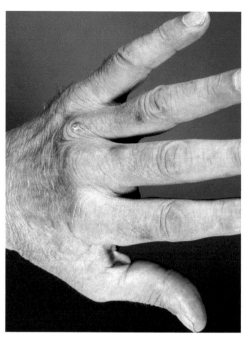

Photograph shows decreased swelling and decreased nodule size after approximately 6 weeks of combination treatment.

therapy for skin and soft tissue infection further indicated that a potentially unusual organism was causing the infection. Furthermore, his consistently negative bacterial tissue cultures and fairly indolent course suggested a more atypical pathogen. Third, the nodularity and location of the involved area (upper extremity, near the area of trauma) were highly consistent with *M marinum* infection. In fact, in a series of 31 patients with confirmed *M marinum* infections, 90% were affected in the upper extremity (1).

As shown by this patient's case, diagnosis of *M marinum* depends heavily on clinical history and physical examination findings, as well as on objective microbiologic data. Patients often initially present with papules on the affected area, and these papules can progress to nodular lymphangitis (also termed *sporotrichoid spread*) (Figure 47.1) (2). Classic histopathologic findings include granulomatous changes and lymphohistiocytic inflammation. Of note, perhaps surprisingly, only a small portion of cases will have a positive result with AFB tissue staining. For example, only 2 of 22 biopsy specimens in the case series of 31 patients were positive for AFB stain (1). Additionally, the final diagnosis frequently relies heavily on tissue culture, which can take several weeks. Cultures should be incubated at 2 different temperatures (28-32°C and 35°C) because *M marinum* typically grows at lower temperatures.

Like other mycobacterial infections, *M marinum* infections generally require prolonged, multidrug antimicrobial therapy. A typical starting regimen could include clarithromycin (500 mg, twice daily), rifampin (600 mg, once daily), and ethambutol (15 mg/kg, once daily). Treatment regimens should be tailored after antimicrobial susceptibilities are known, and other possible agents are trimethoprim-sulfamethoxazole and tetracyclines (doxycycline, minocycline). Therapy should continue for at least 1 to 2 months after symptoms resolve, for a total treatment course of 3 to 4 months. Prognosis is generally quite good with appropriate treatment. For example, in a case series of 63 French patients, 55 (87%) achieved cure with completed treatment (3).

In summary, when treating a patient with a soft tissue infection and history of aquatic-associated trauma, *M marinum* infection should be considered in the differential diagnosis, especially if treatment for more typical infectious organisms fails. Diagnosis is established on the basis of the clinical assessment (indolent course, papules that progress to nodular lymphangitis), histopathologic findings (granulomatous inflammation), and culture results. Treatment should typically include a 3- to 4-month course of at least 2 antimicrobial agents, and frequently used agents include clarithromycin, rifampin, and ethambutol.

References

1. Edelstein H. *Mycobacterium marinum* skin infections: report of 31 cases and review of the literature. Arch Intern Med. 1994 Jun 27;154(12):1359–64.
2. Baddour LM. Soft tissue infections following water exposure [Internet]. [cited 2021 Mar 9]. Available from: https://www.uptodate.com/contents/soft-tissue-infections-following-water-exposure.
3. Aubry A, Chosidow O, Caumes E, Robert J, Cambau E. Sixty-three cases of *Mycobacterium marinum* infection: clinical features, treatment, and antibiotic susceptibility of causative isolates. Arch Intern Med. 2002 Aug 12-26;162(15):1746–52.

Negative Pressure[a,b]

48

Natalia E. Castillo Almeida, MD, and Mary J. Kasten, MD

Case Presentation

A 95-year-old woman from an assisted living facility presented to the emergency department with a 9-day history of left-sided chest pain, progressive dyspnea, and hemoptysis. The initial evaluation showed that she was afebrile and hypoxic (requiring 5 L/min of supplemental oxygen). A computed tomographic angiogram showed several cavitary nodules; the largest nodule measured 1.7 cm and was in the apical right lung. The patient had a positive purified protein derivative skin test in 1996 because of probable exposure to tuberculosis during childhood.

The patient was admitted to the intensive care unit with a suspected diagnosis of active pulmonary tuberculosis, and airborne precautions were taken. Acid-fast bacilli (AFB) smears were negative for 3 consecutive, induced sputum samples. A nucleic acid amplification test (NAAT) on the initial respiratory specimen was positive. An interferon-γ release assay (IGRA) was negative.

The patient started treatment with rifampin, isoniazid, pyrazinamide, and ethambutol (RIPE). Six weeks after the initial sputum sample collection, *Mycobacterium tuberculosis* complex was identified. *M tuberculosis* complex was pansusceptible to RIPE therapy. The patient remained on airborne precautions for 2 weeks and was discharged to a skilled nursing facility after she showed clinical improvement.

Discussion

Tuberculosis is the leading cause of infectious morbidity and mortality worldwide. One-fourth of the world's population is at risk of having tuberculosis disease (1). In the emergency department, patients with suspected or confirmed infectious tuberculosis should be promptly identified, evaluated, and separated from other patients. One of the most critical risk factors for health care–associated transmission of *M tuberculosis* is patients with unrecognized tuberculosis disease who are not promptly isolated with appropriate airborne precautions. Infectious droplet nuclei are generated every time a patient coughs, sneezes, talks, or even sings. Droplet nuclei may be dispersed over long distances by air currents and may be inhaled by susceptible individuals who have not been in contact with the infectious individual (2).

Preventing the spread of aerosol-transmissible pathogens requires the use of airborne infection isolation rooms (AIIRs), which have special air handling and ventilation systems. In addition to AIIRs, respiratory protection with a National Institute for Occupational Safety and Health–certified N95 or higher-level respirator is recommended to prevent acquisition of *M tuberculosis* by health care personnel entering an AIIR (3). Patients with suspected or confirmed respiratory tuberculosis disease should not share rooms.

[a] Portions of this chapter have been published in Introduction to the core curriculum on tuberculosis: what the clinician should know [Internet]. [cited: 2021 Mar 16]. 6th Ed; 2013. Centers for Disease Control and Prevention. Available from: https://www.cdc.gov/tb/education/corecurr/pdf/corecurr_all.pdf.

[b] Portions of this chapter have been published in Lewinsohn DM, Leonard MK, LoBue PA, Cohn DL, Daley CL, Desmond E, et al. Official American Thoracic Society/Infectious Diseases Society of America/Centers for Disease Control and Prevention Clinical Practice Guidelines: Diagnosis of Tuberculosis in Adults and Children. Clin Infect Dis. 2017 Jan 15;64(2):e1-e33. Epub 2016 Dec 8; used with permission.

All respiratory samples from patients suspected of having pulmonary tuberculosis should be assessed by AFB smear microscopy. Three positive AFB smears confirm pulmonary tuberculosis with a sensitivity of 70% when culture-confirmed tuberculosis disease is the reference standard (4). Patients with known or suspected drug-resistant tuberculosis should remain in an AIIR for the duration of their hospital stay. However, airborne precautions may be discontinued if the patient has 3 consecutive sputum smears that are negative for AFB (with samples obtained at a minimum of 8 hours apart and at least 1 sample is an early-morning specimen). Additionally, an alternative diagnosis must be identified that explains the clinical presentation. An early-morning sputum specimen is preferred for the AFB smear because its sensitivity is 12% greater compared with a single-spot specimen (ie, a sputum sample [excluding the early-morning sample] collected in a series of 3 samples) (4). Importantly, a negative result does not completely exclude pulmonary tuberculosis. Therefore, clinical practice guidelines for the diagnosis of tuberculosis also suggest performing a NAAT on the initial respiratory specimen from any patient suspected of having pulmonary tuberculosis.

If a patient has a negative AFB smear and the clinical suspicion for tuberculosis disease is intermediate to high (eg, from cough, weight loss, and cavitation seen on a chest radiograph), a positive NAAT can be used as presumptive evidence of tuberculosis that warrants treatment (5). Our patient also had an IGRA performed. However, IGRAs have high false-negative rates in patients with tuberculosis disease. Patients with a negative IGRA are more commonly older (age ≥60 years), non-Hispanic, white, and infected with HIV. Patients with confirmed tuberculosis diagnoses and negative IGRA may also have poor outcomes (6).

The infectiousness of a person with tuberculosis disease is directly associated with the number of tubercle bacilli that the patient expels in the air. Studies have shown that most patients with pulmonary tuberculosis are no longer infectious after 2 weeks of treatment because of a reduction in coughing and a decrease in viable *M tuberculosis*. Thus, many published guidelines recommend discontinuing airborne precautions in patients with drug-susceptible tuberculosis when the patient has had at least 2 weeks of effective multidrug treatment and shows clinical evidence of improvement. Simple surgical masks are recommended as a source-control measure for patients with tuberculosis when they leave the AIIR because it can prevent viable *M tuberculosis* from being disseminated.

After a patient with pulmonary tuberculosis is medically stable, they may be discharged only if a definitive plan for outpatient therapy has been coordinated with the local tuberculosis control agency. In addition, children younger than 4 years and immunocompromised persons should not live with them, and patients are strictly instructed to leave their home only for medical appointments (3).

Tuberculosis transmission has been documented in health care settings, where health care providers and patients encounter persons with unsuspected, infectious tuberculosis disease who have not been isolated in a timely manner or have not received appropriate treatment. Initial risk assessment for tuberculosis is crucial for determining administrative, environmental, and respiratory protective measures.

References

1. Centers for Disease Control and Prevention (CDC). Decrease in reported tuberculosis cases: United States, 2009. MMWR Morb Mortal Wkly Rep. 2010 Mar 19;59(10):289–94.
2. Jensen PA, Lambert LA, Iademarco MF, Ridzon R; CDC. Guidelines for preventing the transmission of

Mycobacterium tuberculosis in health-care settings, 2005. MMWR Recomm Rep. 2005 Dec 30;54(RR-17):1–141.

3. Sia IG, Wieland ML. Current concepts in the management of tuberculosis. Mayo Clin Proc. 2011 Apr;86(4):348–61.

4. Lewinsohn DM, Leonard MK, LoBue PA, Cohn DL, Daley CL, Desmond E, et al. Official American Thoracic Society/Infectious Diseases Society of America/Centers for Disease Control and Prevention Clinical Practice Guidelines: diagnosis of tuberculosis in adults and children. Clin Infect Dis. 2017 Jan 15;64(2):111–5.

5. Catanzaro A, Perry S, Clarridge JE, Dunbar S, Goodnight-White S, LoBue PA, et al. The role of clinical suspicion in evaluating a new diagnostic test for active tuberculosis: results of a multicenter prospective trial. JAMA. 2000 Feb 2;283(5):639–45. Erratum in: JAMA 2000 Oct 4;284(13):1663.

6. Nguyen DT, Teeter LD, Graves J, Graviss EA. Characteristics associated with negative interferon-γ release assay results in culture-confirmed tuberculosis patients: Texas, USA, 2013-2015. Emerg Infect Dis. 2018 Mar;24(3):534–40.

An Unusual Cause of Prosthetic Joint Infection

49

Caitlin P. Oravec, PA-C, MS, and Douglas R. Osmon, MD

Case Presentation

A 74-year-old man was seen in the orthopedic surgery clinic for a painful right hip. He had undergone a primary hip arthroplasty 14 years ago. The patient did well until 10 months before his presentation, when he had groin pain after working on his deck. Radiographs showed subsidence and loosening of the cemented femoral stem, with a fracture through the cement mantle (Figure 49.1). His inflammatory markers were elevated, with the C-reactive protein level at 31 mg/L (reference range, ≤8.0 mg/L) and the sedimentation rate was 75 mm/h (reference range, 0-22 mm/h).

The patient's history included carcinoma in situ of the urinary bladder, 2 years before the current presentation. He received treatment with 6 weekly bacille Calmette-Guérin (BCG) bladder instillations. He had recently undergone cystoscopy with biopsies to assess for recurrence and had completed a course of oral antibiotics for prophylaxis because he had multiple arthroplasties. His medical history also included urosepsis (5 years before this presentation), dental caries with nonrestorable teeth (but no history of oral infection), diabetes mellitus, hyperlipidemia, and hypertension.

The orthopedic surgeon recommended revision arthroplasty, but because of the patient's history of urosepsis and ongoing dental issues, an ultrasonographically guided aspiration was performed first to rule out prosthetic joint infection. Less than 0.5 mL of serosanguinous fluid was aspirated. A synovial fluid cell count could not be done because of insufficient fluid volume for culture and synovial fluid cell count. Aerobic and anaerobic bacterial cultures were negative.

The patient proceeded to revision arthroplasty. Osteolytic debris was noted, but the joint fluid appeared normal. Three pieces of synovial tissue were submitted for histopathologic examination, and 1 showed acute inflammation (≥10 neutrophils per high-power field). Three tissue samples were sent for aerobic and anaerobic bacteria cultures.

The patient was referred to the infectious diseases clinic for further diagnostic evaluation

Figure 49.1 Radiograph Showing Right Total Hip Arthroplasty

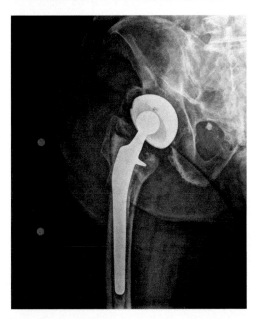

Image shows bone loss along the femoral metadiaphysis and mild lucency around the bone-cement interface of the proximal femoral component.

and guidance about appropriate treatment after the pathologic analysis showed acute inflammation. Bacterial cultures were negative at approximately 1 week after collection. The infectious diseases provider ordered fungal and mycobacterial cultures of the intraoperatively obtained tissue. Treatment with oral cefadroxil was initiated, pending the results of the aerobic and anaerobic cultures.

On day 13 of incubation, the laboratory reported growth of *Mycobacterium tuberculosis* complex, which was identified with nucleic acid hybridization probes. The patient had no known tuberculosis (TB) exposures or risk factors, so he started triple therapy for presumed *Mycobacterium bovis* BCG infection: isoniazid (300 mg daily), rifampin (600 mg daily), and ethambutol (1,600 mg daily). Five-plex real-time polymerase chain reaction (PCR) assays confirmed the diagnosis of prosthetic joint infection with *M bovis* BCG. Urine and blood cultures were negative for mycobacteria. Results of interferon-γ release assays were indeterminate.

Ultimately, he had ongoing drainage from the surgical incision. Eleven days after starting therapy, he underwent a resection arthroplasty (Figure 49.2). Cultures remained positive for *M bovis* BCG. He completed 3 months of treatment with ethambutol, rifampin, and isoniazid and then continued therapy with only isoniazid plus rifampin, to complete a total of 9 months of therapy. He declined reimplantation arthroplasty. He had no obvious evidence of residual or recurrent disease. The C-reactive protein level, 13 months after completion of antibiotic therapy, remained within normal limits (<3.0 mg/L), and the sedimentation rate improved (31 mm/h).

Discussion

The patient's history suggests multiple potential sources for the prosthetic joint infection, including translocation from the recent urologic procedure, transient seeding from poor dentition, or even a skin tear from working on his deck. However, organisms associated with these

Figure 49.2   Radiograph Showing Right Total Hip Arthroplasty Resection

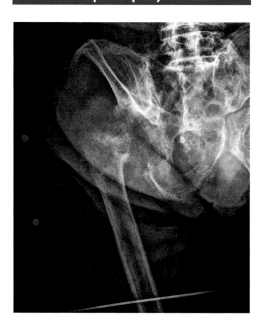

types of infections should grow on routine bacterial cultures. This case shows the importance of obtaining routine mycobacterial cultures in patients with a history of BCG treatment for urologic cancer who present with culture-negative infection during a preoperative evaluation, no matter the amount of time elapsed since BCG therapy. Late-presenting BCG infections have been described up to 13 years after treatments have ended (1).

M tuberculosis complex includes *M tuberculosis, M bovis, M bovis* BCG, *Mycobacterium africanum*, and *Mycobacterium microti*. Distinguishing between *M tuberculosis* and *M bovis* BCG is important for infection control purposes. Although extrapulmonary TB disease is rarely infectious, some patients with extrapulmonary TB disease have unsuspected pulmonary or laryngeal disease, which could spread to others through bacilli-containing respiratory droplets (2). Not distinguishing between TB and BCG also could lead to unnecessary imaging and sputum analyses or inappropriate isolation of the patient.

If 5-plex real-time PCR testing is not available, another way to differentiate between these 2 organisms is susceptibility testing because *M bovis* strains (including the BCG strain) are often pyrazinamide resistant (2). An interferon-γ release assay may also help differentiate between patients infected with *M bovis* BCG and patients infected with *M tuberculosis* because studies have shown that interferon-γ release assays are not affected by bladder BCG treatment (3).

Cancer therapy with BCG has been associated with local and disseminated infections, as well as hypersensitivity reactions. Genitourinary tract complications range from cystitis around the time of instillation to granulomatous prostatitis that may occur months after therapy. The pathogenesis of disseminated disease is not fully understood, but the mycobacteria are thought to gain access to the lymphatic system and blood through disruption of the uroepithelial cells (4).

BCG sepsis syndrome (sometimes termed *BCGosis*) can develop a few days to months after instillations are completed. Presenting features include fever, weight loss, and dyspnea. Computed tomography of the chest may show a miliary pattern of lung nodules. Granulomatous hepatitis has also been reported, with liver function tests showing elevated results. Local infections can occur at sites that are distant from the genitourinary tract, including intravascular infections (eg, mycotic aneurysms) and musculoskeletal infections (eg, vertebral diskitis, osteomyelitis). The diagnosis is usually made by growth of viable *M bovis* from the site of infection, PCR detection of the organism, or histopathologic examination identifying noncaseating granulomas or acid-fast bacilli (1).

Disseminated complications from BCG therapy usually are managed with 3 to 9 months of therapy: the first 2 to 3 months of treatment are with rifampin, isoniazid, and ethambutol, and then therapy is completed with rifampin and isoniazid (4). Glucocorticoids may also have a role in treatment (1).

In the United States, most *M bovis* infections are associated with intravesicular BCG, but *M bovis* is also an important zoonosis. Most zoonotic disease with *M bovis* is seen in developing countries, but it also constitutes about 2% of TB disease in the United States. With *M bovis* being the leading cause of TB in cattle and other large mammals, consumption of infected animal products, such as unpasteurized dairy products, may lead to human disease. *M bovis* is also transmitted from animals to humans and between humans through inhalation of airborne particles. The spectrum of zoonotic *M bovis* disease includes pulmonary infection resembling TB disease, cervical lymphadenitis, and gastrointestinal illness (5). Disseminated and local infections have also been reported, albeit rarely, after BCG vaccination of patients with underlying immune deficiencies (4).

References

1. Gonzalez OY, Musher DM, Brar I, Furgeson S, Boktour MR, Septimus EJ, et al. Spectrum of bacille Calmette-Guérin (BCG) infection after intravesical BCG immunotherapy. Clin Infect Dis. 2003 Jan 15;36(2):140-8. Epub 2003 Jan 3.
2. Core curriculum on tuberculosis: what the clinician should know [Internet]. 6th ed. 2013 [cited 2021 Mar 16]. Atlanta (GA): Centers for Disease Control and Prevention: National Center for HIV/AIDS, Viral Hepatitis, STD, and TB Prevention Division of Tuberculosis Elimination. Available from: https://www.cdc.gov/tb/education/corecurr/pdf/corecurr_all.pdf.
3. Silverman MS, Reynolds D, Kavsak PA, Garay J, Daly A, Davis I. Use of an interferon-gamma based assay to assess bladder cancer patients treated with intravesical BCG and exposed to tuberculosis. Clin Biochem. 2007 Aug;40(12):913-5. Epub 2007 Apr 27.
4. Brown-Elliott BA, Wallace RJ. Infections caused by nontuberculous mycobacteria other than *Mycobacterium avium* complex. In: Bennett JE, Dolin R, Blaser MJ, editors. Mandell, Douglas, and Bennett's principles and practice of infectious diseases. 9th ed. Philadelphia (PA): Elsevier; c2020. p. 3049–58.
5. *Mycobacterium bovis* (bovine tuberculosis) in humans. Centers for Disease Control and Prevention: National Center for HIV/AIDS, Viral Hepatitis, STD, and TB Prevention Division of Tuberculosis Elimination [Internet]. 2011 Aug [cited 2021 Mar 16]. Available from: https://www.cdc.gov/tb/publications/factsheets/general/mbovis.pdf.

HIV and Its Myriad Opportunistic Infections

50

Pooja R. Gurram, MBBS, and Alan J. Wright, MD

Case Presentation

A 36-year-old man presented to the emergency department with concerns about progressively worsening dyspnea, cough, and a 9.1-kg unintentional weight loss during the past 3 months. He had immigrated from Sierra Leone to the United States 3 years ago. His medical history included an episode of herpes zoster affecting the right maxillary nerve distribution of his face. The physical examination showed that he was cachectic, in moderate respiratory distress, and had crackles on auscultation. He also had shallow, painless penile and groin ulcers. He had 3 female sexual partners in his lifetime and had not been sexually active for the past 3 years.

An arterial blood gas analysis showed that the patient's Po_2 was 60 mm Hg, with an alveolar-arterial gradient greater than 35 mm Hg. A chest radiograph was suggestive of bilateral nodular opacities. Computed tomographic imaging of the chest showed bilateral multinodular opacities and ground-glass changes. He was admitted for further evaluation and management. Laboratory tests showed that he had a hemoglobin level of 8 g/dL, white blood cell count of 8×10^9/L, serum creatinine level of 0.9 mg/dL, and alkaline phosphatase level of 414 U/L. His HIV screening and confirmatory tests were positive, with a viral load of 800,000 copies/mL and a CD4 count of 8 cells/mcL. He underwent bronchoscopy with bronchoalveolar lavage. Lavage fluid was tested with polymerase chain reaction (PCR) assays and was positive for *Pneumocystis jirovecii*, and the serum 1,3-β-D-glucan level was 371 pg/mL (reference range, <80 pg/mL). He had positive results with hepatitis screening and hepatitis B surface antigen (HBsAg) tests, and he was also positive for immunoglobulin (Ig) G antibodies against hepatitis B core antigen (HBc). Tests for hepatitis B surface antibody (HBsAb) and HBc IgM were negative. His hepatitis B virus (HBV) load was 15,400 IU/mL. Tuberculosis was excluded after 3 acid-fast bacilli smears and 2 tuberculosis PCR tests of the sputum were negative. A PCR test of the genital ulcers was positive for herpes simplex virus 2, and a syphilis IgG test was negative.

The patient began receiving trimethoprim-sulfamethoxazole (TMP-SMX) and a prednisone taper for treatment of the *Pneumocystis* pneumonia, which improved his symptoms markedly. Within a week after beginning his treatment, he also began combined antiretroviral therapy (cART) with tenofovir disoproxil fumarate, emtricitabine, and dolutegravir. Of note, this program was chosen because it included 2 agents with activity against HBV. Mycobacterial blood cultures came back positive for *Mycobacterium colombiense*, 3 weeks after his hospital discharge. After receiving the *Mycobacterium avium* complex (MAC) diagnosis, he began treatment with azithromycin, ethambutol, and rifabutin. His genital ulcers improved with valacyclovir treatment. This case illustrates the importance of recognizing multiple opportunistic infections and coinfections in patients with advanced HIV infection.

Discussion

Since the introduction of cART for HIV in the United States, AIDS-associated deaths have been reduced by about 50% and new HIV diagnoses have been reduced by about 47%. According to the Centers for Disease Control and Prevention, 1.2 million persons aged 13 years and older were living with HIV in the United States by the end of 2018, and 37,968 persons had new HIV diagnoses in 2018.

The number of persons with end-stage disease and new HIV diagnoses is decreasing in the United States, but HIV/AIDS continues to be a major health concern worldwide. According to the Joint United Nations Programme on HIV/AIDS, about 1.7 million new cases of HIV were diagnosed in 2019, with a prevalence of 38 million. Of these, about 26 million were receiving cART by the end of June 2020. Approximately 690,000 AIDS-associated deaths were reported in 2019, and about 32.7 million AIDS-associated deaths have occurred since its discovery. The incidence and prevalence of HIV/AIDS continue to be very high, with most cases occurring in eastern and southern Africa. Thus, clinicians continue to see patients with AIDS-defining illnesses, particularly in those who are unaware of their diagnosis. Being familiar with HIV/AIDS and its myriad opportunistic infections and coinfections is of utmost importance to clinicians worldwide.

Pneumocystis Pneumonia

Pneumocystis pneumonia is caused by a ubiquitous fungus *P jirovecii*. It is spread through airborne transmission, and by age 4, the majority of the United States population appear to have been exposed to this organism (1). *Pneumocystis* pneumonia has a somewhat subacute onset in patients with HIV/AIDS, and common symptoms are progressive shortness of breath, dry cough, fever, and chest discomfort. Common findings with chest radiography include bilateral reticular interstitial infiltrates, but radiographs show normal findings in 10% to 15% of cases. High-resolution computed tomography is more sensitive than radiography, and it can show a ground-glass pattern, predominantly in the perihilar region, and

the "crazy-paving" pattern, which represents a combination of reticular opacities and septal thickening.

Clinical and radiographic findings are nonspecific in *Pneumocystis* pneumonia, but given the toxicity associated with high-dose TMP-SMX, a definitive diagnosis of *Pneumocystis* pneumonia is essential to justify treatment. Grocott-Gomori methenamine silver (GMS) staining of induced sputum has a sensitivity of less than 50% to 90%, and GMS staining of bronchoalveolar lavage fluid has a sensitivity of 90% to 99%. Histopathologic analysis of lung tissue samples has a sensitivity of 95% to 100%. Even though PCR analysis has greater sensitivity for detecting *Pneumocystis*, it is often difficult to differentiate between colonization and active disease. Thus, although some centers use quantitative PCR to determine fungal load (with higher loads being more consistent with active disease), no standardized threshold value is accepted that confidently differentiates active disease from colonization. Other adjunctive studies of value are lactate dehydrogenase (a marker of cell destruction) and 1,3-β-D-glucan (a component of the cystic cell wall); the latter has high sensitivity but low specificity. With the advent of effective cART and chemoprophylaxis against *Pneumocystis*, the incidence of *Pneumocystis* pneumonia has decreased, but it continues to be seen in patients who are unaware of their HIV diagnosis, who do not have access to HIV care, or who have advanced immunosuppression. Primary prophylaxis is indicated in patients with a CD4 T-cell count less than 200 cells/mcL or patients with a percentage of CD4 T cells less than 14%. A daily double-strength dose of TMP-SMX (160 mg TMP, 800 mg SMX) is preferred for prophylaxis; at this dose, it has prophylactic activity against toxoplasmosis as well. Alternatives for patients with severe allergy to TMP-SMX include dapsone (contraindicated in patients who are deficient in glucose-6-phosphate dehydrogenase), aerosolized pentamidine, and atovaquone. Primary prophylaxis can be discontinued when the CD4 T-cell count exceeds 200 cells/mcL for longer than 3 months while receiving effective cART.

The first-line medication for treating *Pneumocystis* pneumonia also is TMP-SMX, but it is given at a higher dose than that used for prophylaxis. It is administered either intravenously or orally, depending on disease severity and the patient's ability to take and absorb oral medication. Corticosteroids are added to decrease the inflammatory response elicited by dying organisms if the patient's alveolar-arterial gradient is 35 mm Hg or higher and Po_2 is less than 70 mm Hg on ambient (room) air. Alternative medications for patients with severe allergy to the sulfa component of TMP-SMX include dapsone-TMP, clindamycin-primaquine, atovaquone, and intravenous pentamidine. The duration of therapy is 21 days, and then secondary prophylaxis is administered until the CD4 T-cell count exceeds 200 cells/mcL for longer than 3 months while receiving effective cART.

HBV Coinfection With HIV

HBV is one of the leading causes of chronic liver disease worldwide. It is predominantly seen in Asia and Africa, and the major route of transmission continues to be perinatal exposure. In the United States, the most common routes of HBV transmission are sexual and intravenous exposures. According to estimates from the Joint United Nations Programme on HIV/AIDS, approximately 10% of patients with HIV are coinfected with hepatitis B (2). Coinfection with HIV accelerates the progression of hepatitis B liver disease to cirrhosis and hepatocellular carcinoma. However, no clear evidence indicates that patients with an HIV-HBV coinfection have a faster rate of progression to AIDS or an increase in HIV-associated deaths (3).

Every patient with HIV needs to be tested for coinfection with hepatitis B. If an HBsAg test is positive, HBV DNA, hepatitis B e-antigen (HBeAg), and hepatitis B e-antibody (HBeAb) levels must be checked. For patients with HIV-HBV coinfection, the cART regimen must include at least 2 agents that are active against HBV because lamivudine or emtricitabine alone increases the risk of emergence of resistant HBV strains. Thus, for patients with HIV-HBV coinfection, a combination of either lamivudine or emtricitabine plus either tenofovir alafenamide or tenofovir disoproxil fumarate must be used as the nucleoside reverse-transcriptase inhibitor combination.

Disseminated MAC

For patients with HIV, CD4 T-cell counts less than 50 cells/mcL increase the risk of disseminated infection from MAC. MAC comprises multiple subspecies, with *M avium* being the most common. *M colombiense* is a novel strain that was first identified in patients from Colombia. It is phenotypically distinct from other species because it produces urease, and it is genotypically distinct because it has a 16S to 23S rRNA internal transcribed spacer sequence (4).

MAC is ubiquitous in the environment, with the most common routes of transmission being inhalation and ingestion. Common symptoms include fever, weight loss, diarrhea, abdominal pain, and sweating. Common laboratory test abnormalities are anemia and elevated alkaline phosphatase. Primary prophylaxis with either azithromycin or clarithromycin is indicated in patients with HIV/AIDS who have a CD4 T-cell count less than 50 cells/mcL. However, in patients with clinical signs and symptoms suggestive of disseminated infection, primary prophylaxis should be deferred until active disease is excluded, to avoid emergence of resistance if a single-drug regimen is used to treat a disseminated infection.

Common treatment regimens for MAC infection include a 2- or 3-drug regimen with a macrolide (azithromycin or clarithromycin), ethambutol, and possibly rifabutin. In treatment-naive patients, cART is usually started after the first 2 weeks of treatment for MAC, to decrease the risk of immune reconstitution inflammatory syndrome. However, if cART was already initiated before therapy for MAC, it is prudent to continue cART while monitoring for symptoms of immune reconstitution inflammatory syndrome.

References

1. Pifer LL, Hughes WT, Stagno S, Woods D. *Pneumocystis carinii* infection: evidence for high prevalence in normal and immunosuppressed children. Pediatrics. 1978 Jan;61(1):35–41.
2. Spradling PR, Richardson JT, Buchacz K, Moorman AC, Brooks JT; HIV Outpatient Study (HOPS) Investigators. Prevalence of chronic hepatitis B virus infection among patients in the HIV Outpatient Study, 1996-2007. J Viral Hepat. 2010 Dec;17(12):879–86.
3. Hoffmann CJ, Thio CL. Clinical implications of HIV and hepatitis B co-infection in Asia and Africa. Lancet Infect Dis. 2007 Jun;7(6):402–9.
4. Barretto AR, Felicio JS, Sales LHM, Yamada ES, Lopes ML, da Costa ARF. A fatal case of pulmonary infection by *Mycobacterium colombiense* in Para State, Amazon Region, Brazil. Diagn Microbiol Infect Dis. 2016 Jul;85(3):344–6. Epub 2016 Feb 9.

51

A Travel Souvenir

Natalia E. Castillo Almeida, MD, and Mary J. Kasten, MD

Case Presentation

A 33-year-old man presented to the emergency department with a 3-day history of hematuria and fever. His medical history was notable for Wolff-Parkinson-White syndrome after cardiac ablation, and he had previously undergone mitral valve repair because of severe regurgitation. The patient reported recently returning from a 10-day trip to Bali, where he had stayed at a resort and eaten local cuisine, including pork. He denied mosquito bites or freshwater activities but reported 1 episode of self-limited diarrhea. A week before the current emergency department presentation, he had been seen by a local provider after a 5-day history of fever, night sweats, and headaches.

The patient was afebrile, and a physical examination showed right costovertebral angle tenderness. No rebound or guarding was observed. A review of symptoms was negative for dysuria and urethral discharge. A complete blood count and laboratory test results for aspartate aminotransferase, alanine aminotransferase, creatinine, and glomerular filtration rate showed normal findings. Blood smears for *Plasmodium* (malaria) and *Babesia* (babesiosis) were negative. A urinalysis showed gross hematuria, considerable proteinuria, and a trace of leukocytes. A urine Gram stain was negative. Computed tomography of the abdomen and pelvis without contrast showed a congenitally small and atrophic right kidney and no ureterolithiasis or nephrolithiasis. A computed tomographic image from approximately 10 years ago showed similar findings. An evaluation for postinfectious glomerulonephritis indicated that the patient did not have antistreptolysin antibodies. The patient also had a urologic evaluation with cystoscopy, which showed no evidence of lesions within the bladder or kidneys.

The patient was discharged home with close outpatient follow-up. Two days later, the patient was seen at the outpatient infectious diseases clinic with a persistent high fever and hematuria. Further evaluation included a urine examination for *Schistosoma* and a blood test for dengue virus antibodies, and both were negative. A repeat urinalysis showed more than 100 red blood cells and more than 100 white blood cells per high-power field. A bacterial urine culture showed 10,000 to 100,000 colony-forming units (cfu) per mL of pansusceptible *Salmonella enterica* subsp *enterica* serovar Javiana. Peripheral blood cultures were negative.

The patient received the diagnosis of a non-typhoid *Salmonella* (NTS) urinary tract infection (UTI) and was treated with oral levofloxacin (500 mg daily) for 6 weeks. At a follow-up appointment, the patient reported complete resolution of symptoms, and a repeat urinalysis was negative for blood and protein.

Discussion

UTIs are the most common bacterial infections encountered in medicine. UTIs affect 150 million people each year worldwide and account for more than 8 million office visits annually in the United States (1).

Infections of the urinary system may involve the lower urinary tract (confined to the bladder) or the upper urinary tract (pyelonephritis) (1). UTIs can be further categorized as uncomplicated or complicated. A UTI is likely to be classified as uncomplicated if the host patient has no structural or functional abnormalities, is not pregnant, and has not had any urologic instrumentation. Otherwise, UTIs are likely to be considered complicated. The spectrum of urinary conditions ranges from asymptomatic bacteriuria, symptomatic UTI, and sepsis associated with UTI that requires hospital admission.

Asymptomatic bacteriuria is defined as the presence of at least 10^5 cfu/mL of the same uropathogen in 2 consecutive, clean-catch, midstream urine samples for women and in a single sample for men when the person is otherwise asymptomatic (2). In contrast, establishing a UTI diagnosis requires a combination of urinary signs and symptoms (eg, dysuria, hematuria, suprapubic pain) and confirmatory laboratory tests (eg, bacteriuria [$\geq10^5$ cfu/mL], pyuria [≥10 white blood cells per high-power field]). Other indirect methods may be used to detect bacteria or inflammation. Urine dipsticks are commonly used because they can detect nitrite, leukocyte esterase, protein, and blood. If nitrite is detected, the likelihood ratio of a UTI ranges from 2.6 to 10.6, but the sensitivity is relatively low (2). Several diagnostic algorithms for UTI that combine symptoms and dipstick urinalysis results have been proposed, but the sensitivity and specificity of these algorithms vary substantially.

UTIs are caused by gram-negative bacteria (eg, *Escherichia coli*) and gram-positive bacteria (eg, *Staphylococcus saprophyticus*). NTS UTI without gastroenteritis is rare and is usually associated with urologic abnormalities, immunosuppression, and chronic diseases such as diabetes mellitus (3). NTS UTIs accounted for 0.01% to 0.07% of cases of UTI in several studies, but its prevalence has notably increased with time (4). The pathogenesis of NTS UTI includes hematogenous spread or a direct ascending invasion of the genitourinary tract. NTS may be caused by contamination of the urinary tract by stool (eg, in a patient with acute gastroenteritis) or by chronic carriage of NTS in the urine (3). For the patient described above, we hypothesized direct transmission through the consumption of contaminated food that resulted in diarrhea and contamination of the urinary tract. Travelers returning to the United States with the highest risk

of NTS are reported to have visited Africa, Latin America, the Caribbean, and Asia.

An NTS UTI without gastroenteritis presents with typical UTI symptoms, including hematuria (3). In the case described above, hematuria was the only sign of infection. NTS UTIs can occur in the setting of various predisposing factors, including severe immunodeficiency, occult urologic problems, or chronic disease (3). The small and atrophic kidney noted in the patient's evaluation may have contributed to his NTS UTI. In the literature, the most commonly reported genitourinary tract abnormalities associated with NTS UTI are nephrolithiasis, chronic pyelonephritis, rectovesical fistula, urethrorectal fistula, hydrocele, and prior transurethral resection of the prostate (5). It is important to remember that these UTIs can also occur in apparently healthy and immunocompetent individuals.

The treatment of UTIs include antibiotics that can result in long-term alteration of the normal microbiota of the gastrointestinal tract and in the development of multidrug-resistant microorganisms. For this reason, a urine sample should be cultured to identify causative organisms and their antimicrobial susceptibilities.

In patients with acute, uncomplicated cystitis, empiric treatment with nitrofurantoin for 5 days is appropriate because of minimal resistance and a low propensity for altering the normal microbiota of the gastrointestinal tract. An alternative regimen is trimethoprim-sulfamethoxazole for 3 days. Fluoroquinolones are highly efficacious, but they also should be considered an alternative therapy because they can be associated with adverse reactions such as tendonitis, development of aortic aneurysm and dissection, and *Clostridioides difficile*–associated diarrhea (6).

In patients with suspected pyelonephritis, a urine culture with susceptibility testing should always be performed, and the initial empiric therapy should be tailored to the identified pathogen. In this setting, fluoroquinolones are appropriate first-line therapies if the patient does not require hospitalization and if the local prevalence of resistance is low (6).

In patients with NTS UTI, prolonged antibiotic therapy (lasting 2 weeks or longer) is recommended. If a structural abnormality is identified (eg, urolithiasis), we recommend removing the abnormality and providing 1 to 2 weeks of parenteral antibiotics and at least 6 weeks of oral antibiotics (fluoroquinolones or trimethoprim-sulfamethoxazole) (5). The increased duration of treatment is due to the potential for bloodstream infections, the risk of becoming a *Salmonella* carrier with shorter treatment regimens, and concern for antibiotic resistance.

References

1. Foxman B. The epidemiology of urinary tract infection. Nat Rev Urol. 2010 Dec;7(12):653–60.

2. Schmiemann G, Kniehl E, Gebhardt K, Matejczyk MM, Hummers-Pradier E. The diagnosis of urinary tract infection: a systematic review. Dtsch Arztebl Int. 2010 May;107(21):361–7. Epub 2010 May 28.

3. Ramos JM, Aguado JM, Garcia-Corbeira P, Ales JM, Soriano F. Clinical spectrum of urinary tract infections due on nontyphoidal *Salmonella* species. Clin Infect Dis. 1996 Aug;23(2):388–90.

4. Tena D, Gonzalez-Praetorius A, Bisquert J. Urinary tract infection due to non-typhoidal *Salmonella*: report of 19 cases. J Infect. 2007 Mar;54(3):245–9. Epub 2006 Jul 7.

5. Klosterman SA. Salmonella-related urinary tract infection in an elderly patient. BMJ Case Rep. 2014 Sep 5;2014:bcr2014204552.

6. Gupta K, Hooton TM, Naber KG, Wullt B, Colgan R, Miller LG, et al; Infectious Diseases Society of America; European Society for Microbiology and Infectious Diseases. International clinical practice guidelines for the treatment of acute uncomplicated cystitis and pyelonephritis in women: a 2010 update by the Infectious Diseases Society of America and the European Society for Microbiology and Infectious Diseases. Clin Infect Dis. 2011 Mar 1;52(5):e103–20.

Stuck Between a Foot and a Soft Place

52

Matthew J. Thoendel, MD, PhD, and Aaron J. Tande, MD

Case Presentation

A 68-year-old man with an unknown medical history was admitted to the hospital after being found on the floor of his home. His initial evaluation was notable for a hemoglobin level of 5.5 g/dL, platelet count of 164×10^9/L, creatinine level of 1.9 mg/dL, albumin level of 2.0 g/dL, lactate level of 3.7 mmol/L, and N-terminal prohormone brain natriuretic peptide level greater than 30,000 pg/mL. His troponin T level was 2.2 ng/mL and did not show any clinically significant increases after 3 and 6 hours. His erythrocyte sedimentation rate was 5 mm/h, and the C-reactive protein level was 37.9 mg/L. A peripheral blood smear was negative for schistocytes. Subsequent studies were consistent with iron-deficiency anemia. An echocardiogram showed a left-ventricular ejection fraction of 10% to 15%, with moderate to severe left ventricle enlargement and severe generalized hypokinesis. He was initially treated with a red blood cell transfusion and optimization of his cardiac medications.

A physical evaluation showed that he had a purulent ulcer on his left second toe, plus bilateral shallow ulcers on his lower legs. A left foot radiograph showed cortical destruction of the proximal and middle phalanges, indicating osteomyelitis. An orthopedic surgeon and an infectious diseases physician were consulted, and they recommended amputation of the left second toe after medical optimization. Three days after hospitalization, he reported acute, nonbloody diarrhea. A gastrointestinal pathogen stool panel (polymerase chain reaction assays) was positive for Shiga toxin–producing genes but negative

for the *Escherichia coli* O157:H7 serotype. A diagnosis of Shiga toxin–producing *E coli* (STEC) enterocolitis was therefore made. Antibiotics were not recommended because of the concern for developing hemolytic uremic syndrome (HUS), but questions remained about whether and when it would be safe to use perioperative antibiotics for his recommended amputation, as well as possible additional antibiotics, depending on intraoperative findings. The care team and the patient eventually decided to wait until 2 weeks had passed since the onset of symptoms before proceeding with the elective amputation. This approach minimized the risk of HUS developing with perioperative antibiotic use.

Discussion

The potentially increased risk of HUS developing with antibiotic treatment of STEC infections has been reported since STEC was identified as a cause of HUS. HUS is characterized by microangiopathic hemolytic anemia, thrombocytopenia, and acute renal failure. Shiga toxin released by STEC binds to and is taken up by endothelial cells, where it inhibits ribosome function and leads to increased production of procoagulant factors, microthrombosis, and clinical sequelae (1). Shiga toxin is encoded by the *stx1* and *stx2* genes of bacteriophages. Cellular damage, particularly by antibiotics, leads to increased expression of these bacteriophages, which causes upregulation of toxin production, lysis of *E coli* cells, and toxin release, which are thought to contribute to an increased risk of HUS.

The increased risk of HUS development with antibiotic use remains a subject of investigation. Some cohort studies have estimated that the odds ratio increases by as much as 17 fold, although others have shown no relationship (2). A recent meta-analysis that selected the highest-quality studies estimated a 2.2-fold increase in risk (3). The increase in absolute risk depends on predisposing factors, and for the patient described above, it is likely low, given the lower rate of HUS in STEC-infected adults compared with children. In 1 study, adults older than 65 years without bloody diarrhea had a less than 1% risk of HUS without antibiotics; risk increased to approximately 3% for patients receiving antibiotics (4). This 2% to 3% increase in absolute risk is less than the expected reduction in absolute risk when prophylactic antibiotics are used with surgery. However, the relative severity of HUS (compared with a typical postoperative infection) must be factored into the decision to use prophylactic antibiotics.

In the above case, the chronic nature of the patient's osteomyelitis and the lack of surrounding cellulitis meant that the planned surgery was not urgent; thus, the decision to delay surgery and avoid antibiotic use was more straightforward. The use of vancomycin as an alternative antibiotic for surgical-site prophylaxis would theoretically be unlikely to affect E coli toxin production. This approach was discussed but not pursued, given the lack of evidence supporting it. For some patients, surgical intervention may be urgent or emergent, and delaying surgery is not an option. In these situations, the decision to use perioperative prophylactic antibiotics would have to be made on a case-by-case basis. The relative risk of developing HUS (accounting for risk factors such as younger age or the presence of bloody diarrhea) must be weighed against the risks of a surgical site infection, including the likelihood that an infection would occur (eg, clean vs contaminated site), site-specific considerations, and implications of such an infection (eg, central nervous system infection vs soft tissue infection).

The risk of HUS developing with antibiotic use also likely depends on the causative STEC strain. An outbreak in Germany was caused by an O104:H4 STEC strain and was associated with the use of antibiotics, primarily azithromycin used for meningitis prophylaxis during an eculizumab trial; however, azithromycin was not associated with an increased risk of HUS and instead was shown to reduce long-term carriage of the strain (5). In vitro studies also showed no increased toxin release with antibiotic exposure, unlike the outcomes typically observed with O157:H7 STEC strains. In the above case, the STEC isolate was not cultured and the serotype remained unknown. Thus, no treatment decisions could be made on the basis of observations from the O104:H4 outbreak.

References

1. Tarr PI, Gordon CA, Chandler WL. Shiga-toxin-producing *Escherichia coli* and haemolytic uraemic syndrome. Lancet. 2005 Mar 19-25;365(9464):1073-86.
2. Wong CS, Jelacic S, Habeeb RL, Watkins SL, Tarr PI. The risk of the hemolytic-uremic syndrome after antibiotic treatment of *Escherichia coli* O157:H7 infections. N Engl J Med. 2000 Jun 29;342(26):1930–6.
3. Freedman SB, Xie J, Neufeld MS, Hamilton WL, Hartling L, Tarr PI; Alberta Provincial Pediatric Enteric Infection Team (APPETITE), Nettel-Aguire A, Chuck A, Lee B, Johnson D, Currie G, Talbot J, et al. Shiga toxin-producing *Escherichia coli* infection, antibiotics, and risk of developing hemolytic uremic syndrome: a meta-analysis. Clin Infect Dis. 2016 May 15;62(10):1251–8. Epub 2016 Feb 24.
4. Launders N, Byrne L, Jenkins C, Harker K, Charlett A, Adak GK. Disease severity of Shiga toxin-producing *E coli* O157 and factors influencing the development of typical haemolytic uraemic syndrome: a retrospective cohort study, 2009-2012. BMJ Open. 2016 Jan 29;6(1):e009933.
5. Nitschke M, Sayk F, Hartel C, Roseland RT, Hauswaldt S, Steinhoff J, et al. Association between azithromycin therapy and duration of bacterial shedding among patients with Shiga toxin-producing enteroaggregative *Escherichia coli* O104:H4. JAMA. 2012 Mar 14;307(10):1046–52.

Cutaneous Clue to a Fever of Unknown Origin

53

Irene G. Sia, MD, and Carilyn N. Wieland, MD

A 50-year-old man was admitted to the hospital for evaluation of fever and skin lesions. Two months earlier, he had received a diagnosis of lung sarcoma with metastasis to the liver, and he began palliative chemotherapy with doxorubicin and olaratumab. He received a second dose of olaratumab 1 week later, but a week after the second dose of chemotherapy, he felt unwell and started having fevers (temperatures up to 38.9°C). He had a chronic cough but otherwise had no other focal symptoms.

A physical examination showed no localizing findings. His temperature was 38.0°C, and a white blood cell count was $3.7×10^9$/L, with $1.1×10^9$/L neutrophils. His erythrocyte sedimentation rate (ESR) was 61 mm/h, and the C-reactive protein level was 90 mg/L. A computed tomographic (CT) scan showed extensive pulmonary, hepatic, and adrenal metastases and right-sided pleural effusion. Treatment with cefepime and vancomycin was initiated. Blood cultures were negative.

Two days after he was admitted to the hospital, nonpruritic, erythematous plaques and nodules appeared on the right side of his neck (Figure 53.1), and a similar lesion was noted on his right forearm. The lesions became painful. A dermatologist was consulted, and skin punch biopsy specimens were obtained for histopathologic analysis and tissue cultures.

Histopathologic analysis showed diffuse, dermal, and predominantly neutrophilic inflammation. Grocott-Gomori methenamine silver and Gram stains were negative for microorganisms.

Bacterial, fungal, and mycobacterial cultures of the biopsy specimens remained negative. Antibiotics were discontinued. He resumed chemotherapy and began treatment with dexamethasone. The fever and skin lesions resolved. A follow-up CT scan, obtained approximately 6 weeks later, showed a partial tumor response to treatment.

Discussion

Acute febrile neutrophilic dermatosis (also termed *Sweet syndrome*), was first described in

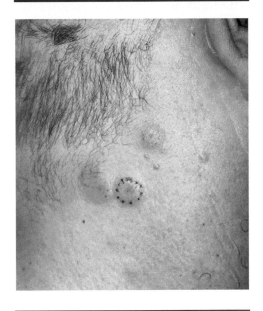

Figure 53.1   Nonpruritic, Erythematous Plaques and Nodules on the Neck

1964 by Robert Douglas Sweet (1). Sweet syndrome is an uncommon inflammatory disorder that is characterized by a constellation of clinical, laboratory, and pathologic findings. Although the cause of Sweet syndrome is unknown, this dermatosis is associated with a broad range of disorders, most commonly hematologic or lymphoid malignancies, solid tumors, or inflammatory bowel disease. The syndrome also can be associated with infections (particularly upper respiratory tract and gastrointestinal infections), pregnancy, other systemic inflammatory disorders, and medications. It is more common in women than in men. Most patients are aged 30 to 60 years.

About 21% to 54% of patients with Sweet syndrome have a concurrent hematologic malignancy or solid tumor (2,3). Acute myelogenous leukemia is the most common hematologic malignancy, and carcinomas of the breast, gastrointestinal tract, and genitourinary tract account for the solid tumors associated with Sweet syndrome. Granulocyte-colony stimulating factor is the drug most commonly associated with Sweet syndrome (3). Other medications linked to Sweet syndrome include azathioprine, trimethoprim-sulfamethoxazole, minocycline, nitrofurantoin, oral contraceptives, and retinoids (4).

The main features of Sweet syndrome are fever, edematous and reddish plaques, neutrophilia, and the histologic finding of diffuse dermal neutrophilic infiltrates. Patients often present with abrupt-onset, tender, and erythematous papules, plaques, or nodules that range in size from several millimeters to several centimeters. Some patients may have pustules, bullae, and central erosion. The skin lesions may occur at any site, although they most frequently involve the face, neck, trunk, and upper extremities. Fever occurs in up to 88% of patients with malignancy-associated Sweet syndrome (2).

Patients with Sweet syndrome may have multisystem involvement with neutrophilic infiltration of other organs, such as the eye, heart, lung, kidney, liver, or spleen, and Sweet syndrome may affect the joints, gastrointestinal system, and central nervous system, resulting in a broad range of clinical manifestations. Leukocytosis with neutrophilia is present in a considerable proportion of patients; ESR and C-reactive protein are also often elevated. The characteristic histopathologic features of Sweet syndrome include prominent superficial dermal edema, diffuse dense neutrophilic infiltrate in the upper dermis and middermis, leukocytoclastic nuclear debris, and absence of vasculitis.

The diagnosis of Sweet syndrome is determined by numerous criteria (5). The 2 major criteria are 1) acute onset of painful, tender, and erythematous plaques or nodules and 2) histopathologic evidence of neutrophilic dermal infiltrates without vasculitis. Additionally, at least 2 of the 4 following clinical features are required for the diagnosis: 1) fever; 2) underlying malignancy, inflammatory disease, pregnancy, or preceding upper respiratory or gastrointestinal tract infection; 3) abnormal laboratory values (elevated ESR or C-reactive protein, leukocytosis, or neutrophilia); and 4) response to treatment with systemic corticosteroids.

The differential diagnosis of Sweet syndrome depends on the morphology of the skin lesions and clinical history. Infection is among the most important considerations. Clinical conditions that mimic Sweet syndrome include entities that may initially present as red macules and then evolve into plaques with pustular or ulcerative features. Prominent central necrosis should increase suspicion for infection, rather than for Sweet syndrome. Ecthyma gangrenosum is associated with *Pseudomonas aeruginosa* sepsis and bacteremia in immunocompromised patients. Lesions commonly begin as painless, red macules that rapidly evolve into areas of induration with pustules or bullae (or both) and then become gangrenous ulcers. Angioinvasive aspergillosis, particularly in patients with hematologic malignancies or hematopoietic cell transplant, can disseminate and have cutaneous manifestations. Cutaneous aspergillosis lesions initially appear as macules, papules, nodules, or plaques and evolve to hemorrhagic bullae or ulcerative nodules. Infection with *Fusarium* species in immunosuppressed patients may present as localized or disseminated skin lesions, with multiple erythematous and tender papular or nodular lesions, frequently with central necrosis. Skin lesions associated with invasive infection by *Candida* species tend to appear as clusters of painless pustules on an erythematous base. In addition, lesions of Sweet syndrome can mimic local bacterial, fungal, and mycobacterial infections.

A skin biopsy should be performed for histopathologic evaluation and tissue cultures to establish the diagnosis of Sweet syndrome. Histopathologic examination must include special stains (eg, Grocott-Gomori methenamine silver, Gram, and acid-fast bacillus stains) to detect microorganisms. Microbial studies such as bacterial, fungal, and mycobacterial cultures of a biopsy specimen should be done to rule out infection.

First-line therapy for Sweet syndrome is systemic corticosteroids, which will promptly improve symptoms and skin lesions. Second-line agents include potassium iodide, colchicine, dapsone, indomethacin, and clofazimine (4). Treatment of the underlying malignancy will result in complete resolution of the skin lesions.

References

1. Sweet RD. An acute febrile neutrophilic dermatosis. Br J Dermatol. 1964 Aug-Sep;76:349–56.
2. Cohen PR, Holder WR, Tucker SB, Kono S, Kurzrock R. Sweet syndrome in patients with solid tumors. Cancer. 1993 Nov 1;72(9):2723–31.
3. Raza S, Kirkland RS, Patel AA, Shortridge JR, Freter C. Insight into Sweet's syndrome and associated-malignancy: a review of the current literature. Int J Oncol. 2013 May;42(5):1516–22. Epub 2013 Mar 28.
4. Cohen PR. Sweet's syndrome: a comprehensive review of an acute febrile neutrophilic dermatosis. Orphanet J Rare Dis. 2007 Jul 26;2:34.
5. Su WP, Liu HN. Diagnostic criteria for Sweet's syndrome. Cutis. 1986 Mar;37(3):167–74.

A Chronic Polyarthritis

54

Douglas W. Challener, MD, Jasmine R. Marcelin, MD,
and Kelly A. Cawcutt, MD

Case Presentation

A previously healthy 55-year-old white man who used to work as a cattle farmer presented with a 1.5-year history of aching joints that was initially limited to his wrists but gradually progressed to involve his fingers and ankles. He had intermittent fevers (up to 38.3°C) that occurred on a daily to weekly basis. He denied nausea, vomiting, abdominal pain, diarrhea, and constipation. After an initial, unsuccessful attempt at symptom management by his primary care doctor, he was evaluated by a rheumatologist for polyarticular arthritis. At that time, his C-reactive protein level was elevated at 27.4 mg/L (reference range, ≤9 mg/L), and results of serologic tests for rheumatoid factor, anticitrullinated protein antibodies, and antinuclear antibodies were negative. The distribution and evolution of joint pain suggested the diagnoses of palindromic rheumatism and seronegative rheumatoid arthritis, and he was treated with methotrexate and prednisone for nearly a year.

Despite treatment, the patient continued to have intermittent fevers, night chills, and joint pain. A computed tomographic (CT) scan of the chest, abdomen, and pelvis showed retroperitoneal lymphadenopathy and mesenteric inflammation. A CT-guided lymph node biopsy showed lymphoid hyperplasia with scattered fibrohistiocytic areas that suggested granulomatous inflammation. Serologic evaluation for *Histoplasma* and *Brucella* species were negative. A serologic polymerase chain reaction (PCR) assay for *Tropheryma whipplei* was negative, as was an interferon-γ release assay.

With these negative test results, his care team resolved to continue treatment for presumed rheumatologic disease. He was switched from methotrexate to hydroxychloroquine because of concern of methotrexate-induced fever. However, with the continued lack of response, he was then transitioned to tocilizumab. Ultimately, during the following months, the joint symptoms progressed to involve his knees, and diarrhea also developed. The diarrhea began more than a year after he first sought medical evaluation for his syndrome. A joint aspirate of his right knee was obtained, and a PCR test of the aspirate was positive for *T whipplei*. A subsequent small-bowel aspirate was also positive for *T whipplei* (PCR test).

He was treated for 4 weeks with intravenous ceftriaxone. After this course was completed, he began maintenance therapy with low-dose trimethoprim-sulfamethoxazole (TMP-SMX). He had some initial improvement but then had symptom recurrence plus additional symptoms of shortness of breath, chest pain, and blurry vision. Multisystem Whipple disease (WD) was subsequently diagnosed and included right eye vitritis and pericarditis. The patient restarted treatment with intravenous ceftriaxone for 4 weeks. He also received intravitreal ceftazidime because of ophthalmologic evidence of inflammatory lesions in both eyes. The intravenous treatment course was then followed by a regimen of high-dose TMP-SMX and oral doxycycline. His joint symptoms, shortness of breath, and chest pain completely resolved; however, he had several rounds of waxing and waning visual blurriness in both eyes and repeated the 4-week course of intravenous ceftriaxone and intravitreal ceftazidime on 3 occasions. He was ultimately transitioned to oral suppressive TMP-SMX (1 double-strength dose, twice daily) and rifampin

(600 mg daily) and successfully completed a year of therapy without relapse.

Discussion

WD is a rare, systemic illness first described in 1907 by George H. Whipple. It is classically characterized by weight loss, diarrhea, abdominal pain, and arthralgias. The infectious organism, *T whipplei*, is a gram-positive, intracellular bacillus. Although *T whipplei* was not successfully cultured in vitro until the late 1990s, its bacterial morphology was confirmed approximately 30 years earlier with light microscopy. The organism is universally present in the environment, and contaminated soil has been identified as a possible source of infection. The bacteria also are prevalent in seawater sediments and influxes to sewage treatment areas, and unsurprisingly, this organism has been detected in stool samples from sewage plant workers (1). Humans are the only known host of *T whipplei*, and up to 11% of healthy persons may have *T whipplei* present in their stool. Asymptomatic carriage seems to be as common as WD is rare, with up to 70% of Europeans having positive serologic findings (2). Nevertheless, it can also cause acute infection, rare chronic infection, and WD (3).

T whipplei may be transmitted through the stool and saliva of infected patients. The bacteria are phagocytosed by macrophages in the digestive lumen, and after being ineffectively degraded, they subsequently replicate within mucosal macrophages and mononuclear cells in the blood (4). Thus, any organ system can be affected in WD (5). *T whipplei* have been found in cardiac valves, duodenal samples, blood, stool, saliva, synovial fluid, and cerebrospinal fluid of affected individuals. The skin also may serve as a reservoir for *T whipplei*, even in patients without evidence of WD, and skin darkening may occur (6).

The multitude of presentations, the lack of growth of the organism in standard cell culture media, and the long-term nature of WD make diagnosis challenging. Classically, WD affects middle-aged, white men living in rural areas. The prodromal stage of WD usually starts with arthralgia and lasts for months or even years before gastrointestinal problems manifest (3). Common features at presentation are colicky abdominal pain and watery diarrhea that lead to weight loss, plus arthralgia and arthritis. Patients less frequently have occult intestinal blood loss or steatorrhea. The disease can ultimately progress into cachexia, ascites, and peripheral edema caused by severe malnutrition. Additionally, patients may have low-grade fever, adenopathy, and anemia. Neurologic symptoms may be present in up to 25% of patients. Patients may present with involvement of the central nervous system and have headaches, cognitive dysfunction, ataxia, seizures, insomnia, and meningismus. Some patients will have oculofacial myorhythmia (rhythmic convergence of the eyes with contraction of the muscles of mastication), which is pathognomonic for WD (7). Ocular WD is an example of central nervous system involvement and is usually a late finding. It can manifest as visual acuity changes with uveitis, retinitis, or choroiditis (8).

Diagnosis is often established with a small-bowel examination and biopsy. During an upper endoscopy, the small bowel in WD will appear as a pale-yellow mucosal surface with dilated villi, but this appearance is nonspecific. Histologically, foamy macrophages with particles that are positive for periodic acid–Schiff (PAS) stain are detected in the lamina propria of the duodenum. Ziehl-Neelsen staining can be used to differentiate between these inclusions and inclusion bodies associated with *Mycobacterium avium intracellulare* infection (1). If a small-bowel biopsy cannot be performed or is nondiagnostic, WD may be diagnosed by using alternative methods, such as a PCR test, PAS staining, or immunohistochemistry assay of affected tissue. Typically, either multiple test sites or multiple different assays are required to positively establish a diagnosis in the absence of a small-bowel biopsy (2).

WD usually is curable, but successful treatment requires prolonged courses of antibiotics. The treatment of choice for many years was tetracycline, although relapse rates approached 40%. Currently, effective treatment of long-term classic or localized WD consists of induction therapy with intravenous ceftriaxone or penicillin G for 2 weeks, followed by 1 year of maintenance therapy with TMP-SMX. No consensus guidelines exist regarding the treatment of ocular disease, although combination therapy with TMP-SMX and rifampin for at least 1 year has been reported to be highly effective. Rifampin and TMP-SMX have favorable penetration of the blood-brain barrier compared with tetracycline (8). Although neurologic deficits caused by structural brain damage are irreversible, most nonneurologic symptoms will resolve in several weeks. Immune reconstitution inflammatory syndrome is a complication of WD treatment that may occur with eradication of the organism, and patients who have been treated with immunosuppressants for presumed rheumatologic disorders before antimicrobial therapy are particularly at risk. Clinical relapse occurs in approximately a quarter of patients and should be treated with reinduction therapy followed by maintenance therapy. PCR assays can be used to confirm cure because of its high sensitivity. For patients with continued symptoms despite therapy, repeat testing should be performed (2).

References

1. Schneider T, Moos V, Loddenkemper C, Marth T, Fenollar F, Raoult D. Whipple's disease: new aspects of pathogenesis and treatment. Lancet Infect Dis. 2008 Mar;8(3):179–90.
2. Fenollar F, Lagier JC, Raoult D. *Tropheryma whipplei* and Whipple's disease. J Infect. 2014 Aug;69(2):103–12. Epub 2014 May 28.
3. Fenollar F, Puechal X, Raoult D. Whipple's disease. N Engl J Med. 2007 Jan 4;356(1):55–66.
4. Schoniger-Hekele M, Petermann D, Weber B, Muller C. *Tropheryma whipplei* in the environment: survey of sewage plant influxes and sewage plant workers. Appl Environ Microbiol. 2007 Mar;73(6):2033–5. Epub 2007 Feb 2.
5. Angelakis E, Fenollar F, Lepidi H, Birg ML, Raoult D. *Tropheryma whipplei* in the skin of patients with classic Whipple's disease. J Infect. 2010 Sep;61(3):266–9. Epub 2010 Jun 19.
6. Lagier JC, Lepidi H, Raoult D, Fenollar F. Systemic *Tropheryma whipplei*: clinical presentation of 142 patients with infections diagnosed or confirmed in a reference center. Medicine (Baltimore). 2010 Sep;89(5):337–45.
7. Maiwald M, Relman D. Whipple's disease and *Tropheryma whippelii*: secrets slowly revealed. Clin Infect Dis. 2001 Feb 1;32(3):457–63. Epub 2001 Jan 18.
8. Touitou V, Fenollar F, Cassoux N, Merle-Beral H, LeHoang P, Amoura Z, et al. Ocular Whipple's disease: therapeutic strategy and long-term follow-up. Ophthalmology. 2012 Jul;119(7):1465–9. Epub 2012 Mar 13.

Questions and Answers

Questions

Multiple Choice (choose the best answer)

II.1. A 60-year-old male horse rancher from the Midwest presented to the emergency department with a 2-week history of malaise, progressive cough with green sputum, dyspnea, and pleuritic chest pain. His medical history included nonalcoholic liver cirrhosis for which he underwent orthotopic liver transplantation 3 years ago. His medications included tacrolimus, mycophenolate mofetil, and prednisone. Computed tomography of his chest showed right upper-lobe necrotizing pneumonia. Blood cultures grew gram-positive bacteria that appeared rod shaped in liquid media and coccoid in solid media, with salmon-pink colonies. Which of the following statements describes the best treatment approach?

a. Empiric antimicrobial therapy should include trimethoprim-sulfamethoxazole

b. Combination oral antimicrobial therapy is recommended initially

c. Monotherapy with vancomycin is the treatment of choice

d. Combination of oral and intravenous antimicrobial therapy is indicated in this case

e. Surgical intervention is immediately recommended

II.2. A 40-year-old bisexual man from Florida presents to his primary physician's office because of a nonresolving, viral-like illness and worsening fatigue for the past 2 weeks, despite symptomatic treatment. He had presented to an urgent care facility 3 days earlier, when an HIV serologic screen and a test for infectious mononucleosis were negative. Which of the following diagnostic tests is most appropriate at this time?

a. Rapid molecular test for influenza A and B viruses

b. Repeat HIV serologic screen

c. HIV RNA test

d. Cytomegalovirus serologic test

e. Epstein-Barr virus antibody test

II.3. A 24-year-old man with a history of HIV infection presents with a 1-month history of progressive headache, photophobia, and nausea. His most recent laboratory tests showed a CD4 level of 156 cells/mcL and a viral load of 2,900 copies/mL. He notes occasional noncompliance with his regimen of abacavir, dolutegravir, and lamivudine. Computed tomography (CT) of the head shows no abnormalities. His condition is diagnosed as cryptococcal meningitis on the basis of cerebrospinal fluid (CSF) and serum antigen titers that are positive for *Cryptococcus* and a CSF profile that is consistent with fungal infection. He begins treatment with liposomal amphotericin B and flucytosine and easily tolerates this regimen. He is dismissed on hospital day 4 and is scheduled to have an outpatient follow-up evaluation after 2 weeks of induction therapy. What testing is important to obtain at the 2-week follow-up appointment?

a. Head CT and serum CD4 and HIV RNA level

b. Head CT and electrocardiogram

c. Lumbar puncture and serum creatinine, potassium, and magnesium

d. Magnetic resonance imaging of the brain and spine

e. Echocardiogram and CT of the chest

II.4. A 52-year-old man received the diagnosis of ocular syphilis. He reported a history of a mild allergic reaction to penicillin. He asks if there are other treatment options that are not as frequent as intravenous penicillin or whether he can avoid penicillin altogether. What do you advise?

a. Treat with intramuscular benzathine penicillin, 2.4 million units, once per week

b. Treat with oral doxycycline, 100 mg, twice daily, for 7 days

c. Treat with oral azithromycin, 250 mg for 10 days

d. Treat with intravenous ceftriaxone, 2 g, once a day, for 10-14 days

e. Treat with intravenous azithromycin, 500 mg daily for 10 days

II.5. A 32-year-old man reported 3 weeks of blurry vision. Funduscopic examination findings were consistent with right-sided panuveitis. A fourth-generation HIV screening test was positive, with a CD4$^+$ T-cell count of 58 cells/mcL and a viral load of 68,000 copies/mL. A rapid plasma reagin test was positive, with a titer of 1:128. He denied headache, neurologic weakness, or cognitive changes. What is the next best step in the management of this patient?

a. Treat with intravenous penicillin G for confirmed ocular syphilis

b. Obtain a lumbar puncture and send the cerebrospinal fluid sample for venereal disease research laboratory testing

c. Perform a vitrectomy

d. Treat with outpatient ceftriaxone as a convenient alternative to penicillin

e. Treat with oral doxycycline, 100 mg, twice daily, for 7 days for convenience

II.6. A 50-year-old man from New Mexico presented to his physician with new skin nodules, 3 months after a respiratory illness. He did not have headaches. Skin biopsy showed noncaseating granulomas and spherules on Gomori methenamine silver staining. Which of the following is NOT recommended to diagnose his condition?

a. *Coccidioides* serology

b. Fungal blood cultures

c. Lumbar puncture

d. Skin biopsy with culture and histopathologic examination

e. *Coccidioides* polymerase chain reaction of clinical specimens

II.7. A 50-year-old man from New Mexico presented to his physician with new skin nodules, 3 months after a respiratory illness. He did not have headaches. Skin biopsy showed noncaseating granulomas and spherules on Gomori methenamine silver staining. What is the preferred treatment for this condition?

a. Oral flucytosine

b. Oral fluconazole

c. Intravenous amphotericin B

d. Intravenous caspofungin

e. Oral terbinafine

II.8. A 66-year-old white woman presented to the emergency department with right lower extremity cellulitis. She had not had cellulitis previously. Her body mass index (BMI) was 27 kg/m^2, and she had a history of coronary artery disease (with coronary artery bypass graft and right saphenous venectomy, 5 years earlier), eczema affecting her elbows, and breast cancer (with left mastectomy and lymph node dissection, 20 years earlier). Her cellulitis was treated with a 5-day course of oral cefadroxil. Which of the following is the most important risk factor for development of cellulitis in this patient?

a. BMI of 27 kg/m^2

b. Coronary artery bypass graft, 5 years earlier

c. Eczema

d. Breast cancer

e. White race

II.9. A 66-year-old woman had 4 episodes of right lower extremity cellulitis. Her body mass index was 27 kg/m^2, and she had a history of coronary artery disease with coronary artery bypass graft (requiring right saphenous venectomy), eczema affecting her elbows, and left mastectomy and lymph node dissection for breast cancer. What is the best strategy to avoid future episodes of lower extremity cellulitis in this patient?

a. Daily oral penicillin V potassium

b. Daily oral erythromycin

c. Monthly intramuscular benzathine penicillin

d. Weekly intravenous cefazolin

e. Twice-monthly intravenous dalbavancin

II.10. A 62-year-old man presents with an 8-month history of fatigue and dry cough. Chest imaging shows bilateral cavitating lung lesions. A computed tomography–guided biopsy of one of the lesions shows gram-positive filamentous bacilli. A sputum culture grows *Nocardia* after 22 days of incubation. Which of the following statements is true about this case?

a. *Nocardia asteroides* is the most common species that causes human disease

b. Blood cultures are likely to be positive for *Nocardia*

c. Modified acid-fast staining will identify *Nocardia*

d. Special culture media is required for *Nocardia* growth

e. The main site of primary infection is the central nervous system

II.11. A 47-year-old woman from Arkansas presents with a 6-month history of low-grade fevers and purpuric rash bilaterally on her lower extremities. Laboratory evaluation showed pancytopenia, elevated liver function, and elevated inflammatory markers. Skin biopsy findings were consistent with leukocytoclastic vasculitis. An extensive evaluation yielded no evidence of inflammatory or neoplastic disease. Her medical history included a bicuspid aortic valve requiring replacement with a bioprosthesis. A transesophageal echocardiogram showed a large abscess surrounding the aortic prosthesis. A serologic test for Q fever was positive, and Q fever

endocarditis was diagnosed. Which of the following statements are true?

a. Echocardiography is not necessary after acquiring an acute infection for patients with preexisting valve lesions because the disease is self-limited

b. The treatment of choice for Q fever endocarditis is oral doxycycline, taken daily for 12 months

c. The treatment of choice for Q fever endocarditis is oral doxycycline plus hydroxychloroquine, taken daily for 18 months

d. The infection is more common in females

e. Extensive exposure to the Q fever pathogen is necessary to acquire the infection

II.12. A 45-year-old woman with a history of acute myeloid leukemia presented with altered mental status of 3 days' duration. Her family reported a change in her behavior and inability to remember anything. She had an allogeneic hematopoietic stem cell transplant 28 days earlier. A physical examination showed that she was afebrile and hemodynamically stable, and she had anterograde amnesia without focal neurologic deficits. Her absolute neutrophil count had been greater than 0.5×10^9/L for the past 7 days. A lumbar puncture was performed, and the cerebrospinal fluid analysis showed a white blood cell count of 14 cells/mcL with 90% lymphocytes, protein level of 90 mg/dL, and glucose level of 45 mg/dL. Results of polymerase chain reaction (PCR) tests for human herpesvirus (HHV) 6 in the plasma and cerebrospinal fluid are pending. Which of the following statements is true regarding her diagnosis?

a. Magnetic resonance imaging will mostly show changes in the frontal lobes

b. A negative PCR test result for HHV-6 in the plasma will exclude HHV-6 encephalitis

c. Empiric treatment with cidofovir is indicated

d. Her current illness most likely represents reactivation of an HHV-6 infection acquired during early childhood

e. Patients with umbilical cord blood transplants have lower risk of HHV-6 infection than patients receiving peripheral blood stem cell transplants

II.13. A 39-year-old heterosexual man with a 20-year history of HIV infection presented to a new infectious diseases physician for consideration of restarting antiretroviral treatment. The patient was treatment experienced and had been exposed to nucleoside reverse transcriptase inhibitors, nonnucleoside reverse transcriptase inhibitors, protease inhibitors, and integrase inhibitors. He had a history of long-term medication noncompliance for multiple reasons, including medication intolerance, loss to follow-up, and denial. He was not currently receiving any antiretroviral therapy. Laboratory tests showed a $CD4^+$ helper T-cell count of 150 cells/mcL and HIV-1 viral load of 50,000 copies/mL. Genotypic drug-resistance testing identified the following mutations: M184V, K101H, G190A, Q148S, G140S, G163R, and S230N. Which antiretroviral drug class does the virus show susceptibility to?

a. Nucleoside reverse transcriptase inhibitors

b. Nonnucleoside reverse transcriptase inhibitors

c. Protease inhibitors

d. Integrase strand transfer inhibitors

e. These genes do not confer clinically significant resistance to any class

II.14. A 39-year-old heterosexual man with a 20-year history of HIV infection and a history of long-term medication noncompliance underwent genotypic drug-resistance testing. The following mutations were identified: M184V, K101H, G190A, Q148S, G140S, G163R, and S230N. Given his

resistance testing results, what antiretroviral regimen is likely to be most effective?

a. Tenofovir-emtricitabine, abacavir, ritonavir-boosted darunavir, etravirine

b. Abacavir-lamivudine-dolutegravir

c. Tenofovir-emtricitabine-cobicistat-elvitegravir

d. Maraviroc, raltegravir, tenofovir-emtricitabine

e. Tenofovir-emtricitabine-rilpivirine

II.15. A 29-year-old patient with diabetes mellitus presents with erythema, edema, and severe pain in his left leg. He recently had been treated for cellulitis but said that he had not noticed any improvement. The area that he had previously noticed was now turning blue. His blood pressure was 120/85 mm Hg, his heart rate was 105 beats/min, his respiratory rate was 18 breaths/min, and his temperature was 38.1°C. What is the most appropriate next step?

a. Superficial skin swab

b. Empiric antibiotics and surgical consultation

c. Computed tomographic scan of the left leg

d. Ultrasound of the left leg

e. Observation

II.16. A 29-year-old patient with diabetes mellitus presents with erythema, edema, and severe pain in his left leg. He recently had been treated for cellulitis but said that he had not noticed any improvement. The area that he had previously noticed was now turning blue. The patient was taken to the operating room, and leg findings were consistent with necrotizing fasciitis. A débridement was completed. What antibiotic therapy should be initiated, assuming that he has no relevant allergies?

a. Vancomycin

b. Piperacillin-tazobactam plus clindamycin plus vancomycin

c. Clindamycin plus piperacillin-tazobactam

d. Vancomycin plus piperacillin-tazobactam

e. Oritavancin

II.17. A 48-year-old black man with HIV and diet-controlled type 2 diabetes mellitus presented to his physician for a general medical examination after not receiving medical care for 3 years. He was previously prescribed antiretroviral therapy (ART) that consisted of elvitegravir, cobicistat, emtricitabine, and tenofovir, but he was only intermittently taking these medications. He noted worsening lower extremity edema and foamy urine. His blood pressure was elevated at 148/95 mm Hg, serum creatinine was elevated at 2.8 mg/dL, and urinalysis showed nephrotic-range proteinuria. His estimated glomerular filtration rate was 37 mL/min per 1.73 m². A kidney biopsy specimen had findings consistent with HIV-associated nephropathy. He was informed of the diagnosis, and his blood pressure was still elevated (152/96 mm Hg). Which of the following medication changes should be made?

a. Change ART to abacavir, dolutegravir, and lamivudine if an HLA-B*5701 test is negative; add aspirin, atorvastatin, and lisinopril

b. Change ART to emtricitabine, rilpivirine, and tenofovir; add aspirin, atorvastatin, and amlodipine

c. Continue ART with elvitegravir, cobicistat, emtricitabine, and tenofovir; add amlodipine

d. Change ART to darunavir, cobicistat, emtricitabine, and tenofovir

e. No medication change

II.18. A 52-year-old man from Minnesota is planning to undergo dental extraction for a cracked tooth (right first upper molar). He had a bioprosthetic aortic valve replacement about 2 years ago and has no known drug allergies. Which of the following is the most appropriate management option for endocarditis prophylaxis?

a. Amoxicillin

b. Cephalexin

c. Clindamycin

d. No antibiotic prophylaxis

e. Intravenous vancomycin

II.19. A 57-year-old woman from Brazil presented with a severe headache and jaw claudication. She was diagnosed with temporal arteritis and received 3 doses of methylprednisolone, 1 g each, followed by a prolonged taper. Three weeks after her initial diagnosis, she was readmitted with a fever, confusion, headache, and neck stiffness. Computed tomography of the head was negative for mass lesions, and a cerebrospinal fluid analysis showed elevated protein, low glucose, and neutrophilic pleocytosis. Cerebrospinal fluid cultures grew *Escherichia coli*. The patient was treated intravenously with high-dose ceftriaxone for 2 weeks and showed marked improvement. What is the next appropriate step in management?

a. Start suppressive therapy with oral cefadroxil because she is immunocompromised

b. Repeat the lumbar puncture before discontinuing therapy, to document clearance of the infection

c. Perform a colonoscopy to assess for malignancy as a source of *E coli* meningitis

d. Obtain *Strongyloides* serology and stool cultures

e. Order an abdominal or pelvic computed tomographic scan with contrast to assess for intestinal obstruction

II.20. A 50-year-old man presented with sudden-onset shortness of breath. He was recently diagnosed with pancreatic adenocarcinoma. His blood pressure was in the normal range, but his heart rate was slightly elevated. He was afebrile. An emergency department physician ordered a D-dimer test, and results were within normal limits. A chest radiograph was equivocal for an infiltrate. He was diagnosed with community-acquired pneumonia and admitted to a medicine ward for treatment. He required supplemental oxygen at the time of admission to maintain saturation. His oxygen requirements continued to increase over the next days, despite appropriate antibiotic therapy. A computed tomographic angiogram of the thorax showed a large saddle pulmonary embolism. Anticoagulation therapy was initiated and he improved. Which diagnostic error(s) was/were made?

a. Anchoring bias
b. Availability heuristic
c. Observation bias
d. Framing effect
e. Referral bias

II.21. A 47-year-old woman with a 10-year history of HIV, most recently treated with tenofovir, emtricitabine, and efavirenz, presents for a general medical examination and notes that she is sexually active with a male partner who is unaware of her HIV status. What is your next step in management regarding partner notification?

a. Have the public health department assist in partner notification
b. Encourage the patient to notify her partner
c. Call her partner to notify him of her HIV status
d. Make no recommendation at this time. Schedule a follow-up appointment with the patient and her partner
e. Advise her to secure legal assistance to determine whether she has violated state laws.

II.22. A 65-year-old man with a recent vancomycin-resistant *Enterococcus* infection presented with new-onset fever and dyspnea, 2 weeks after initiation of daptomycin treatment. He had increased work of breathing that required emergent intubation. Laboratory studies showed an elevated white blood cell count with neutrophil predominance. A chest radiograph showed bilateral pulmonary infiltrates and pleural effusion. Bronchoscopy was performed. Differential cell count of the bronchoalveolar lavage showed 29% eosinophils. Which of the following statements is true regarding his diagnosis?

a. This patient does not have daptomycin-induced acute eosinophilic pneumonia (AEP) because he does not have peripheral eosinophilia
b. This patient requires a lung biopsy to confirm the diagnosis of daptomycin-induced AEP
c. This patient should be rechallenged with daptomycin to confirm the diagnosis of daptomycin-induced AEP
d. Management includes empiric therapy with ivermectin
e. Management with corticosteroids is indicated

II.23. A 20-year-old HIV-positive homosexual man was referred to the HIV clinic with a new diagnosis of hepatitis C virus (HCV) genotype 1 coinfection that was identified with routine screening. He is otherwise healthy. His current antiretroviral therapy (ART) consists of efavirenz, emtricitabine, and tenofovir disoproxil fumarate. He has an undetectable viral load and a CD4 T-cell count of 440 cells/mcL. After appropriate laboratory evaluation and imaging studies are performed, what is the next step?

a. Temporarily discontinue his current ART to begin HCV therapy
b. Initiate anti-HCV therapy with sofosbuvir-velpatasvir
c. Initiate anti-HCV therapy with ledipasvir-sofosbuvir
d. Initiate anti-HCV therapy with peg-interferon and ribavirin
e. Consider changing his ART regimen with initiation of HCV treatment

II.24. A 25-year-old man was diagnosed with HIV. He had a CD4 count of 89 cells/mcL and a viral load of 80,000 copies/mL. He was started on combination antiretroviral therapy (cART). Three months after initiation of cART, he presented with a purple, nonblanching, patchy skin rash on a lower extremity. AIDS-related Kaposi sarcoma (KS) was diagnosed via skin biopsy and was thought to be due to immune reconstitution inflammatory syndrome. His CD4 count had a dramatic increase to 375 cells/mcL, and his viral load was <500 copies/mL. The patient denied any signs of visceral organ involvement, and his oral mucosa appeared normal during the physical examination. What should be the next step in the management of KS?

a. Discontinue cART

b. Apply a corticosteroid ointment

c. Continue cART and monitor closely

d. Switch to a different kind of antiretroviral therapy

e. Add valacyclovir

II.25. A 56-year-old man with end-stage renal disease attributable to type 2 diabetes mellitus underwent deceased-donor kidney transplant 2 years before presentation; his allograft was maintained with prednisone, mycophenolate mofetil, and tacrolimus. He was admitted with fever, headache, and altered mental status. A computed tomographic scan of the brain did not show any abnormalities, and a lumbar puncture was performed. Cryptococcal antigen testing on the cerebrospinal fluid was positive, with a titer greater than 1:2,560. Combined antifungal therapy was initiated with liposomal amphotericin B and flucytosine; mycophenolate mofetil was discontinued. He recovered well and was discharged home on consolidation therapy with fluconazole (800 mg daily). He presented 1 week after discharge with diffuse tremors, confusion, and acute renal failure. The most appropriate next step is:

a. Discontinue fluconazole and resume liposomal amphotericin B and flucytosine

b. Obtain a computed tomographic scan

of his head and proceed with lumbar puncture if negative

c. Start treatment with broad-spectrum antimicrobial agents

d. Withhold tacrolimus and check serum level

e. Start corticosteroids for immune reconstitution inflammatory syndrome

II.26. A 27-year-old woman, originally from southern Japan, presents to the clinic for a general medical examination. She is a known carrier of human T-lymphotropic virus (HTLV) 1. Which of the following would be an appropriate statement to counsel the patient regarding transmission of HTLV-1?

a. HTLV-1 is not transmitted through blood transfusions

b. She does not need to use a protective barrier for sexual intercourse

c. Breast milk can transmit HTLV-1

d. HTLV-1 is transmitted through plasma

e. HTLV-1 status is not assessed before tissue donation

II.27. A 34-year-old man with diabetes mellitus presented with a headache, epistaxis, and decreased vision. Three days before presentation, he had seen his primary care physician, who initiated treatment for bacterial sinusitis with oral amoxicillin and clavulanic acid. Despite taking the antibiotics, his headache worsened. A physical examination showed that he had bilateral proptosis and a palatal eschar in the oropharynx. Laboratory testing showed a blood glucose level of 450 mg/dL, anion gap of 25 mEq/L, and bicarbonate of 14 mmol/L. His white blood cell count was 16×10^9/L. In addition to surgical débridement, what is the best therapy?

a. Intravenous (IV) liposomal amphotericin B

b. Oral posaconazole

c. IV voriconazole

d. Hyperbaric oxygen

e. IV amphotericin B plus deferoxamine

II.28. Which of the following tests is required to diagnose rhinocerebral mucormycosis?

a. Blood cultures

b. Histopathologic examination and culture of surgical tissue

c. Urinary antigen testing

d. Serum immunoglobulin M and immunoglobulin G to zygomycetes

e. Magnetic resonance imaging of the head

II.29. A 20-year-old man from Bukavu, on the southern part of Lake Kivu in the Democratic Republic of the Congo, presents with a 9-month history of leg edema. Extensive evaluations yield no evidence of filarial disease, and a skin biopsy identifies a sarcoma, with special stains showing positivity for human herpesvirus 8 (HHV-8). The patient is HIV negative. Which of the following statements are true about this case?

a. The patient most likely has epidemic Kaposi sarcoma (KS)

b. Chemotherapy is unlikely to be a major part of this patient's treatment

c. The area where the patient is from suggests that he has endemic KS

d. This presentation of disease is more common in females

e. Antiviral therapy directed at HHV-8 is the cornerstone of treatment

II.30. A 41-year-old man who recently emigrated from Brazil presents with a 1-week history of fever, right-sided upper-quadrant abdominal pain, and nausea. He has osteoarthritis, for which he takes acetaminophen (1,000 mg, 4 times daily). He has had 3 sexual partners (male and female) in the past year but denies any history of sexually transmitted infection. A physical examination shows a fever of 38.1°C, scleral icterus, and tenderness on palpation of the right upper abdominal quadrant. The Murphy sign is negative. Clinically significant laboratory findings are as follows: white blood cell count, 15.5×10^3/mcL; international normalized ratio, 1.1; creatinine, 1.1 mg/dL; aspartate transaminase, 1,325 U/L; alanine transaminase, 1,592 U/L; alkaline phosphatase, 623 U/L; total bilirubin, 5.6 mg/dL; and direct bilirubin, 3.4 mg/dL. Serologic tests are positive for hepatitis A virus (HAV) immunoglobulin (Ig) G; negative for HAV IgM; positive for anti–hepatitis B core (HBc) IgM; negative for anti-HBc IgG; positive for hepatitis B surface antigen (HBsAg); negative for anti-HBs antibodies; and negative for hepatitis C virus antibodies. Given his positive HBsAg result, a test for anti–hepatitis D virus (HDV) total antibodies is ordered and shows positive results. A subsequent HDV RNA test shows detectable levels. What is his most likely diagnosis?

a. Acute hepatitis B virus (HBV) and HDV coinfection

b. Acute HDV infection and acetaminophen-induced hepatotoxicity

c. Acute HDV infection and immunity to HBV from a prior vaccination

d. HDV superinfection of chronic hepatitis C virus infection

e. HDV superinfection of chronic HBV infection

II.31. A 70-year-old woman with a history of essential hypertension presented to the emergency department with a 3-day history of nausea, vomiting, and severe headache that was suggestive of meningitis. She had visited her primary care doctor 3 days earlier and received a pneumococcal vaccine. A computed tomographic scan of her head showed no intracranial lesions. A lumbar puncture was performed, and the findings of the cerebrospinal fluid (CSF) analysis were consistent with bacterial meningitis. Blood and CSF cultures were ordered, and empiric treatment was initiated with antibiotics and dexamethasone. Which of the following is true?

a. Invasive pneumococcal disease is mainly caused by vaccine serotypes

b. The *Streptococcus pneumoniae* vaccine can cause false-positive *S pneumoniae* immunochromatographic antigen test results

c. The accuracy of the *S pneumoniae* immunochromatographic antigen test has not been proven in children

d. The *S pneumoniae* immunochromatographic antigen test is not useful in patients who have received antibiotics for more than 24 hours

e. Blood cultures are rarely positive in patients with pneumococcal meningitis

II.32. A 67-year-old man with no relevant medical history presents to the infectious diseases clinic to inquire about pneumococcal vaccination and prevention of meningitis. Which of the following is false regarding pneumococcal immunization?

a. The pneumococcal polysaccharide vaccine protects against 23 serotypes

b. The pneumococcal conjugate vaccine (PCV13) protects against 13 serotypes

c. Both vaccines provide protection against pneumonia

d. Only PCV13 provides protection against pneumonia, meningitis, and bloodstream infection

e. PCV13 and the pneumococcal polysaccharide vaccine cannot be given at the same clinic visit

II.33. A 67-year-old man is diagnosed with Good syndrome. He begins treatment with intravenous immunoglobulin infusions. He says that he is planning a trip to Angola. Which of the following vaccinations are indicated?

a. Measles, mumps, rubella

b. *Haemophilus influenzae* type B

c. Varicella-zoster virus

d. Yellow fever

e. Human papillomavirus

II.34. A 67-year-old man is diagnosed with Good syndrome. He receives the appropriate vaccinations, and after thymectomy, he begins receiving intravenous

immunoglobulin. His immunoglobulin levels normalize, but his CD4+ count remains at 157 cells/mcL. What additional therapy, if any, could be considered?

a. No additional therapy is necessary

b. Trimethoprim-sulfamethoxazole

c. Azithromycin

d. Acyclovir

e. Amoxicillin

II.35. A 42-year-old man was seen in a primary care clinic with concerns about a sore throat, fever, headache, and myalgia. Three days ago, the patient had visited a whirlpool spa with work colleagues. He noted that 2 of his colleagues did not come to work on the day that he went to the clinic. A chest radiograph was negative for pneumonia. A urine *Legionella* antigen assay was positive. What is the best treatment option for this patient?

a. Oral azithromycin

b. Oral cephalexin

c. Intravenous erythromycin

d. Intravenous aminoglycosides

e. No treatment

II.36. A 57-year-old woman was admitted to the hospital with a fever, dry cough, and fatigue of 1 week's duration. A chest radiograph showed extensive bilateral consolidation. A test for *Legionella* urine antigen was positive. A sputum culture grew *Legionella* species after 5 days. She is currently receiving inpatient therapy with oral levofloxacin. She had a history of early-onset dementia and lived at a long-term care facility. Further investigation identified an ongoing outbreak of Legionnaires disease at that facility. What is the appropriate follow-up for this patient?

a. Obtain a chest radiograph every month

b. Obtain a monthly sputum culture to document clearance of bacteria from the respiratory tract

c. Repeat the *Legionella* urine antigen test every 4 months

d. Follow clinically

e. Perform monthly blood cultures for *Legionella* species

II.37. A 33-year-old man from Minnesota presents to the emergency department with fever, malaise, and a painful lesion on his right arm. A physical examination shows that his vital signs are stable but his temperature is 38.2°C. A tender, ulcerative lesion with central black eschar is noted on his right arm. He also has tender lymphadenopathy in the right axilla. He reports that a stray cat bit him on the right arm 5 days ago. What is the most likely cause of his symptoms?

a. Herpes simplex virus infection
b. *Sporothrix* infection
c. *Francisella* infection
d. *Ehrlichia* infection
e. *Leptospira* infection

II.38. An 18-year-old man from Wisconsin presented with a fever, productive cough, and pleuritic chest pain 2 days after he pulverized a squirrel while mowing the lawn. He was diagnosed with right-sided, lower-lobe, community-acquired pneumonia. He began treatment with ceftriaxone and azithromycin but showed no clinical improvement. Sputum cultures grew small, gram-negative coccobacilli on chocolate agar; no growth was seen with eosin methylene blue agar. The culture isolate was identified by matrix-assisted laser desorption/ionization–time of flight mass spectrometry (MALDI-TOF MS) as a *Francisella* species. Which of the following is an acceptable option for treating his pneumonia?

a. Vancomycin
b. Gentamicin
c. Cefepime
d. Ceftaroline
e. Meropenem

II.39. What isolation precautions should be used for a patient with tularemia?

a. Contact
b. Droplet
c. Standard
d. Airborne
e. Contact plus airborne

II.40. A 48-year-old man with paraplegia and long-term use of a suprapubic catheter was hospitalized with a 2-day history of fever, pelvic pain, and bladder spasms. He previously had multiple catheter-associated urinary tract infections (UTIs) and was known to be colonized with multidrug-resistant, gram-negative organisms. Urine and blood samples taken at admission were cultured and grew *Escherichia coli* that was resistant to meropenem. Results of screening tests for carbapenem-resistant *Enterobacteriaceae* (CRE) were positive for *Klebsiella pneumoniae* carbapenemase and negative for New Delhi metallo–β-lactamase. Which of the following choices describes the best option for management?

a. Ceftazidime-avibactam should be considered as a potential therapeutic option
b. Polymyxin B is pharmacologically less reliable than colistin for treating CRE and should not be used
c. Tigecycline is appropriate monotherapy for bloodstream infections with CRE
d. Colistin should not be used for UTIs
e. Polymyxin B has been proven to be more nephrotoxic than colistin and should be avoided

II.41. A 55-year-old man was undergoing treatment for a prosthetic joint infection with methicillin-resistant *Staphylococcus aureus*. He had completed 6 weeks of therapy with intravenous vancomycin plus rifampin and was currently receiving levofloxacin and rifampin. His platelet count had gradually decreased from $200,000\times10^6$/L before the infection to $55,000\times10^6$/L after 10 weeks of therapy. The other parameters of his complete blood count were within normal limits, and the only medications he received on a regular basis were antibiotics. Which of the following is correct regarding his diagnosis?

a. The thrombocytopenia is related to direct myelosuppression from levofloxacin

b. The decreased platelet count is mostly from antibody-mediated thrombocytopenia due to the infection

c. Resolution of the thrombocytopenia after discontinuing the offending agent would confirm the suspicion of drug-induced thrombocytopenia

d. The patient will have a 100% chance of thrombocytopenia development if his treatment is switched from rifampin to rifabutin

e. The decreased platelet count is unlikely to be due to his active antibiotic therapy

II.42. Which of the following solid-organ transplant recipients has the highest risk of having primary cytomegalovirus (CMV) disease if the donor (D) is CMV seropositive and the patient (recipient [R]) is CMV seronegative (CMV D$^+$/R$^-$ mismatch)?

a. A 30-year-old kidney transplant recipient, CMV D$^+$/R$^-$, with good allograft function, after completing 6 months of valganciclovir prophylaxis

b. A 35-year-old heart transplant recipient, CMV D$^+$/R$^-$, with no history of allograft rejection, after completing 6 months of valganciclovir prophylaxis

c. A 40-year-old lung transplant recipient, CMV D$^+$/R$^-$, with a history of acute graft rejection 3 months after transplantation, after completing 3 months of valganciclovir prophylaxis

d. A 45-year-old liver transplant recipient, CMV D$^+$/R$^-$, whose immunosuppression regimen was tapered to tacrolimus monotherapy, after completing 3 months of valganciclovir prophylaxis

e. A 50-year-old kidney transplant recipient, CMV D$^+$/R$^-$, with a history of acute graft rejection, and is currently restarted on valganciclovir prophylaxis

II.43. A 23-year-old man presented with a 2-month history of an ulcerative forearm lesion. Four months ago, he had spent 2 weeks in Costa Rica doing mostly outdoor activities. He initially noticed a papule 1 month after his return, which gradually increased in size and then ulcerated. He did not have any pain, and he did not recall any recent injuries. He is afebrile. What is true regarding testing for suspected cutaneous leishmaniasis (CL)?

a. Serology remains the best test to diagnose CL

b. Polymerase chain reaction has poor sensitivity but high specificity

c. Histopathology examination alone is sufficient to distinguish between different species

d. *Leishmania* cultures can take up to 4 weeks to grow

e. Blood agar plate cultures are the preferred culture method for leishmaniasis

II.44. A 52-year-old transgender woman receiving hormonal therapy presents to an HIV clinic for consideration of HIV pre-exposure prophylaxis (PrEP). She engages in transactional sex and has about 5 male partners monthly. She reports receptive-anal intercourse and uses condoms with approximately 30% of her encounters. She gets tested monthly for sexually transmitted infections (STIs) and has never been diagnosed with an STI. She has no other medical conditions and states that she feels well today. Her last unprotected sexual encounter was 2 weeks ago. She tells you that several other transgender women in her community have started HIV PrEP, and she is wondering whether she might also benefit from it. She should be informed of which of the following?

a. Although tenofovir disoproxil fumarate/emtricitabine alone is the most commonly prescribed PrEP regimen, you will prescribe a 3-drug program for her because she is taking hormones

b. Although she has high risk of HIV acquisition, no data suggest that PrEP is effective for HIV prevention in transgender women, so you will not prescribe it for her

c. She is a candidate for PrEP but will need baseline testing to evaluate the risk of treatment, including HIV testing (antigen-antibody test and HIV RNA), estimate of renal function, and hepatitis B screening

d. She will require monthly follow-up visits while receiving PrEP to ensure that she is adherent and tolerating PrEP

e. She can be started on PrEP today and seen annually for follow-up visits to ensure that she is adherent and tolerating PrEP

II.45. A 53-year-old woman with rheumatoid arthritis (treated with infliximab) presented with a 3-week history of painful skin lesions on her right arm. She denied any fever or chills. She reported spending weekends outside hiking and recalled several tick bites. She also reported having rashes in the past from poison ivy. She worked at the local fish store. A physical examination also showed nodular lesions with ulcerations on both legs. What is the next best step in management?

a. Start doxycycline

b. Prescribe topical corticosteroids

c. Obtain a skin biopsy

d. Prescribe oral corticosteroids

e. Reassure and schedule a follow-up assessment in 1 week

II.46. Which statement is true regarding organ transplant for patients with HIV?

a. These patients have a higher incidence of opportunistic infections after transplant because of enhanced immunosuppression, in addition to HIV

b. Survival rates of transplant recipients coinfected with HIV and hepatitis C virus (HCV) are the same as those of patients with monoinfection

c. Patients who receive protease inhibitor–based antiretroviral therapy and patients who receive integrase inhibitor–based antiretroviral therapy have similar drug-drug interactions

d. For recipients of solid-organ transplants, rejection rates are higher for patients who are HIV positive compared with patients who are HIV negative

e. Rates of graft loss are similar for patients with HIV or HCV monoinfection compared with patients with HIV-HCV coinfection

II.47. A 30-year-old man presented in July with a severe headache, blurred vision, and severe pain in his right upper back and left midabdomen that wrapped around the trunk to the midline. In May, he had spent 5 days hunting turkey in wooded areas of northern Wisconsin. He did not recall any tick bites. The symptoms began 3 weeks after he had an erythematous skin rash on his left arm and right thigh that eventually resolved. A physical examination showed that the patient had a left seventh nerve palsy and a stiff neck, but he had no motor or sensory deficits. Which of the following studies is most likely to lead to the diagnosis in this patient?

a. Serum *Borrelia burgdorferi* immunoglobulin (Ig) M levels

b. Brain magnetic resonance imaging

c. Cerebrospinal fluid (CSF) and serum *B burgdorferi* IgG levels

d. CSF *B burgdorferi* polymerase chain reaction (PCR)

e. Serum Lyme PCR

II.48. A 43-year-old man with HIV presents to the clinic with ongoing viremia (HIV viral load, 13,480 copies/mL) and a CD4 count of 142 cells/mcL. He is intermittently nonadherent with his medication regimen of coformulated darunavir (800 mg) and cobicistat (150 mg) plus coformulated tenofovir disoproxil fumarate (300 mg) and emtricitabine (200 mg), once daily. He has gastrointestinal disturbances (nausea, diarrhea, and vomiting) that he associates with the coformulated darunavir-cobicistat. He also has intermittent nonadherence with the boosted protease inhibitor (darunavir-cobicistat) because it interacts with his psychiatric medications. The fluctuant levels of his psychiatric medications make titration difficult; consequently, his major depression and schizophrenia are poorly controlled. The patient previously was receiving raltegravir, but he was nonadherent because of alcohol abuse and the therapy failed. His current and historical genotypes show that he has reverse transcriptase (K103N) and integrase mutations (N155H, Q148H). No protease mutations are identified. Which would be the best antiretroviral therapy option for this patient?

a. Coformulated bictegravir/emtricitabine/tenofovir alafenamide (50 mg/200 mg/25 mg, once daily)
b. Tipranavir (500 mg, twice daily) boosted with ritonavir (200 mg, twice daily) plus maraviroc (300 mg, twice daily)
c. Dolutegravir (50 mg, twice daily) plus coformulated tenofovir alafenamide/emtricitabine (25 mg/200 mg, once daily)
d. Raltegravir (1,200 mg, once daily) plus coformulated tenofovir alafenamide/emtricitabine (25 mg/200 mg, once daily)
e. Coformulated efavirenz/emtricitabine/tenofovir disoproxil fumarate (600 mg/200 mg/300 mg, once daily)

II.49. A 43-year-old woman with congenital tetralogy of Fallot and a complex cardiac surgical history has a disseminated *Mycobacterium chelonae* pacemaker infection. She is treated with imipenem-cilastatin (1,000 mg, intravenous [IV], every 12 hours), amikacin (500 mg, IV, every 24 hours), and azithromycin (500 mg, oral, once daily). After several months of antimycobacterial treatment, she reports bilateral tinnitus, left-sided hearing loss, and ongoing dizziness. Apart from these new concerns, she is doing

well, and weekly laboratory monitoring does not identify any concerns. Amikacin troughs have been undetectable for the past month on a stable dose. Which of the following statements about this case is true?

a. Ordering a serum creatinine test and a urinalysis could help determine whether the patient has amikacin-related ototoxicity
b. The time course indicates that her hearing changes are strongly associated with azithromycin
c. There is concern for loss of hair cells in the cristae ampullares
d. Ordering a pharmacogenomic panel would help determine whether the patient has a CYP2C19 allele that increases her risk of aminoglycoside-related ototoxicity
e. Amikacin should be given with ampicillin for synergistic activity against *Mycobacterium* species

II.50. A female Somali immigrant presented to a travel clinic with a 3-month history of intermittent fevers, severe fatigue, joint pain, epigastric pain, and unexplained weight loss. She had taken a 3-month trip to visit family in Somalia, and her symptoms began 1 week after she returned. She did not receive any pre-travel vaccinations, nor did she take anti-malarial chemoprophylaxis. She reported frequent ingestion of unpasteurized camel milk during her trip. Testing identified a microcytic anemia. She was unresponsive to 14 days of oral cefdinir. Chest radiography and abdominal ultrasonography showed normal findings. Two months into her illness, she started having asymmetric, painful swelling of her ankles bilaterally and in the proximal interphalangeal joints of her right hand. A blood malaria multiplex polymerase chain reaction test and an HIV screening test showed negative findings. What is this patient's most likely diagnosis?

a. Typhoid fever

b. Dengue fever

c. Chikungunya viral infection

d. Brucellosis

e. Falciparum malaria

II.51. A 64-year-old man presented with a 5-month history of fever, night sweats, and back pain. He started having symptoms 1 week after returning from a 4-week trip to Qatar. He reported consuming unpasteurized cheese during his travel. Two months after symptom onset, he had severe low back pain. An examination showed that he had a normal heart rate and normal blood pressure. Pertinent examination findings included palpable splenomegaly and point tenderness at the L4 to L5 spinal level. Blood cultures grew *Brucella melitensis*. Magnetic resonance imaging of the lumbar spine showed L4 and L5 vertebral osteomyelitis with diskitis. What is the most appropriate first-line treatment regimen?

a. Rifampin plus doxycycline for 6 weeks

b. Trimethoprim-sulfamethoxazole plus doxycycline for 12 weeks

c. Doxycycline for at least 12 weeks plus intravenous or intramuscular streptomycin for 2 to 3 weeks

d. Doxycycline plus ciprofloxacin for 12 weeks

e. Doxycycline monotherapy for 6 weeks

II.52. A 55-year-old woman with a history of diabetes mellitus and recurrent urinary tract infections presented to her primary care physician with burning during urination and a low-grade fever. A urine culture grew *Escherichia coli*. She was prescribed a 1-week course of cephalexin.

Three days after starting treatment, she presented with a high-grade fever, nausea, vomiting, worsening dysuria, and urinary hesitancy. She also had a new rash that was associated with skin tenderness. A physical examination showed that she was hypotensive and tachycardic.

The rash was diffuse and erythematous, with pustules. Laboratory tests showed a white blood cell count of 15,000/mcL with normal differential, aspartate transaminase of 356 U/L, alanine aminotransferase of 289 U/L, and creatinine of 1.2 mg/dL. Given the patient's presentation, which of the following statements is correct regarding her diagnosis?

a. Penicillin skin testing in the future can be useful

b. The presentation is mostly consistent with toxic shock syndrome

c. The patient likely has drug rash with eosinophilia and systemic symptoms, given her symptoms and the duration between drug exposure and presentation

d. A skin biopsy will show mostly neutrophilic infiltrates, subepidermal edema, and subcorneal pustules

e. The patient should be screened for strongyloidiasis

II.53. A 64-year-old man presented with memory impairment. He was previously healthy but began having memory loss and intermittent confusion 9 weeks earlier. In the past few weeks, he had difficulty performing activities of daily living. A physical examination showed that he had considerable psychomotor retardation with aphasia and apraxia. A laboratory evaluation included a basic metabolic profile, rapid plasma reagin, an HIV screen, and assessment of thyroid-stimulating hormone, vitamin B_{12}, and folate levels; all results were negative or in the reference range. Computed tomographic imaging of the brain showed normal results. However, magnetic resonance imaging of the brain showed abnormal signal hyperintensity at several cortical locations. An analysis of the cerebrospinal fluid showed a normal cell count, glucose level, and protein level, but the protein 14-3-3 level was elevated. A brain biopsy was performed because prion disease (Creutzfeldt-Jakob disease) was suspected. What is true regarding the processing of instruments after the biopsy procedure?

a. Heat-resistant instruments should only be autoclaved

b. Instruments that came in contact with low-infectivity tissues should undergo the usual disinfection procedures before reuse

c. Disposable instruments that came in contact with high-infectivity tissues should be incinerated

d. Heat-sensitive, reusable instruments should be incinerated

e. Instruments should be treated in a standard manner, similar to any other procedure

II.54. A 42-year-old man with alcoholic liver disease presents with a dog bite on his leg. At presentation, he has a temperature of 38.2°C, heart rate of 120 beats/min, and blood pressure of 95/62 mm Hg. Blood samples are obtained for cultures. A physical examination of his leg shows swelling around his calf, with erythema extending to the proximal knee, plus purulence at the puncture wound site. A radiograph of his leg does not show any fractures, but a small abscess beneath the puncture wound is identified. He undergoes irrigation and débridement of the wound. Which of the following medications is the first-line antibiotic?

a. Oral amoxicillin-clavulanate

b. Intravenous cefepime

c. Intravenous ampicillin-sulbactam

d. Oral azithromycin

e. Intravenous vancomycin

II.55. A 45-year-old man with a history of hypertension, HIV positivity, and renal transplant presented to the travel clinic before a trip to Brazil for a summer vacation. He planned to stay in Rio de Janeiro for 10 days and to take a 3-day cruise on the Amazon River. He had previously traveled to the same region in 2013 and did not receive a yellow fever vaccine (YFV) at that time. For the current trip, he planned to stay in air-conditioned cabins, to apply insect repellent, and to wear permethrin-impregnated clothing. The patient had HIV diagnosed in 1992 but had an undetectable viral load with antiretroviral therapy. His CD4 count was stable (450-550 cells/mm^3 during the past 2 years and 524 cells/mm^3 2 months ago). He received a kidney transplant 1 year earlier for HIV-associated nephropathy and did not have any rejection episodes. His current immunosuppressive regimen included prednisone (5 mg daily). What would be considered a contraindication for YFV for this individual?

a. HIV infection

b. Plans to stay in air-conditioned environments and use insect repellents

c. Renal transplant status

d. Travel to an area that is nonendemic for yellow fever

e. Previous travel to the same region without infection

II.56. A 30-year-old man comes to your clinic to establish care. He has an unremarkable medical history but reports having 10 male and 5 female sexual partners in the past year. He has receptive and insertive anal intercourse and oral intercourse with all his sexual partners. He does not have any medical concerns today. What screening tests for sexually transmitted infections would you recommend for this patient?

a. HIV screening test and urine nucleic acid amplification tests (NAATs) for gonorrhea and chlamydia

b. HIV screening test, urine, rectal, and oropharyngeal NAATs for gonorrhea and chlamydia, hepatitis screening test, and syphilis serologic test

c. HIV screening test only

d. HIV and hepatitis screening tests

e. Hepatitis screening test only

II.57. A 25-year-old woman comes for a follow-up visit 1 month after treatment of urogenital gonorrhea with oral cefixime and oral azithromycin. She has no symptoms at this visit. What would you recommend at this time?

a. No further testing

b. Another course of oral cefixime and oral azithromycin

c. One dose of intravenous ceftriaxone and oral azithromycin

d. Repeat urine nucleic acid amplification test

e. Gram stain and culture of the urine

II.58. A 62-year-old woman with uncontrolled diabetes mellitus presents with worsening right-sided shoulder and chest pain. She had hit her shoulder on a post 1 week earlier and had erythema that gradually developed around a small, superficial wound. A physical examination shows that her right shoulder and chest are exquisitely tender and edematous, almost "wood hard," with pain that is disproportionately high for the apparent lesion. An urgent computed tomographic image of the chest suggests possible necrotizing fasciitis with emphysematous changes, and she undergoes extensive surgical resection. She starts treatment with piperacillin-tazobactam plus vancomycin, and a preliminary histopathologic analysis of bacteria taken from the incision shows branching, non–spore-forming, gram-positive bacilli. Which of the following is the best next step in management?

a. Administer a dose of intravenous immunoglobulin

b. Continue piperacillin-tazobactam and discontinue vancomycin

c. Administer clindamycin intravenously, every 6 hours

d. Start hyperbaric oxygen treatment

e. Administer a dose of methylprednisolone

II.59. A 65-year-old married man from central Arkansas presented with a 5-month history of a large, painful gingival ulcer (Figure II.Q59). He had a history of moderate smoking and a recent unintentional weight loss of 15 kg. He owned a jewelry store and had a pet Moluccan cockatoo. He denied high-risk sexual activity or outdoor activities. Laboratory tests showed mildly elevated alkaline phosphatase and a normochromic, normocytic anemia (hemoglobin, 12.7 g/dL; reference range, 13.5-17.5 g/dL). A biopsy of the gingival ulcer showed benign oral mucosa with acute and chronic inflammation and noncaseating granulomas. A polymerase chain reaction test for herpes simplex virus was negative.

Figure II.Q59.   Large Gingival Ulceration

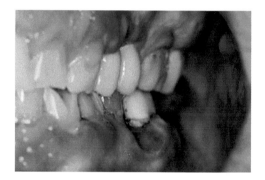

A computed tomographic scan of the abdomen and pelvis showed new nodular enlargement of the bilateral adrenal glands (not seen in a scan that was obtained 2 years prior). No appreciable adenopathy was noted. A repeat biopsy of the gingival lesion was ordered (results pending). Which of the following is the most likely diagnosis?

a. Lymphoma

b. Disseminated histoplasmosis

c. Invasive candidiasis

d. Behçet syndrome

e. Disseminated blastomycosis

II.60. A 55-year-old woman with an unremarkable medical history presents with a 1-month history of right forearm pain, swelling, and erythema. She is an avid fish tank enthusiast and cares for her fish on a daily basis. She underwent a biopsy and débridement and then received a course of cephalexin and later trimethoprim-sulfamethoxazole, but her symptoms persisted. Bacterial cultures were negative. She has remained afebrile and clinically stable but reports ongoing, considerable discomfort in her right upper extremity. She now has new nodules tracking proximally up her arm. Which of the following is the best next step for establishing the diagnosis?

a. No further testing
b. Repeat débridement and have the tissue cultured for bacteria and fungi
c. Serum immunoglobulin G testing for *Mycobacterium marinum*
d. Repeat débridement and have the tissue cultured for mycobacteria
e. Magnetic resonance imaging of the right upper extremity

II.61. A 70-year-old woman presented to the emergency department with a 9-day history of hemoptysis and pleuritic chest pain. She previously had a positive purified protein derivative test for suspected tuberculosis exposure during childhood. An initial computed tomographic angiogram showed several cavitary nodules. The patient was admitted to the intensive care unit with a suspected diagnosis of pulmonary tuberculosis that was later confirmed by cultures to be positive for *Mycobacterium* species. She started treatment with rifampin, isoniazid, pyrazinamide, and ethambutol. This patient can be considered noninfectious when she meets which of the following criteria?

a. She is adherent to an adequate regimen for 2 weeks or longer and shows evidence of clinical improvement
b. She is adherent to an effective multi-drug treatment and has no adverse events during the first 2 days of therapy
c. She has 3 consecutive sputum smears that are negative for acid-fast bacilli (obtained at a minimum of 8 hours apart, with at least 1 sample being an early-morning specimen)
d. She wears a surgical mask that covers her mouth and nose when coughing or sneezing
e. She has a negative result with the interferon release assay

II.62. A 67-year-old man with bladder cancer is currently receiving intravesical treatment with *Mycobacterium bovis* bacille Calmette-Guérin (BCG). He presents to the emergency department in septic shock. Computed tomography of the chest shows miliary opacities, and blood tests show markedly elevated liver enzyme levels. BCG sepsis is suspected, and the patient starts treatment with rifampin, isoniazid, and ethambutol. Which of the following statements is false regarding the suspected diagnosis?

a. Rifampin, isoniazid, and ethambutol therapy can be discontinued if myco-bacterial blood cultures are negative
b. Traumatic catheterization before the patient's last BCG instillation is a risk factor in the development of this infection
c. Growth of *Mycobacterium tuberculosis* complex in a culture from the affected site confirms the diagnosis
d. *M bovis* BCG is often pyrazinamide resistant
e. Most infections associated with *M bovis* BCG are caused by BCG therapy for bladder cancer

II.63. A male patient has a new diagnosis of HIV. His CD4 T-cell count is 8 cells/mcL, and the HIV viral load is 800,000 IU/mL. He also has *Pneumocystis jirovecii* pneumonia, which is being treated with trimethoprim-sulfamethoxazole. When is the best time to initiate combined antiretroviral therapy (cART)?

a. Start cART 3 weeks after he finishes treatment for *P jirovecii* pneumonia

b. Start cART after 8 weeks

c. Start cART after he finishes secondary prophylaxis for *P jirovecii* pneumonia

d. Start cART as soon as possible, within 2 weeks of initiating treatment against *P jirovecii*

e. Start cART after 12 weeks

II.64. In a patient with a newly diagnosed HIV infection and chronic hepatitis B, which of the following medication regimens must be avoided?

a. Tenofovir alafenamide, emtricitabine, and dolutegravir

b. Tenofovir disoproxil fumarate, emtricitabine, and dolutegravir

c. Abacavir, lamivudine, and dolutegravir

d. Emtricitabine, raltegravir, and tenofovir alafenamide

e. Tenofovir alafenamide, emtricitabine, bictegravir

II.65. A 25-year-old woman with an unremarkable medical history is evaluated during a routine office visit. She is pregnant and at 36 weeks' gestation. She reports no urinary symptoms such as dysuria or urgency, and she does not have a fever. Her only medication is a prenatal vitamin. Her abdominal examination findings are consistent with her stage of pregnancy, and no costovertebral tenderness is noted. Her urine culture shows greater than 100,000 colony-forming units per mL of *Escherichia coli*; further testing indicates that it is susceptible to ampicillin, trimethoprim-sulfamethoxazole, and ciprofloxacin. Which of the following is the most appropriate treatment?

a. Amoxicillin

b. Observation

c. Repeat urine culture

d. Trimethoprim-sulfamethoxazole

e. Vitamin C

II.66. A 54-year-old man with severe degenerative osteoarthritis was seen in the clinic before a left knee arthroplasty procedure that was scheduled for later that week.

He reported the recent onset of bloody diarrhea, and an infectious diarrhea panel (polymerase chain reaction assays) was performed. It was positive for the presence of a Shiga toxin gene (*stx1* or *stx2*) and an *Escherichia coli* O157:H7 strain. The orthopedic surgeon asked for recommendations regarding management of the diarrhea, given the planned surgery. Which of the following would be the best recommendation for management?

a. Treat with ciprofloxacin for 7 days and proceed with surgery at the end of treatment

b. Treat with azithromycin for 3 days and proceed with surgery at the end of treatment

c. Treat with azithromycin for 3 days but delay surgery until subsequent stool testing shows elimination of the Shiga toxin–producing *E coli* strain

d. Treat with supportive measures (no antibiotics) and postpone surgery until 2 weeks after resolution of symptoms

e. Proceed with surgery as planned but add azithromycin to cefazolin for preoperative prophylaxis

II.67. A 52-year-old woman was evaluated for fever and a rash. She had recently received a diagnosis of acute myelogenous leukemia. A long-term central venous catheter was placed. She received induction chemotherapy with daunorubicin (90 mg/m² per day) for 3 days and cytarabine (100 mg/m² per day) for 7 days. Severe neutropenia and fever developed after 10 days. She responded to antibiotic treatment and her marrow recovered. She was well at home until 3 days before her presentation, when she had a fever without localizing symptoms. A complete blood count showed a white blood cell count of 11.5×10^9/L with 35% band cells. She was admitted to the hospital and started treatment with cefepime. Her temperature was 38.9°C, her pulse was 97 beats/min, and her respiratory rate was 22 breaths/min. A chest radiograph showed no infiltrates. Results of blood cultures, urine cultures, and viral studies were negative. On the second hospital day, the patient had an acute onset of nonpruritic, painful papules on her face and hands, and red-purple, tender nodules appeared on her neck. A dermatologist was consulted, and a punch biopsy was obtained from a skin lesion. The patient's fever continued, despite antibiotic treatment. On hospital day 4, the biopsy report indicated dense dermal infiltration of neutrophils, with no evidence of vasculitis. Stains for microorganisms were negative. Which of the following is the most likely diagnosis?

a. Leukemia cutis
b. Disseminated fusariosis
c. Sweet syndrome
d. Pyoderma gangrenosum
e. Ecthyma gangrenosum

II.68. A 59-year-old white man presents with a 7-month history of diarrhea and consequent 6.8-kg weight loss. He attempted various diets (gluten free, lactose free, etc) without a change in stool characteristics. His family notes that he is increasingly forgetful and absentminded. A small-intestine biopsy is performed. What might you expect to see in the biopsy specimen?

a. Macrophages positive for periodic acid–Schiff stain
b. Intraepithelial lymphocytosis with flattening of villi
c. Variable villous atrophy with crypt hyperplasia
d. Transmural lymphoid aggregation with nonnecrotizing granulomas
e. Pseudomembrane formation

II.69. A 59-year-old white man presents with a 7-month history of diarrhea and consequent 6.8-kg weight loss. He attempted various diets (gluten free, lactose free, etc) without a change in stool characteristics. His family notes that he is increasingly forgetful and absentminded. What skin finding might you expect in this patient?

a. Actinic keratosis
b. Scleroderma
c. Vitiligo
d. Melanoderma
e. Seborrheic keratosis

Answers

II.1. Answer d.

Combination antimicrobial therapy that includes either vancomycin or carbapenem plus 1 or 2 oral agents should be offered in the initial therapy phase, before transitioning to maintenance therapy. This approach is particularly useful for patients with bacteremia or severe infectious presentations. Use of agents with intracellular activity (eg, macrolides) is important in the treatment of *Rhodococcus equi* because its ability to survive within macrophages is a key aspect of its virulence. For patients who do not respond to medical management alone, the addition of a surgical approach should be considered. Trimethoprim-sulfamethoxazole should not be considered a reliable active agent because of resistance, and empiric antimicrobial treatment generally includes a combination of either vancomycin or carbapenem with a macrolide, fluoroquinolone, or rifampin.

II.2. Answer c.

Given the patient's risk of acquiring HIV, his symptoms resembling an acute retroviral syndrome, and the negative HIV screen, the most appropriate test is the RNA viral load to screen for acute HIV infection. Repeating the HIV screen at this point (only 3 days after a negative HIV screen) is unlikely to yield a positive result because the median time to HIV antibody production is approximately 21 days (RNA viral replication can be detected as early as 10 days after infection). Cytomegalovirus and Epstein-Barr virus antibody tests could detect infectious mononucleosis, but these infections are less likely, given the negative infectious mononucleosis test result and the patient's risk for HIV infection.

II.3. Answer c.

After 2 weeks of induction therapy, a lumbar puncture is needed to determine whether the cerebrospinal fluid is sterile. Once or twice weekly, serum creatinine, potassium, and magnesium should be measured to assess for acute kidney injury, hypokalemia, and hypomagnesemia due to amphotericin B treatment. Head-spine computed tomography (CT) and magnetic resonance imaging are unnecessary because imaging findings cannot be used reliably to monitor treatment response. An electrocardiogram may be useful to assess for QT prolongation before initiation of fluconazole therapy, but it is not absolutely necessary in a young patient with no history of cardiac disease. Echocardiography and CT imaging of the chest have no role in assessing the response to cryptococcal meningitis therapy.

II.4. Answer d.

Macrolide resistance has been documented in syphilis; therefore, azithromycin is not recommended for treatment (MMWR Recomm Rep. 2015 Jun 5;64[RR-03]:1-137). Doxycycline (200 mg, twice daily, for 21 days) has been used by some authors (Antimicrob Agents Chemother. 1985 Aug;28[2]:347-8), but this treatment is not recommended by the Centers for Disease Control and Prevention. Ocular syphilis is treated like neurosyphilis. Intramuscular benzathine penicillin does not penetrate to the cerebrospinal fluid in appropriate concentrations and is not recommended. Intravenous ceftriaxone has been used as an alternative to intravenous penicillin G, and it is the best answer choice for this question, but the evidence supporting use of ceftriaxone is not as robust as that supporting penicillin G. If penicillin G can be tolerated, it should be the first option (Clin Infect Dis. 2000 Mar;30[3]:540-4).

II.5. Answer b.

Ocular syphilis can develop at any stage of syphilis, and this finding should prompt an evaluation for neurosyphilis with a lumbar puncture and additional testing (MMWR Recomm Rep. 2015 Jun 5;64[RR-03]:1-137). A positive result with the cerebrospinal fluid venereal disease research laboratory test would confirm neurosyphilis and also help establish a definitive diagnosis of ocular syphilis. For patients with neurosyphilis, a lumbar puncture needs to be repeated every 6 months until cell counts are normal. Repeat treatment for neurosyphilis can be considered if the cell counts have not decreased after 6 months or if they have not normalized after 2 years.

II.6. Answer c.

The patient has no headaches or additional central nervous system symptoms. Therefore, he has a very low likelihood of having coccidioidomycosis meningitis. Furthermore, the diagnosis can be established with a biopsy of the skin nodules. Lumbar puncture is not recommended because it is unlikely to contribute to the diagnosis or affect prognosis, and it can potentially contribute to additional morbidity from the procedure.

II.7. Answer b.

Fluconazole is the treatment of choice for disseminated coccidioidomycosis, and for a patient who can tolerate oral therapy, it does not need to be administered intravenously.

Oral flucytosine is used in combination with amphotericin B products for induction therapy of disseminated cryptococcosis, and it would not be used in this setting. Liposomal amphotericin B can be used as salvage therapy for coccidioidomycosis that does not respond to fluconazole. Caspofungin and terbinafine do not have any activity against *Coccidioides immitis* or *Coccidioides posadasii*.

II.8. Answer b.

The patient's coronary artery bypass graft procedure required harvesting her right saphenous vein via saphenous venectomy, and her episode of cellulitis involved the right lower extremity. Prior saphenous venectomy has been associated with increased risk of ipsilateral lower extremity cellulitis. Patients with a body mass index (BMI) greater than 30 kg/m^2 have an increased risk of cellulitis; however, this patient's BMI is only 27 kg/m^2, and although her weight may still contribute to overall comorbidity, it is not the most important risk factor. Eczema and dry skin can provide portals of entry for bacteria that lead to cellulitis, but this patient's problem areas were her elbows and not her lower extremities. The mastectomy and lymph node dissection for breast cancer likely have resulted in some measure of lymphedema, which is a known risk factor for cellulitis; however, these typically upper extremity procedures are not risk factors for lower extremity cellulitis. White race is not considered a risk factor for development of lower extremity cellulitis.

II.9. Answer a.

Oral penicillin V potassium is efficacious for preventing recurrent cellulitis. This recommendation is based on the largest clinical trial to date that described 6- and 12-month prophylaxis regimens for recurrent cellulitis. Smaller studies have described success with oral erythromycin and intramuscular benzathine penicillin, but these studies lack the power of the oral penicillin V potassium studies. Additionally, erythromycin can have markedly adverse gastrointestinal effects, and unlike penicillin V potassium, erythromycin resistance occurs among some strains of β-hemolytic streptococci. Intramuscular benzathine penicillin can be expensive, making oral penicillin V potassium more cost effective. Intravenous dalbavancin has been studied for treatment of acute skin and soft tissue infections, but it is cost prohibitive even in this context and cannot be reasonably considered as a prophylaxis regimen. Weekly cefazolin is inappropriate because, despite being an effective intravenous treatment for active cellulitis, no clinical trial has shown its efficacy and safety for cellulitis prophylaxis.

II.10. Answer c.

Historically, *Nocardia asteroides* was thought to be the main *Nocardia* species that caused human disease, but recent data indicate that many of these species were misidentified. The term *N asteroides* is no longer used to represent isolates from human nocardiosis. The lungs are the most common target organ for primary infection by *Nocardia*, whereas the central nervous system is the most common organ involved in extrapulmonary spread. Although *Nocardia* spreads hematologically, blood cultures are rarely positive. *Nocardia* is capable of growth on different culture media but may take more than 14 days to grow. Acid-fast staining should always be used in conjunction with Gram stain because the acid-fast characteristic of *Nocardia* is heavily dependent on the growth media used and the age of the culture.

II.11. Answer c.

A combination of doxycycline (100 mg, twice daily) and hydroxychloroquine (20 mg, 3 times a day) for at least 18 months is the standard therapy for Q fever endocarditis, but therapy may need to be prolonged. This treatment regimen shows bactericidal activity in vitro and has been associated with lower mortality and relapse rates compared with other treatments. An alternative regimen for patients who cannot tolerate hydroxychloroquine is doxycycline plus a fluoroquinolone for 3 to 4 years. Monotherapy with doxycycline is often ineffective and has been associated with a 50% mortality rate. Patients with acute infection and preexisting valve lesions should undergo echocardiography and receive doxycycline and hydroxychloroquine treatment for 12 months to prevent infective endocarditis. The infection is more common in males, who have a 5-fold increased risk of acquiring the disease. *Coxiella burnetii* is highly infectious and can cause large outbreaks.

II.12. Answer d.

This case description is consistent with human herpesvirus (HHV) 6 encephalitis, which can occur in patients soon after allogeneic hematopoietic stem cell transplant. Most people acquire a primary HHV-6 infection by age 2 to 3 years, and 90% will have a latent infection. The patient likely has a reactivated infection. Magnetic resonance imaging will typically show changes in the bilateral medial temporal lobes. A higher HHV-6 viral load in the plasma is associated with a higher risk of encephalitis, but patients can have negative plasma HHV-6 polymerase chain reaction test results and still have central nervous system disease. Ganciclovir or foscarnet are first-line choices for therapy. Patients receiving umbilical cord blood transplants have a higher risk of disease development.

II.13. Answer c.

M184V is a nucleoside reverse transcriptase inhibitor resistance mutation. K101H and G190A are nonnucleoside reverse transcriptase inhibitor resistance mutations. Q148S, G140S/G163R, and S230N are major, minor, and insignificant integrase strand transfer inhibitor resistance mutations, respectively. The patient has not shown any protease inhibitor resistance mutations.

II.14. Answer a.

M184V is a nucleoside reverse transcriptase inhibitor resistance mutation that confers high-level resistance to lamivudine and emtricitabine. M184V may confer low-level resistance to abacavir, and tenofovir susceptibility is not affected; therefore, both can be included in the treatment regimen. K101H and G190A are nonnucleoside reverse transcriptase inhibitor resistance mutations that confer high-level resistance to efavirenz and nevirapine and low-level resistance to etravirine and rilpivirine. Rilpivirine has a lower genetic barrier to resistance; in a patient with compliance issues, etravirine would be the more appropriate nonnucleoside reverse transcriptase inhibitor. Q148S, G140S/G163R, and S230N are major, minor, and insignificant integrase strand transfer inhibitor (INSTI) resistance mutations, respectively. Together, these mutations confer resistance to all INSTIs, and thus, INSTIs should not be included in the treatment regimen. The patient has not shown any protease inhibitor resistance mutations; therefore, any of these could be included in the regimen. There is no evidence of CCR5 tropism; therefore, maraviroc would not be appropriate without this information.

II.15. Answer e.

The patient likely has early stage necrotizing fasciitis. Empiric initiation of antibiotics and prompt surgical consultation are critical for successful management. In situations such as this, when the diagnosis is clear, surgical consultation should not be delayed for imaging. Wound cultures are likely to only delay definitive therapy, and observation alone is contraindicated.

II.16. Answer b.

The empiric antimicrobial regimen for necrotizing fasciitis should include agents that are active against gram-negative, gram-positive, and anaerobic bacteria, including group A β-hemolytic *Streptococcus* and *Clostridium* species. The ideal regimen includes a carbapenem or a β-lactam and β-lactamase combination, clindamycin, and another drug with activity against methicillin-resistant *Staphylococcus aureus*. When tissue and blood culture results are available, antibiotic therapy should be tailored to treat the identified bacteria.

II.17. Answer a.

Because of the patient's kidney dysfunction, the antiretroviral therapy regimen ideally should not include tenofovir, cobicistat, rilpivirine, or atazanavir. A regimen of abacavir, dolutegravir, and lamivudine may be the least nephrotoxic. However, abacavir can increase risk of cardiovascular disease. The patient should initiate treatment with aspirin and atorvastatin because his cardiovascular risk is increased by chronic kidney disease, diabetes mellitus, and abacavir. Lisinopril would be beneficial for management of hypertension and proteinuria. Although amlodipine is beneficial for hypertension, it may worsen lower extremity edema.

II.18. Answer a.

Antibiotic prophylaxis to prevent bacterial endocarditis is recommended only for patients with the highest risk. Such patients may have the following risk factors:

- History of infective endocarditis
- Prosthetic cardiac valve or prosthetic material used for valve repair
- Cardiac transplant and subsequent cardiac valvulopathy
- Congenital heart disease (CHD)

- Unrepaired cyanotic CHD, including palliative shunts and conduits
- History of a complete repair of a congenital heart defect in the past 6 months, with the repair involving prosthetic material or a device (placed surgically or by catheter)
- Repaired CHD (via prosthetic material or device) with residual defects at or adjacent to the repair site

For high-risk patients undergoing dental procedures, antibiotic therapy is appropriate and should be directed against viridans group streptococci (Circulation. 2007 Oct 9;116[15]:1736-54). The preferred antibiotic is amoxicillin because it has lower rates of resistance and is well absorbed in the gastrointestinal tract. Cephalexin and clindamycin are options for patients who are allergic to penicillins (without immunoglobulin E–mediated allergy, if cephalexin is used), but these drugs have higher rates of resistance compared with amoxicillin.

II.19. Answer d.

Spontaneous bacterial meningitis with Enterobacteriaceae (including *Escherichia coli*) is an infrequent condition in adults and is usually associated with predisposing factors, including severe *Strongyloides stercoralis* infection. Serology and stool cultures are the most appropriate tests to diagnose a *Strongyloides* infection.

Suppressive therapy is not indicated after a single episode of gram-negative meningitis. Although a repeat lumbar puncture to document clearance of infection is indicated for syphilis or cryptococcal meningitis, it is not necessary for meningitis due to *E coli*. Colonic malignancy has a known association with *Streptococcus gallolyticus* (formerly *Streptococcus bovis*) but not with *E coli* bacteremia. No clinical features in the patient's presentation suggest an intestinal obstruction.

II.20. Answer a.

This scenario describes anchoring bias. The team focused on the diagnosis of community-acquired pneumonia and failed to consider the possibility of a pulmonary embolism until the patient's condition deteriorated. The availability heuristic refers to one's tendency to more readily access recently encountered information. If the physicians had seen a dozen community-acquired pneumonia cases presenting this same way, perhaps they could have made this error. Observation bias (the Hawthorne effect) occurs when results are changed by the act of observing. This effect is relevant in many research studies but not the clinical scenario at hand. The framing effect is the different interpretation of the same data, depending on how they are presented. Referral bias is specific to research and is a variant of selection bias.

II.21. Answer b.

The best choice is to first encourage the patient to notify her partner personally. If the patient does not follow through with partner notification, the health care provider or health department can notify the partner after a domestic violence screen is performed.

II.22. Answer e.

This patient meets the criteria for daptomycin-induced acute eosinophilic pneumonia (AEP). Diagnosis is made on the basis of his clinical, laboratory, and radiologic findings. The absence of peripheral eosinophilia does not exclude the diagnosis. Lung biopsy is not indicated because the differential cell count from bronchoalveolar lavage showed an excess of eosinophils. Rechallenging with daptomycin is not appropriate, given the concern of worsening symptoms. Initiating antihelminth therapy is not indicated because it will not address the underlying cause. Management of daptomycin-induced AEP includes withdrawal of daptomycin and initiation of corticosteroids, given his respiratory failure.

II.23. Answer c.

Antiretroviral therapy (ART) should never be discontinued to treat hepatitis C virus (HCV) in a coinfected individual. Sofosbuvir-velpatasvir should not be used in regimens containing efavirenz. HCV therapy with peginterferon and ribavirin results in inferior sustained viral response rates compared with direct-acting anti-HCV agents. Ledipasvir-sofosbuvir can be used with most ART regimens, although caution should be exercised in regimens containing tenofovir disoproxil fumarate. Concurrent administration of ledipasvir-sofosburvir and tenofovir disoproxil fumarate may increase the risk of nephrotoxicity. However, with appropriate monitoring, his ART regimen does not need to be changed if it is currently working. If the patient requests a change, transition to a tenofovir alafenamide–containing regimen could be considered in the future.

II.24. Answer c.

Discontinuation of combined antiretroviral therapy (cART) is not appropriate because he is responding well and appears stable, except for the manifestation of cutaneous Kaposi sarcoma (KS). At this time, cART is the most important intervention because it provides long-term benefits and survival free of opportunistic infection. Applying a corticosteroid ointment is not indicated because that will not address the KS. The patient should continue cART and be monitored closely for a clinical response of his KS. If it does not respond in the setting of improving CD4 counts, then another treatment could be considered. However, cART should be continued, irrespective of the therapy for KS. Given that the patient's HIV load is responding well to the current cART regimen, changing the regimen is unlikely to be helpful.

II.25. Answer d.

This patient likely is presenting with tacrolimus toxicity due to failure to decrease the dose when fluconazole was initiated. The most appropriate intervention is to withhold tacrolimus and check the serum level. The fluconazole dose should be adjusted to renal clearance at the time of presentation, but it should not be discontinued.

II.26. Answer c.

Breast milk can transmit human T-lymphotropic virus (HTLV) 1. Transmission of HTLV-1 can also occur sexually and through blood transfusion, injection drug use, and tissue donation. Plasma transfusion is not an effective means of HTLV-1 transmission.

II.27. Answer a.

This patient appears to have rhinocerebral mucormycosis. The diagnosis will be confirmed with surgical débridement and histologic examination. Treatment with intravenous liposomal amphotericin B is indicated, in addition to surgical débridement. Posaconazole is a reasonable option if the patient cannot tolerate amphotericin B. Voriconazole has no action against zygomycetes. Hyperbaric oxygen may be an option for adjunct therapy, but it should not replace adequate surgical débridement and antifungal therapy. Deferoxamine should be avoided in patients with zygomycosis because it can exacerbate the infection.

II.28. Answer b.

Blood cultures are usually negative in mucormycosis. Histopathologic examination of surgical tissues can confirm the characteristic broad, aseptate hyphae and right-angle branching of Mucorales fungi. In addition to the characteristic histopathology findings, culture growth of Mucorales fungi is diagnostic. Urinary antigen testing or serology has no role in the diagnosis of an acute infection. Magnetic resonance imaging can be helpful for identifying involved structures and possible invasion, but it is not sufficient for establishing a diagnosis in the absence of a biopsy.

II.29. Answer c.

The patient has endemic Kaposi sarcoma (KS), which is hyperendemic in the volcanic region south of Lake Kivu. Epidemic KS describes the form of sarcoma that more typically is associated with HIV, but this patient is HIV negative. The cornerstone of treatment is chemotherapy, not antiviral medications. The patient's age is consistent with this diagnosis, as is his sex.

II.30. Answer a.

This patient's fever, right-sided upper-quadrant abdominal pain, sexual history, and transaminitis all suggest acute viral hepatitis. His positive test results for anti–hepatitis B core (HBc) immunoglobulin (Ig) M, and hepatitis B surface antigen (HBsAg) are consistent with acute hepatitis B virus (HBV) infection. The positive test results for anti–hepatitis D virus (HDV) total antibodies and HDV RNA suggest acute HDV and HBV coinfection. HDV monoinfection cannot occur (HBV infection is required). Although the patient is taking acetaminophen, his dose is within the recommended range. The patient's serologic test results do not suggest prior vaccination (a patient with a prior vaccination would be negative for HBsAg, positive for anti-HBs antibodies, and negative for anti-HBc IgM). Although a patient can have concurrent infection with HDV and hepatitis C virus, for HDV to be pathogenic, HBV coinfection is required. HDV superinfection of chronic HBV infection would show test results that are negative for anti-HBc IgM and positive for anti-HBc IgG.

II.31. Answer b.

Streptococcus pneumoniae vaccine may cause false-positive pneumococcal antigen test results in patients who received the vaccine within 5 days before having the test performed (South Med J. 2011;104[8]:593-7). Invasive pneumococcal disease is usually caused by nonvaccine serotypes with greater antimicrobial resistance. The *S pneumoniae* latex antigen tests are not recommended for use in children because of the high rate of false-positive results, which is thought to arise from nasopharyngeal colonization. However, the immunochromatographic antigen test is very sensitive and specific for diagnosing pneumococcal meningitis in children. These tests can be useful in establishing the bacterial pathogen, even for patients who have received antibiotic therapy and are therefore culture negative. Blood cultures are positive for 75% of patients with pneumococcal meningitis, and they are a useful diagnostic tool for establishing the pathogen and determining susceptibilities when cerebrospinal fluid cannot be obtained.

II.32. Answer c.

Although both vaccines provide protection against meningitis and bacteremia, only the pneumococcal conjugate vaccine also provides protection against pneumonia (MMWR Morb Mortal Wkly Rep. 2012;61[21]:394-5). Both vaccines are named after the number of serotypes covered.

II.33. Answer b.

The only vaccine that is indicated for this patient is *Haemophilus influenzae* type B. Patients with defects in cellular immunity should not receive live vaccines because of a risk of disseminated infection, and vaccines for measles, mumps, rubella, varicella-zoster virus, and yellow fever are all live. *H influenzae* type B and pneumococcal vaccinations are indicated for patients with primary immunodeficiency and are safe in these situations. Human papillomavirus vaccination is not indicated for a 67-year-old man.

II.34. Answer b.

Although no consensus guidelines exist, the current practice is to provide antibiotic prophylaxis to patients with Good syndrome, similar to what is provided to patients with HIV. This patient's CD4+ count is less than 200 cells/mcL; he should receive trimethoprim-sulfamethoxazole for prophylaxis against *Pneumocystis* pneumonia.

II.35. Answer e.

The patient's symptoms are consistent with Pontiac fever. It is important to note that the *Legionella* urine antigen assay can be positive in patients with Pontiac fever. Most patients do not seek medical attention. The illness usually resolves within 3 to 5 days.

II.36. Answer d.

Clinical follow-up is required because there is no test that will show that the patient is cured. Patients with extensive bilateral Legionnaires disease may excrete urine antigen for weeks to months after recovery. Abnormal radiographic findings are slow to resolve and may persist for up to 4 months. Repeat sputum cultures are not required, and blood cultures are positive in only 10% of critically ill patients. In this case, the facility used an automated biocide delivery system to clean the cooling tower. This system automatically turned off the cooling tower pumps during low-demand periods, and the disinfectant was not delivered. Thus, *Legionella* bacteria could multiply in the cooling tower.

II.37. Answer c.

The stray cat is likely to have ingested a small rodent that is infected with *Francisella tularensis*. The bacteria may have been inoculated from the cat's mouth when the cat bit the patient. None of the other agents are associated with cat bite and the clinical presentation.

II.38. Answer b.

Aminoglycosides, such as gentamicin, are the drugs of choice for treating tularemia.

II.39. Answer c.

Patients with tularemia should be placed on standard isolation precautions because person-to-person transmission of *Francisella tularensis* has not been documented.

II.40. Answer a.

Ceftazidime-avibactam is a newly approved antibiotic that offers unique activity against organisms producing *Klebsiella pneumoniae* carbapenemase and should be considered as an option for treating this infection. Polymyxin B has recently been shown to be more reliable than colistin in terms of pharmacokinetics, given that it does not need to be converted to an active form and is not renally cleared. Thus, therapeutic concentrations of polymyxin B are more rapidly achieved. Tigecycline has a large volume of distribution and is unlikely to achieve high enough serum concentrations to be effective for bloodstream infections. Compared with colistin, polymyxin B does not achieve high concentrations in the urine; thus, colistin is the recommended polymyxin for treating urinary tract infections. No strong evidence suggests that polymyxin B is more nephrotoxic than colistin.

II.41. Answer c.

Resolution of the thrombocytopenia after stopping the offending agent is a strong argument for the diagnosis; a drug rechallenge is not always feasible or needed, especially with high-risk medications. The decreased platelet count is mostly an immune-mediated thrombocytopenia due to rifampin. In many case series, patients who cannot tolerate rifampin are successfully transitioned to rifabutin (72% of the patients in 1 case series [J Antimicrob Chemother. 2014 Mar;69{3}:790-6]).

II.42. Answer c.

All transplant recipients described in the question have a high risk of cytomegalovirus (CMV) disease because of the CMV serologic mismatch between donor and recipient. Solid-organ transplant recipients do not have an inherent ability to mount an immediate pathogen-specific immune response against reactivated CMV. The risk of CMV disease varies by transplant type, probably because of the intensity of immunosuppression and because risk is directly associated with the amount of CMV-harboring lymphoid tissue in the transplanted allograft (lung allograft > heart = liver > kidney). The risk of primary CMV disease therefore is highest among lung transplant recipients because a lung allograft likely harbors the most CMV. In addition, lung transplant recipients are given a more intense immunosuppression regimen, especially if a patient shows allograft rejection. The 3-month duration of antiviral prophylaxis is also insufficient for the prevention of CMV disease in lung transplant recipients; for these patients, at least 12 months of antiviral prophylaxis is recommended.

II.43. Answer d.

Leishmania cultures are typically incubated in liquid culture medium for 4 weeks; culturing is performed at the Centers for Disease Control and Prevention (CDC; Atlanta, Georgia), at the Walter Reed Institute for Research (Silver Spring, Maryland) for US military personnel, or at McGill University (Montreal, Canada) for Canadian patients. Several culture media, including liquid media (eg, Schneider drosophila) and solid media (eg, Novy-MacNeal-Nicolle) are used. These may be requested from the CDC before the planned

biopsy. Serology may remain negative in cutaneous leishmaniasis because of poor antibody response with cutaneous disease alone. In cases of visceral leishmaniasis, serology may sometimes be helpful if biopsy and polymerase chain reaction (PCR) are negative and if the disease is clinically suspected, but positive serology alone does not distinguish between active or past infection. PCR has high sensitivity (up to 97%) and somewhat lower specificity (67%). PCR can also be used to accurately identify different species. Typical amastigotes with kinetoplasts are seen on biopsy specimens, but the appearance is similar for all *Leishmania* species, and histopathology alone cannot be used to distinguish between different species.

II.44. Answer c.

Before prescribing preexposure prophylaxis (PrEP), the risk of HIV acquisition needs to be determined by sexual risk behaviors. Higher risk is associated with condomless receptive penile-anal or penile-vaginal sex, serodiscordant relationships, a higher number of partners or frequency of encounters, a history of sexually transmitted infections, and sex while using drugs. If a high-risk patient is identified, the next step is to determine the risk of treatment by evaluating for preexisting HIV infection (due to the risk of resistance developing with 2 drugs), estimate of renal function (PrEP is approved for use only in patients with an estimated glomerular filtration rate greater than 60 mL/min per 1.73 m^2), and screening for hepatitis B (due to the risk of a hepatitis flare if therapy is discontinued). Multiple studies have shown that PrEP with daily tenofovir disoproxil fumarate/emtricitabine can prevent the acquisition of HIV infection in patients who are highly adherent. The risks and benefits of a PrEP program with 3 drugs has not been studied and is not recommended. Data suggest that PrEP is protective for cisgender and transgender individuals, provided that they are adhering to therapy. If baseline testing is negative and PrEP is prescribed, an initial 1-month follow-up visit should be scheduled to evaluate for adverse effects, with follow-up every 3 months thereafter. The need to continue PrEP should be reassessed at least annually, and therapy should be continued for 1 month after the last high-risk exposure.

II.45. Answer c.

For this immunocompromised patient, the next best step would be to obtain a skin biopsy. Skin lesions in immunocompromised individuals can have various causes, including infection, vasculitis, autoimmune disease, or drug reactions. Possible infectious agents include *Treponema pallidum*, *Nocardia*, rapidly growing nontuberculous mycobacteria, *Mycobacterium marinum*, *Mycobacterium tuberculosis*, *Sporothrix schenckii*, and *Blastomyces*, *Coccidioides*, *Aspergillus*, and *Cryptococcus* species. Although the patient was exposed to ticks, her clinical presentation does not correspond to tick-borne illness. Corticosteroid treatment is inappropriate because the underlying cause of skin lesions is not known, and administration of corticosteroids may lead to worsening of lesions. Watchful waiting is not correct because the patient clearly has progression of skin lesions and likely will not improve without specific treatment.

II.46. Answer d.

Patients with HIV and hepatitis C virus coinfection have a much higher rate of acute cellular rejection. This increased rate is thought to be due to multiple factors, including drug-drug interactions, immune dysregulation inherent to HIV infection, and more T cells with a memory phenotype.

II.47. Answer c.

The patient's clinical presentation is consistent with Bannwarth syndrome, a rare manifestation of Lyme neuroborreliosis that is associated with lymphocytic meningitis, cranial neuropathy, and inflammatory radiculopathy. The recent erythematous skin rash likely was erythema chronicum migrans. In this setting, a serum screening test for Lyme disease (enzyme immunoassay [EIA]) should be positive and can be confirmed with an immunoglobulin (Ig) G Western blot (WB). For the cerebrospinal fluid (CSF), an EIA should be positive, but no standards for confirmatory WB of the CSF have been established. Comparison of simultaneously performed quantitative EIAs of the serum and CSF can be used to calculate the antibody index, defined as the ratio of *Borrelia burgdorferi*–specific IgG antibodies in the CSF and serum. The antibody index is the test most likely to yield the diagnosis of neuroborreliosis in the setting of Bannwarth syndrome, with antibody index levels greater than 1.5 suggesting intrathecal synthesis of Lyme antibodies.

Serum Lyme IgM antibodies may be positive in neuroborreliosis and in acute Lyme disease without neurologic involvement, and their presence is not indicative of intrathecal antibody synthesis. Brain magnetic resonance imaging can show nonenhancing or enhancing lesions of cranial nerves affected by neuroborreliosis, but these findings are nonspecific. A CSF polymerase chain reaction (PCR) test for *B burgdorferi* is less likely to yield a diagnosis of neuroborreliosis because the test has a reported median sensitivity of 22.5% for neuroborreliosis. Serum Lyme PCR is unlikely to be positive in the setting of Lyme neuroborreliosis caused by *B burgdorferi*. Serum Lyme PCR would be reasonable to assess for a *Borrelia mayonii* infection, which is a recently recognized rare cause of Lyme disease acquired in Minnesota and Wisconsin.

II.48. Answer c.

Dolutegravir (DTG) (50 mg, twice daily, with a dual-nucleoside regimen of anticipated activity) would be appropriate treatment. The patient had intermittent noncompliance that contributed to the failure of his raltegravir (RAL)–based regimen. The identified mutations of N155H and Q148H likely represent separate clonal populations of the virus because these pathways tend to be mutually exclusive for the development of RAL resistance. Thus, antiviral activity with DTG is anticipated. Furthermore, the VIKING-3 study showed that DTG has clinical activity, virologic success, and tolerability at a dose of 50 mg (twice daily). DTG avoids drug-drug interactions between the protease inhibitor and the patient's psychiatric medications, and the patient may have relief from the gastrointestinal disturbances associated with his boosted protease inhibitor. Relief of gastrointestinal intolerance and enabling titration of medications to control his psychiatric conditions could translate into more effective adherence.

Although bictegravir (BIC) has activity against first-generation integrase strand transfer inhibitor (INSTI) mutations in vitro, we do not have clinical data for patients whose first-generation INSTI therapy has failed, nor do we have an appropriately established clinical dosing scheme for BIC in the setting of first-generation INSTI failure.

Tipranavir may well have activity against the patient's viral isolate, but it will affect adherence because it poses a similar adverse effect profile (with likely even more gastrointestinal adverse effects because of the increase in ritonavir needed with tipranavir). It likely also will interact with his psychiatric medication. Furthermore, we do not have a tropism assay showing an R5-tropic virus, which would be necessary to justify use of maraviroc.

The patient has resistance to a first-generation INSTI, making RAL an inappropriate option. Continuing a first-generation INSTI in this setting could lead to additional

sequence mutations and evolution that could compromise the effectiveness of second-generation INSTIs and eliminate the option of INSTI-class drugs for this patient.

Efavirenz would be inappropriate for 2 primary reasons. First, the patient has the K103N mutation, which would eliminate the activity of efavirenz. Second, efavirenz is well known to exacerbate psychiatric illness and could contribute to suicidal ideation in a patient with uncontrolled depression.

II.49. Answer c.

The patient is experiencing signs of vestibular toxicity (ie, ongoing dizziness), which has been associated with the loss of hair cells in cristae ampullares. A serum creatinine test and urinalysis are not useful in this setting because studies have shown that renal dysfunction and ototoxicity are independent adverse effects of aminoglycosides. Aminoglycoside ototoxicity tends to occur later in the course of exposure (>72 hours) and thus cannot be ruled out on the basis of the time course. The mitochondrial sequence variant A1555G in the 12S ribosomal RNA gene (not the pharmacogenomic CYP2C19 variant) is genetically associated with aminoglycoside-related ototoxicity. Synergy of aminoglycosides (eg, amikacin) with ampicillin increases activity against gram-positive bacteria, but it is not known to affect activity against *Mycobacterium* species.

II.50. Answer d.

Brucellosis should be suspected in a febrile, returned traveler who drank unpasteurized camel milk in a highly *Brucella*-endemic country. Although *Salmonella typhi* and *Salmonella paratyphi* also are endemic in Somalia and the patient did not receive a typhoid fever vaccination (which is only 70% effective), clinical improvement should have occurred with cefdinir therapy. The incubation period for dengue is 7 to

10 days, and the milder forms of dengue fever are self-limited and have a short illness duration. Although chikungunya viral infection may be associated with prolonged postinfection inflammatory arthritis, the persistent systemic symptoms do not fit this condition. Although falciparum malaria should always be considered as a possible cause of fever in a traveler returning from Somalia, a malaria multiplex polymerase chain reaction test was negative.

II.51. Answer c.

Doxycycline for 12 weeks plus streptomycin for 2 to 3 weeks is the regimen of choice for spondylitis, with cure rates of up to 92%. The combination of rifampin and doxycycline is an alternative treatment option, but the minimum treatment duration for *Brucella* spondylitis and vertebral osteomyelitis is 12 weeks. Trimethoprim-sulfamethoxazole is not a preferred antibiotic for brucellosis therapy. Doxycycline plus ciprofloxacin for 12 weeks may be an alternative regimen for spondylitis. Monotherapy is not appropriate for treatment of brucellosis.

II.52. Answer d.

Skin testing is useful for immediate hypersensitivity reactions, but this patient had a reaction 3 days after starting treatment. The type of skin rash and the temporal association with drug exposure do not support the diagnoses of toxic shock syndrome or drug rash with eosinophilia and systemic symptoms. A skin biopsy will confirm the clinical suspicion of acute generalized exanthematous pustulosis and will likely show mostly neutrophilic infiltrates, subepidermal edema, and subcorneal pustule.

II.53. Answer c.

Creutzfeldt-Jakob disease (CJD) infection control guidelines from the World Health Organization (WHO) provide valuable guidance for health care personnel involved in the care of patients with suspected or confirmed CJD. Incineration is recommended for disposable instruments and waste that were in contact with high-infectivity tissues from patients with suspected or confirmed CJD. For patients with suspected CJD, reusable instruments that were in contact with low-infectivity tissues should be quarantined until the diagnosis is confirmed pathologically. Instruments should then be processed according to the pathology results. Usual sterilization processes may be inadequate for prions, but special processes depend on the instrument's heat sensitivity. Sterilization protocols may include immersion in sodium hydroxide or sodium hypochlorite (for heat-sensitive and heat-resistant instruments) and autoclaving (for heat-resistant instruments only). The WHO guidelines include recommendations for processing reusable, heat-sensitive instruments.

For more information, see WHO infection control guidelines for transmissible spongiform encephalopathies: report of a WHO consultation; Geneva, Switzerland, 23-26 March 1999. World Health Organization [cited 2021 Jan 29]. Available from: https://www.who.int/csr/resources/publications/bse/whocdscsraph2003.pdf?ua=1.

II.54 Answer c.

Given his presentation with an abscess plus a fever and underlying liver disease, initial intravenous therapy with an extended-spectrum β-lactam such as ampicillin-sulbactam is advised because it would cover *Pasteurella* species and oral anaerobes that are found in a dog's mouth. The severity of the patient's injury precludes use of oral antibiotics. Neither cefepime nor azithromycin cover the full spectrum of organisms, particularly oral anaerobes that are common to animal bites.

II.55. Answer c.

The patient's renal transplant status is a contraindication for the yellow fever vaccine

(YFV). The Centers for Disease Control and Prevention (CDC) identifies the following contraindications for YFV:

- Allergy to a vaccine component
- Age <6 months
- HIV infection with symptoms, or CD4 T-lymphocyte count of <200 cells/mm³, or <15% of total in children aged <6 years
- Thymus disorder or removal, if associated with abnormal immune function
- Primary immunodeficiency of any kind
- Recent bone marrow or solid-organ transplant (<2 years since transplant) or receiving immunosuppressive therapy at any time after transplant
- Any immunosuppressive or immunomodulatory therapy, including radiotherapy
- Malignancy

The patient's CD4 count was more than 500 cells/mm³, and he had an undetectable HIV load. Although risks and benefits should be considered for certain individuals, HIV infection is not a contraindication for YFV for this individual. The CDC also cautions that risks of YFV may outweigh benefits in the following situations:

- Patient age 6 to 8 months
- Patient age 60 years or older
- Asymptomatic HIV infection and CD4 T-lymphocytes 200-499 cells/mm³ (15%-24% of total for children aged <6 years)
- Pregnancy
- Breastfeeding (rare case reports describe YFV-associated neurologic disease in breastfeeding infants of recently vaccinated mothers)

Air-conditioned environments and insect repellents may be protective, but they do not provide complete protection against yellow fever (YF) infection. Previous travel to a YF-endemic region does not confer immunity to YF infection. YFV is the most effective intervention to prevent YF in travelers to high-risk areas. The patient is traveling to the Amazon River region, an area known to have high risk of YF infection. In addition, YFV has been recommended for travelers to the Rio de Janeiro and São Paulo regions of Brazil since 2017, after those areas had outbreaks of sylvatic YF from December 2016 through March 2017. Before travel, it is always advisable to check the current travel vaccination recommendations from the World Health Organization and CDC because disease epidemiology may vary with time.

For more information, see Gershman MD, Staples JE. Travel-related infectious diseases: yellow fever [Internet]. Atlanta (GA): Centers for Disease Control and Prevention [cited 2021 Mar 10]. Available from: https://wwwnc.cdc.gov/travel/diseases/yellow-fever; and Centers for Disease Control and Prevention (CDC). Fatal yellow fever in a traveler returning from Amazonas, Brazil, 2002. MMWR Morb Mortal Wkly Rep. 2002 Apr 19;51(15):324-5.

II.56. Answer b.

An HIV screening test, urine, rectal, and oropharyngeal nucleic acid amplification tests for gonorrhea and chlamydia, hepatitis screening test, and syphilis serologic test are recommended, given the patient's risk factors and exposure history. The other options listed would miss several important infections, which increases risk for the patient and his sex partners.

II.57. Answer d.

A repeat urine nucleic acid amplification test is recommended because the patient had a nontraditional therapy regimen. It is important to confirm cure or resolution because the patient otherwise would risk having a remnant infection that increases risk for herself and her sex partners.

II.58. Answer b.

The presence of branching, non–spore-forming, gram-positive bacilli plus the gradual worsening of the patient's condition for more than a week most likely represents infection due to *Actinomyces* species. Broad coverage with piperacillin-tazobactam is appropriate because other associated bacteria (termed *companion pathogens*) are commonly present. Clinical data for intravenous immunoglobulin and hyperbaric oxygen treatments are mainly derived from necrotizing fasciitis caused by streptococci, and their value in this setting remains controversial. Evidence supporting the use of clindamycin in necrotizing fasciitis is mainly derived from experimental studies, and clindamycin has not been tested clinically with actinomycosis. Corticosteroids might be considered only for patients with severe cellulitis who do not have diabetes mellitus.

II.59. Answer b.

The most likely diagnosis is disseminated histoplasmosis with bilateral adrenal involvement in a patient with considerable exposure to bird guano. Lymphoma is unlikely because the biopsy showed benign mucosa and computed tomographic imaging did not show bulky adenopathy. Invasive candidiasis is incorrect because the patient has signs and symptoms of a systemic disease, the lesions do not match the fluffy white appearance of oral candidiasis, and the patient does not have a beefy, red tongue. Behçet syndrome is unlikely because it often presents with concurrent genital or eye lesions, and lesions can spontaneously regress. Disseminated blastomycosis is unlikely because it typically does not present with oral lesions. Disseminated blastomycosis may present with skin lesions (ulcers or exophytic lesions), brain infection (mass, meningoencephalitis, or abscess), bone lesions (lytic lesions), or prostate involvement (in men).

II.60. Answer d.

The clinician should have high clinical suspicion for infection with *Mycobacterium*
marinum because of the patient's history of repeated fish tank exposure, the skin and soft tissue infection's lack of response to appropriate standard antibiotic therapy, and the negative bacterial cultures. The development of nodular lymphangitis makes this diagnosis even more probable. To definitively diagnose the infection, débridement with mycobacterial culture is preferred. There is no clear role for repeat bacterial cultures, and serum antibody testing does not currently have a meaningful role in diagnosing *M marinum* infection, although positive results with interferon-γ release assays have been reported. Finally, magnetic resonance imaging is not indicated because *M marinum* rarely involves the bone and imaging likely would show only nonspecific soft tissue swelling.

II.61. Answer a.

Any patient with confirmed pulmonary tuberculosis can be considered noninfectious when the patient has had at least 2 weeks of effective multidrug treatment and shows clinical evidence of improvement. For all patients with suspected (not confirmed) pulmonary tuberculosis, 3 consecutive sputum smears must be negative for acid-fast bacilli before discontinuing use of an airborne infection isolation room. Surgical masks are respiratory protection controls designed to stop droplet nuclei from being spread (exhaled) by the patient. Interferon release assays do not have a role in decisions about isolation.

II.62. Answer a.

Diagnosis of disseminated *Mycobacterium bovis* bacille Calmette-Guérin (BCG) infection is not always established with positive cultures, and lack of mycobacterial growth does not exclude BCG infection. Tissue biopsies positive for acid-fast bacilli or histopathologic examination showing noncaseating granulomas have been reported for patients with negative culture results. The disseminated nature of BCG infection may be attributable to disruption of uroepithelial cells and could be caused by traumatic catheterization. The *M bovis* BCG strain is a member of the *Mycobacterium tuberculosis* complex. Finally, most strains of *M bovis* are resistant to pyrazinamide, and BCG infections in the United States most commonly occur after bladder cancer treatment with BCG.

II.63. Answer d.

Studies have shown that starting combined antiretroviral therapy within 2 weeks of starting treatment for *Pneumocystis jirovecii* pneumonia decreases the risk of mortality and rate of progression to AIDS (PLoS One. 2009;4[5]:e5575). Immune reconstitution inflammatory syndrome is rare with *Pneumocystis* pneumonia, but when it occurs, it is usually mild to moderately severe and improves with conservative management.

II.64. Answer c.

Because the combination has only 1 agent that is active against hepatitis B virus (lamivudine), this regimen increases the risk of emerging strains that are resistant to lamivudine and emtricitabine because of their structural similarities.

II.65. Answer a.

Asymptomatic bacteriuria should be treated in patients who are pregnant. Asymptomatic bacteriuria during pregnancy increases the risk of pyelonephritis and is associated with preterm birth and low birthweight. Amoxicillin is safe to use in the third trimester, but trimethoprim-sulfamethoxazole is a category C drug in pregnancy. Observation only, vitamin C, and repeating the culture are inappropriate actions.

II.66. Answer d.

Waiting for the diarrhea to resolve while providing supportive care decreases the risk of complications before a planned, nonurgent surgery. The use of antibiotics to treat diarrhea caused by *Escherichia coli* O157:H7 is associated with an increased risk of hemolytic uremic syndrome.

II.67. Answer c.

The patient's clinical assessment offers valuable clues to the diagnosis of Sweet syndrome. The rapid onset of painful skin lesions associated with fever in a patient with a condition known to be associated with Sweet syndrome (eg, acute myelogenous leukemia) should raise clinical suspicion for the diagnosis.

Leukemic involvement of the skin can occur in patients with acute myelogenous leukemia; a biopsy will show cutaneous infiltration by malignant, immature leukocytes. Disseminated *Fusarium* infection typically presents as refractory fever in a profoundly neutropenic patient with multiple skin lesions; a blood culture may grow a mold. Pyoderma gangrenosum is an uncommon neutrophilic dermatosis that typically presents as a rapidly developing, painful, and purulent ulcer with an undermined border. It is often associated with an underlying systemic disease, most commonly inflammatory bowel disease, arthritis, and hematologic disease or malignancy. A biopsy of the ulcer edge will show dermal necrosis and neutrophilic infiltrates. Ecthyma gangrenosum, classically associated with *Pseudomonas aeruginosa* septicemia, commonly begins with painless, red macules that rapidly evolve into areas of induration, then develop into pustules or bullae (or both), and ultimately become gangrenous ulcers. Histopathologic analysis will show perivascular hemorrhage, neutrophilic infiltration with central necrosis, and an abundance of gram-negative rods.

II.68. Answer a.

This patient has clinical symptoms consistent with Whipple disease, and the biopsy specimen would be expected to show macrophages that are positive for periodic acid–Schiff stain. Intraepithelial lymphocytosis with villi flattening would be seen in celiac disease, as would variable villous atrophy with crypt hyperplasia. Central nervous system involvement is not expected in celiac disease. Transmural lymphoid aggregation with non-necrotizing granulomas would be seen in Crohn disease. Pseudomembrane formation would be unusual in Whipple disease.

II.69. Answer d.

Interestingly, *Tropheryma whipplei* can be detected commonly in the skin of patients with Whipple disease, even if the patient has no skin lesions. The most common cutaneous manifestation of Whipple disease is melanoderma (abnormal darkening of the skin). The pathogenesis of this finding remains unknown.

Index

Figures and tables are indicated by *f* and *t* following a page number.